Hospice and Palliative Care Handbook

Quality, Compliance, and Reimbursement

About the Author

Tina M. Marrelli, MSN, MA, RN, is President of Marrelli and Associates, Inc., a health care consulting and publishing firm. Ms. Marrelli is the author of *The Handbook of Home Health Standards and Documentation Guidelines for Reimbursement*, "The Little Red Book" (Fourth edition, Mosby, 2001), *The Nurse Manager's Survival Guide* (Third edition, Mosby, 2004) *The Handbook of Home Health Orientation* (Mosby, 1997), *The Nursing Documentation Handbook* (Third edition, Mosby, 1996), *The Hospice and Palliative Care Handbook* (Mosby, 1999), and *Mosby's Home Care & Hospice Drug Handbook* (Mosby, 1999). She is also the co-author of *Home Health Aide: Guidelines for Care* (Marrelli, 1996), *Home Care and Clinical Paths: Effective Care Planning Across the Continuum* (Mosby, 1996), *Home Health Aide: Guidelines for Care Instructor Manual* (Marrelli, 1997), *The Manual of Home Health Practice* (Mosby, 1998), and *Home Care Therapy: Quality, Documentation, and Reimbursement* (Marrelli, 1999). Ms. Marrelli is also an editorial board member of *The Journal of Community Health Nursing* and *Geriatric Nursing* and contributes specialty articles for the monthly home health newsletter, *Clinical Supervisor Alert*.

Ms. Marrelli received a Bachelor's degree in Nursing from Duke University School of Nursing in 1975. She has directed various health care programs and has extensive experience in home care, hospice, and hospital settings. She has a Master of Arts in Management and Supervision, Health Care Administration and a master's in nursing. Ms. Marrelli worked at the central office of the Health Care Financing Administration (HCFA), now the Centers for Medicare and Medicaid Services (CMS), for four years in the areas of home care and hospice policy and operations, where she received the Bureau Director's Citation. She is a member of Sigma Theta Tau, and is certified by the American Nurses Association (ANA) credentialing center as a home health nurse. Ms. Marrelli serves on the National Hospice and Palliative Care Organization's (NHPCO) Standards and Accreditation Committee, has been the recipient of the Arizona Association for Home Care's 1998 Genie Eide Award, and has served as a member of the Hospice and Palliative Nurses Association's "National Competency Project."

Marrelli and Associates, Inc. provides consultative services to hospitals, universities, publishers, home health agencies, hospices and other programs in the areas of management, compliance, accreditation, and other quality initiatives, daily operations, retention and recruitment initiatives, clinical documentation systems and written product development, case management models, and numerous other areas. Tina can be contacted via e-mail at *news@marrelli.com* or through the web site *www.Marrelli.com.*

Hospice and Palliative Care Handbook

Quality, Compliance, and Reimbursement

SECOND EDITION

Tina M. Marrelli
MSN, MA, RN
Health Care Consultant
Boca Grande, Florida

with assistance from Maureen A. Williams
MED, RN, BC
Director of Staff Development
The Institute for Education and Leadership
Capital Hospice
Fairfax, Virginia

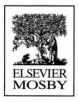

ELSEVIER
MOSBY

ELSEVIER
MOSBY

11830 Westline Industrial Drive
St. Louis, Missouri 63146

HOSPICE AND PALLIATIVE CARE HANDBOOK   ISBN 0-323-02479-3
Copyright © 2005 by Mosby, Inc.

Notice

Hospice/Palliative Care and Home Health Care are ever-changing fields. Standard safety precautions must be followed, but as new research and clinical experience broaden our knowledge, changes in treatment and drug therapy may become necessary or appropriate. Readers are advised to check the most current product information provided by the manufacturer of each drug to be administered to verify the recommended dose, the method and duration of administration, and contraindications. It is the responsibility of the licensed prescriber, relying on experience and knowledge of the patient, to determine dosages and the best treatment for each individual patient. Neither the publisher nor the author assumes any liability for any injury and/or damage to persons or property arising from this publication.

Previous edition copyrighted 1999

International Standard Book Number 0-323-02479-3

Executive Editor: Loren S. Wilson
Managing Editor: Linda Thomas
Publishing Services Manager: John Rogers
Project Manger: Kathleen L. Teal
Design Manager: Bill Drone

Printed in the United States of America.

Last digit is the print number: 9 8 7 6 5 4 3 2 1

REVIEWERS

Barbara Cary, MSN, FNP-BC
Clinical Coordinator
Maplecrest Living and Rehabilitation Center
Madison, Maine

Karen Crain Cote, RN, MSN
Director
Hallmark Health Hospice
Malden, Massachusetts

Barbara J. Edlund, PhD, RN, ANP
Associate Professor
College of Nursing
Medication University of South Carolina
Charleston, South Carolina

Pat M. Gibbons, BSN, CHPN
Director
Beacon Place
Greensboro, North Carolina

Susan P. Ladue, RN
Assistant Clinical Director
Unique Nurses (Home Health Agency)
Annandale, Virginia

Sharon Peterson, RN, BSN
Manager
Health Care for the Homeless Program
Crusader Clinic
Rockford, Illinois

PREFACE

This book was written to facilitate the integration of care, standards, and planning for hospice into clinical documentation and forms. The interdisciplinary documentation described in this book will assist health care professionals in providing quality hospice care that meets regulatory standards, such as those of Medicare. Although the Medicare program is a medical model, the Medicare framework can lend itself to effectively providing quality hospice care. The interdisciplinary hospice team members have the clinical skills and the information required to identify and address patient and family needs holistically. This book facilitates the integration of hospice team members, such as nursing, physical and occupational therapy, spiritual and psychosocial counseling, nutritional counseling, volunteer support, and speech-language pathology, into a usable format to assist in planning and providing care.

The priority for hospice clinicians and managers is to meet the unique and multifaceted needs of patients and their families. The format of this book lends itself to the integration of assessed patient and family needs into a plan consistent with accurate completion of hospice clinical records that support compliance and quality while managing complex care plans. This book assists in the documentation of that process and analysis (e.g., documentation of the care planning process).

This book contains 30 care guidelines that include direction for assessment, documentation, and reimbursement to assist in meeting quality and regulatory standards. These care guidelines give new and experienced hospice clinicians examples of interventions and documentation that may assist in supporting the presence of and continuous need for hospice care. The text is also a way to standardize care, documentation, and care processes across an organization and among team members. These standards can be reviewed and practiced in orientation, in hospice care sites and during clinical case conferences. The generation of appropriate, quality and reimbursable documentation is a learned process. Like any new skill learning and improvement occur with practice and positive feedback toward the desired outcome. This book integrates the documentation needed to support covered care and reimbursement while listing the care considerations for patients and their families by clinical problem or diagnosis.

Special features have been included to make this book easy to use. *Queries for Quality* is a new feature in this edition and is found in all the clinical care guidelines. In the clinical care guidelines sections (Parts Four and Five) standard abbreviations are used to simplify the descriptions of hospice care. If any abbreviation is confusing, its meaning can be checked in Part Eight. In addition, the Table of Contents is alphabetized in the care guidelines sections, and cross-referenced materials are found under the associated or other heading. For example, the care guideline "Breast Cancer and Mastectomy Care" is also listed under "Mastectomy Care," for easier identification and retrieval of needed information. This feature should help you find material quickly. Furthermore, each specific care guideline cross-references related care guidelines to assist the reader in accessing additional information. For example, in the guideline for "Depression and Other Psychiatric Care," the reader is also referred to "Alzheimer's Disease and Other Dementias," should that be a related or complicating problem for the patient and his or her family. For a more detailed discussion of how to use this book for planning, delivering, evaluating, and documenting hospice care, see the section "Guidelines for Use," which details additional features of this revised edition.

ACKNOWLEDGMENTS

A heartfelt thank you to all the hospice clinicians and managers, of all disciplines and professions, who have provided insight and practice examples from their own special hospice experiences. All of this information helps keep the focus practical while providing skillful and compassionate hospice care.

Lynda S. Hilliard deserves an award for her ready ear and detail-oriented recommendations for the process and manuscript. Special thanks to Bill and L.B. Glass for humor and support, respectively, and always understanding when deadlines loomed and schedules were out of control.

Tina M. Marrelli, MSN, MA, RN

GUIDELINES FOR USE

The goal of this book is to assist hospice clinicians and managers meet quality, coverage, and reimbursement standards and requirements through their daily practice, operations, and documentation activities. The Hospice Care Guidelines, or topics, are organized alphabetically for easy retrieval and review of information.

There may be more than one case scenario that is appropriate for your hospice patient. For example, for care of a patient with cancer and an open wound, the following two Care Guidelines could be referred to: "Cancer Care" and "Wound/Pressure Ulcer Care." Depending on the type of cancer, "Brain Cancer," "Breast Cancer," "Head and Neck Cancer," or "Prostate Cancer" could also be appropriate. The information can be individualized for your patients/families, used throughout the clinical record, and serve as a basis for a common glossary in interdisciplinary team or group (IDG) discussions. It is formatted for easy review for care and care planning.

The following information refers to the specifically numbered entries in each of the 30 Hospice Care Guidelines.

1. **General considerations.** This entry contains general information on the designated topic in relation to hospice care. The diagnostic information would be used generally for supporting the medical necessity of hospice care and the reason that the patient was admitted to hospice.
2. **Needs for visit.** This information lists what is generally needed prior to making a hospice visit and supports planning and the securing of physician orders and clinical information needed for the assessment prior to the provision of hospice care.
3. **Safety considerations.** This section lists the general kinds of safety concerns that may impact hospice care, based on the diagnoses or care guidelines problems listed. The information in safety considerations is to be used upon assessment and throughout the care and care planning among the team.
4. **Potential diagnoses and codes.** Depending on the model of hospice provided, the ICD-9 codes may be used on the plan of care, on Health Care Financing Administration (HCFA) form 485, or for billing purposes. They are alphabetized to assist in identification and location.

The source for all codes was the current edition of the ICD-9-CM published by the Commission on Professional and Hospital Activities. The ICD-9-CM system sometimes requires secondary codes for a complete description of the diagnostic entity. For example, pneumonia in the presence of AIDS is coded as both 486 (pneumonia) and 042 (AIDS). It is important, in such instances, to use all the codes given and in the order presented, with or without decimals as listed in the text. If your hospice is a Medicare-certified hospice (or home health agency), your Regional Home Health Intermediary (RHHI) may have preferred or recommended codes, and those codes should be used when appropriate for your patient. These RHHI code updates are usually communicated to your manager through the RHHI's newsletters.

Codes for associated operations or postoperative care are listed, as appropriate, and surgical codes are marked (surgical) in the text after the ICD-9 number listed. Operation codes may be recognized by their two-digit structure. Diagnosis codes always have three digits before the decimal point and in some cases have no decimal point at all. Operation codes have only two digits before the decimal and are always followed by one or two digits, following the decimal:

Diagnosis: Osteomyelitis, lower leg, 715.96

Surgical procedure: S/P BKA, 84.15

Certain essential assumptions have been made regarding hospice services. These assumptions are that if the patient is a beneficiary of a medical insurance program, such as Medicare, the patient meets recognized hospice and insurer standards and is therefore appropriate for hospice admission and care and justified for reimbursement. Remember that modifiers to diagnosis terms may be important. Modifiers such as acute/chronic, unilateral/bilateral, upper/lower, and adult/juvenile frequently require differentiation in the ICD-9 codes. Similarly, slight variations in terminology may be significant. Please note that the ICD-9 system contains more than 10,000 diagnosis code categories and more than 40,000 cross-referenced diagnosis terms. We have attempted to clearly illustrate such distinctions in the text. Your intermediary may have other or additional specific ICD-9 codes they prefer for you to use. In those cases, use the intermediary's recommended codes. For further information, consult the ICD-9 codes books or a qualified coder.

5. **Skills and Services identified.** This section lists and identifies the hospice team members and some of their specialized functions or interventions, based on the patient's/family's diagnoses or problems and unique circumstances. The skills and services identified in this section include those of the nurse; home health aide; social worker; volunteer(s); spiritual counselor, dietitian/nutritional counselor; physical or occupational therapist; speech-language pathologist; bereavement counselor; pharmacist (for some diagnoses); and music, massage, art and other therapists.

Hospice nursing has been listed as the first service. Because of the multifaceted interventions and complex coordination activities that must occur with skillful hospice nursing care, the nursing section is subcategorized into eight areas. These are: (a) Comfort and Symptom Control, (b) Safety and Mobility Considerations, (c) Emotional/Spiritual Considerations, (d) Skin Care, (e) Elimination Considerations, (f) Hydration/Nutrition, (g) Therapeutic/Medication Regimens, and (h) Other Considerations. This specificity should assist in the identification and prioritization of patient/family care interventions.

Interventions for nursing and other services often use verbs in the description of care and to support holistic, skillful interventions. These services may also be used, where appropriate, as the orders for the plan of care. It is important to note that the patient/family care plan must be individualized and based on the assessed needs. This information is provided as a list to assist in the identification of needed hospice care and assists all hospice team members by providing a baseline for services based on the specialized team member's education and professional scope of practice.

6. **Outcomes for care.** Outcomes are quantifiable or measurable goals for care across a time span. The outcomes listed are not lengthy or complex but should be able to be identified generally as met or not met. The outcomes are based on the hospice patient's/family's assessed findings and unique situation. These outcomes are utilized in the interdisciplinary care planning process, planning records, and clinical documentation.

7. **Patient, family, and caregiver educational needs.** This section addresses the unique educational needs of patients, their families, and caregivers. The most common types of information that patients need to safely remain at home are listed in this section. Please keep in mind that this is a handbook, and the listing is by no means intended to be all-inclusive. Your patient and family may have needs that are as varied as their history, with unique learning styles and barriers.

8. **Specific tips for quality documentation and reimbursement.** These tips are often based on diagnoses that contribute to concise, specific documentation assisting in supporting quality, coverage, and reimbursement. This information may be used in the assessment form, visit notes, IDG minutes, care coordination, and planning of activities. Remember that all services need to be based on your patient's/family's unique medical condition and history as determined on the assessment visit(s) and throughout the patient's/family's length of care. Regardless of payor, the documentation must demonstrate the hospice care provided and the patient's/family's response to that care. A more in-depth discussion about the level and specificity of documentation needed in hospice care and the many requirements that effective documentation meets are addressed in Part Two.

9. **Queries for Quality.** The questions in *"Queries for Quality"* were created to assist clinicians and managers identify that they are asking specific questions related to quality and reimbursement. Some of the questions help support medical necessity, while others seek to help in achieving more disease-specific hospice and palliative care goals. These questions could be incorporated into educational sessions or other opportunities to improve care and documentation of care.

10. **Resources for hospice care and practice.** Informational resources are listed to assist the clinician and patients/families with educational and other needs, based on the unique care diagnosis. For example, under this section in the "Renal Care (End Stage)" guideline, there are resources listed from the National Kidney Foundation brochure entitled *When Stopping Dialysis Treatment Is Your Choice* and other patient education materials available through their 800 number. Similarly, in the "Care of the Child with Cancer" guideline, resources listed include *Radiotherapy Days,* a colorful book that explains radiation to young patients and specialized pain resources, as well as supportive organizations such as the Make-A-Wish Foundation and the Candlelighters Childhood Cancer Foundation. These resources have been specially chosen to support patient and clinician education needs. Readers are encouraged to write to the author should they have

additional resources they believe should be included in a subsequent edition. Send the resource or the information about the resource to the following address: P.O. Box 629, Boca Grande, FL 33921-0629 or FAX to (941) 697-2901 or send via e-mail to news@marrelli.com.

Notice

NOTE TO THE READER: The author and publisher have diligently verified the considerations discussed for accuracy and compatibility with officially accepted standards at the time of publication. With continual advancements in health care practice and great variety in particular patient needs, we recommend that the reader consult the latest literature and exercise professional judgment in using the guidelines in this book. In addition, the assumption is made that the clinical professional is functioning under physician orders and adheres to other regulatory guidelines or laws.

CONTENTS

PART ONE **HOSPICE: A UNIQUE PRACTICE SPECIALITY,** 1

What is Hospice? 2
Hospice Care, 3
The Growth of Hospice, 3
Hospice Settings, 6
Patients Seen in Hospice, 6
Types of Hospice Organizations, 6
The Interdisciplinary Team, 7
   Roles of Hospice Team Members, 9
Defining Hospice Nursing, 22
Hallmarks of Effective Hospice and Palliative Care, 22
Identified Differences Between Home Care and Hospice Nursing, 28
Medicare Hospice 101, 31
Skills and Knowledge Needed in Hospice Care, 35
The Hospice Orientation, 38
   Hospice Orientation Considerations, 39
   Defining the Hospice Orientation, 40
   Competency Assessment and Validation, 40
   Organizational Orientation Topics, 41
Safety in Hospice, 51
Map Reading: Update of an Important Skill, 53
Summary, 54
Review Exercises, 55

PART TWO **AN OVERVIEW OF HOSPICE
          DOCUMENTATION,** 56

Hospice Documentation, 57
   Why Is the Clinical Record So Important? 57
   Factors Contributing to More Emphasis on Documentation, 60
   Importance of the Hospice Record, 64
   Documentation: The Key to Coverage, Compliance, and Quality, 65
Hospice Documentation 101, 65
   Medicare Hospice Documentation: A Checklist Approach, 72
   Effective Hospice Documentation: A Checklist Approach, 72
   Clinical Path Considerations, 74
   Defining Clinical Paths, 74
   Automation: Effectively Integrating Care and Documentation, 75
   Summary, 75
   Review Exercises, 77

PART THREE   **PLANNING AND MANAGING CARE IN HOSPICE,** 78

Planning and Managing Care in Hospice, 79
Hospice Care Examples, 83
Summary, 85
Review Exercises, 86

PART FOUR   **MEDICAL-SURGICAL CARE GUIDELINES: SPECIAL PATIENTS AND FAMILIES,** 87

Acquired Immune Deficiency Syndrome (AIDS) Care, 89
Alzheimer's Disease and Other Dementias Care, 105
Amyotrophic Lateral Sclerosis (ALS) and Other Neuromuscular Care, 117
Bedbound Care, 129
Brain Tumor Care, 144
Breast Cancer Care, 157
Cancer Care, 170
Cardiac Care (End Stage), 185
Catheter Care, 352
Cerebral Vascular Accident (CVA) Care, 200
Chronic Obstructive Pulmonary Disease (*see* Lung Care), 291
Colostomy Care (*see* Supportive Care: Catheter, Feeding Tube, and Ostomy Care), 352
Constipation Care, 215
Dementia Care, 115
Depression and Psychiatric Care, 227
Diabetes Mellitus and Other Vascular Conditions Care, 241
Dialysis Therapy (*see* Renal Disease Care), 336
Enteral-Parenteral Care (see Infusion Care or Supportive Care), 273
Gastrostomy and Other Feeding Tube Care (*see* Supportive Care: Catheter, Feeding Tube, and Ostomy Care), 352
Head and Neck Cancer Care, 258
Immobility Care (*see* Bedhound Care), 129
Impaction Care (*see* Constipation Care), 215
Infusion Care, 273
IV Care (see Infusion Care), 273
Laryngectomy Care (*see* Head and Neck Cancer Care), 258
Lung Care (End Stage), 291
Mastectomy Care, 169
Nasogastric Tube Feeding Care (*see* Supportive Care: Catheter, Feeding Tube, and Ostomy Care), 352
Organic Brain Syndrome Care (*see* Alzheimer's Disease and Other Dementias Care), 105
Ostomy Care, 352

Pain Care, 307
Parenteral Therapy (*see* Infusion Care), 273
Peripheral Vascular Disease Care (*see* Diabetes Mellitus and Other Vascular Conditions Care), 256
Pressure Ulcer Care, 382
Prostate Cancer Care, 321
Psychiatric Care, 227
Pulmonary Disease Care (*see* Lung Care), 305
Renal Disease Care (End Stage), 336
Stroke Care (*see* Cerebral Vascular Accident Care), 200
Supportive Care: Catheter, Feeding Tube, and Ostomy Care, 352
Tracheostomy Care (*see* Head and Neck Cancer Care), 258
Tumor Care (*see* Cancer Care), 170
Urinary Catheter Care, (*see* Supportive Care: Catheter, Feeding Tube, and Ostomy Care), 352
Vascular Access Device Care (*see* Infusion Care), 273
Wound and Pressure Ulcer Care, 382

PART FIVE   **HOSPICE CARE OF CHILDREN: SPECIAL PATIENTS AND FAMILIES,** 400

Acquired Immune Deficiency Syndrome (AIDS) (Care of the Child With), 402
Cancer (Care of the Child With), 414
Care of the Medically Fragile Child, 426

PART SIX   **PAIN: ASSESSMENT AND MANAGEMENT RESOURCES,** 443

Pain Assessment Monitor, 444
Initial Pain Assessment Tool, 445
Pain Intensity Scales, 446
FACES Pain Rating Scale, 447
Pain Control Record, 448
Nurse's Power and Responsibility in Relation to Medication for Pain Relief, 449
Barriers to the Assessment and Treatment of Pain, 450
Harmful Effects of Unrelieved Pain, 452
Classification of Pain by Inferred Pathology, 454
Routes of Opioid Administration, 455
Rectal Administration of Opioid Analgesics, 459
Immediate Help for Pharmaceutical Control of Pain, 461
How to Use Oral Analgesics Rectally in an Emergency, 461
Quick Alternatives to Liquid Form of Rectal Administration, 463
Immediate Help for Pharmacological Control of Pain, 464
    Maximal Pain Relief with Nonprescription Drugs, 464

PART SEVEN   **HOSPICE DEFINITIONS, ROLES, AND ABBREVIATIONS,** 467

Key Hospice Definitions and Roles, 468
Key Hospice Abbreviations, 480

PART EIGHT   **DIRECTORY OF RESOURCES,** 483

Resources, 484
Administration, 485
Advance Directives (See also "End-of-Life Issues"), 485
Aides (Hospice Aide, Home Health Aide, Certified Nursing Assistant [CNA]), 485
AIDS/HIV, 486
Book Resources, 486
Clinical Resources, 487
End-of-Life Issues, 488
Ethics, 488
Fraud and Abuse, 488
Government, 489
Hospice Nursing Certification, 489
Internet Sites, 489
Journals, 490
Medicare, 491
National Organizations, 492
Nutrition Resources, 493
Orientation, 493
Other Resources, 493
Pain, 494
Patient Resources, 495
Pediatric, 496
Spiritual, 497
Volunteers, 498

APPENDIX   **NANDA INTERNATIONAL-APPROVED NURSING DIAGNOSES,** 499

PART ONE

HOSPICE
A Unique Practice Specialty

1

When I was first introduced to hospice, I remember thinking this is how we should care for all patients—truly individualized care; comfort and symptom relief; a collaborative, caring team effort; special volunteers; and spiritual support.

TINA M. MARRELLI

Hospice is a special kind of care and support that is primarily provided in the privacy and comfort of the patient's home. According to the National Hospice Palliative Care Organization (NHPCO), 25% of hospice patients died in their own personal residences.[1] For this reason and others, hospice is a special type of home care. Simply put, hospice is an organized method of providing care, directed toward comfort and support, to patients with a limited life expectancy. Hospice focuses on making every remaining day the best it can be.

Approximately 28% of *all* Medicare costs goes toward care of people in their last year of life; almost 50% of those costs are expended in the last 2 months of life.[1] Significant savings are seen when terminally ill cancer patients are cared for at home.[2]

The hospice focus, very different from the curative-focused rescue medicine mentality of the U.S. health care system, is causing a groundswell of support for palliative care and hospice services. As a result, hospice is projected to grow significantly in the coming years.

Part 1 provides an overview of hospice care, explaining the special aspects that contribute to the high-quality care given to patients and their families. Part 1 also defines the hospice specialty for those wishing to move into this unique and satisfying professional career.

WHAT IS HOSPICE?

Hospice has strong roots in history. *Hospice* is derived from a term used historically to designate a resting place for weary travelers. Today, hospice is a multidimensional and interdisciplinary package that provides rest for weary patients and their families. Hospice patients have usually been through different treatments for curative purposes, including any combination of chemotherapeutic protocols, radiation therapy, and surgeries, and may have been on multiple regimens. Some patients have been battling cancer, AIDS, cardiac disease, pulmonary disease, or other diseases for years and have come to hospice when the medical model could no longer in good conscience continue curative treatment.

Hospice then moves in to help patients focus their limited time on themselves, their partners, and their loved ones while optimizing quality of life in the manner that they and their families choose. The NHPCO sets out standards, including the following[3]:

Hospice provides support and care for persons in the last phases of incurable diseases so that they may live as fully and comfortably as possible. Hospice recognizes dying as part of the normal process of living and focuses on maintaining the quality of remaining life.

Hospice affirms life and neither hastens nor postpones death.
Hospice exists in the hope and belief that through appropriate care
and the promotion of a caring community sensitive to their needs,
patients and families may be free to attain a degree of mental and
spiritual preparation for death that is satisfactory to them.

These standards provide the framework for hospices as they seek to provide the best possible care for patients and their families.

HOSPICE CARE

Hospice is a special approach to caring for terminally ill patients that stresses palliative care (relief of pain and uncomfortable symptoms) as opposed to curative care. In addition to meeting the patient's medical needs, hospice care addresses the physical, psychosocial, and spiritual needs of the patient's family/caregiver. The emphasis of the hospice program is on keeping the patient at home with family and friends. It is important to note that although some hospices are located in hospitals, skilled nursing facilities (SNFs), and home health agencies (HHAs), Medicare requires that hospices meet specific Medicare Conditions of Participation (COPs) and be separately certified and approved for Medicare participation. With this definition and structure come requirements that may be a part of the organization's orientation program and of the roles and nuances of coverage provided throughout the care guidelines that follow.

THE GROWTH OF HOSPICE

Many changes have occurred in the external health environment that continue to make home care and hospice two of the fastest-growing segments of the health care industry for professional clinicians and managers (see Figure 1-1 for illustrations of the growth of hospice). Some of the most appealing aspects are the interdisciplinary focus, the clinician and family/caregiver interactions, the range and diversity of skills and knowledge employed, and the sense of satisfaction that accompanies caring for patients and their families as equal partners in care and care planning.

The following list contains some of the factors contributing to the rapid growth of hospice:

- The changing health care delivery system
- The shift from inpatient care to outpatient and community-based care, such as home care
- The search for alternative methods of care and treatment
- The growth of managed care and lower cost-setting implications
- Technological advances
- Legal and risk-management issues
- Ethical dilemmas relating to end-of-life issues

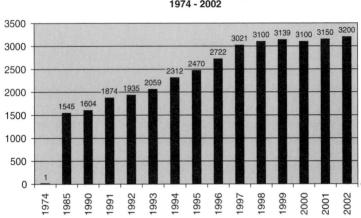

Figure 1-1, A Number of hospice programs in the United States by year (multiple locations). (Courtesy The National Hospice and Palliative Care Organization, www.nhpco.org. *Link:* Provider Graph.)

- The patient's emergence as an educated consumer seeking value and service
- General dissatisfaction with end-of-life care
- The changing belief systems of patients and their families relating to death and illness
- The renewal of spirituality as an important part of life and illness
- The grassroots efforts contributing to hospice's being seen as a valuable and caring alternative for many patients and families
- The desire of patients and families to make their limited time valued and affirming
- Demographic changes, including:
  The growing number of the frail and elderly
  The growing number of AIDS patients seeking hospice
- Cost savings
- The trend toward improving quality of life, an ethic that hospice espouses and actualizes in communities across the country

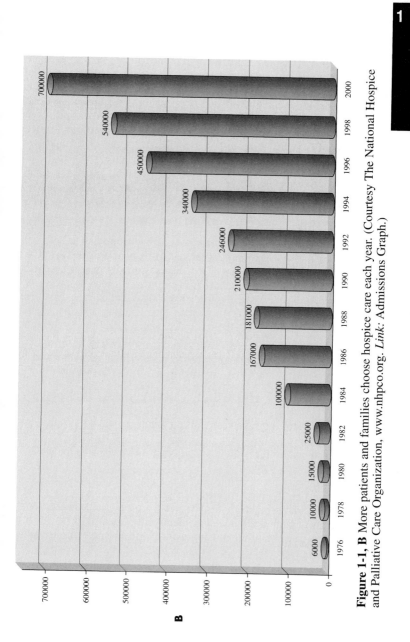

Figure 1-1, B More patients and families choose hospice care each year. (Courtesy The National Hospice and Palliative Care Organization, www.nhpco.org. *Link:* Admissions Graph.)

1

HOSPICE SETTINGS

Hospice can be provided to patients and their families in any setting and transcends traditional care settings and boundaries. Because most hospice care is provided in the privacy and comfort of the patient's home, the emphasis of this book is on home hospice care, although the care and standards addressed apply to all care settings. The term *hospice* is used in its broadest sense and includes community-based free-standing hospices, home health agency–based hospices, volunteer hospices, facility-based hospices, and other organizational models providing or supporting hospice care services. Regardless of care site, hospice is a special kind of care that emphasizes making each day the best it can be for patients and their loved ones.

PATIENTS SEEN IN HOSPICE

The problems of patients seen in hospice care are in many ways similar to those of the general home care patient population. Admission to hospice is predicated on the poor prognosis of the patient; a poor prognosis is generally stated as "6 months or less if the disease runs its expected course." Infants, children, and adults are cared for by hospice. Some hospices, such as a pediatric hospice, may have a specialized focus, but most hospices generally have admission policies that state their mission and the specific patient populations served. Diseases of patients cared for by hospices include various cancers; AIDS; end-stage renal, cardiac, and lung diseases; dementia; and other diseases that are associated with a limited life expectancy.

TYPES OF HOSPICE ORGANIZATIONS

The different types or "auspices" of programs providing hospice care include the following:
- An inpatient hospice unit at a facility such as a hospital, nursing home, or subacute unit
- A community-based hospice, such as a not-for-profit volunteer organization serving a defined rural geographical area
- A free-standing inpatient hospice, such as a hospice that cares for patients through death in a large metropolitan area
- A home care organization that provides hospice care with specially trained home care hospice nurses, volunteers, and other team members
- Corporations that provide hospice care
- Continuing care retirement community (CCRC) hospice program
- Other models, such as health maintenance organizations (HMOs)

As managed care continues to grow, other systems, such as alliances or network hospices, are expected to emerge to provide this special care to patients.

THE INTERDISCIPLINARY TEAM

The interdisciplinary team (IDT) is a key component of hospice care. This team and its members' roles are explained in depth in this section. The hospice and palliative care team members include the following:

Patients and families
Clinician
Social workers
Physicians (including hospice medical directors)
Dietitians/Dietary counselors
Bereavement counselors
Spiritual counselors/Chaplains
Volunteers
Physical therapists
Occupational therapists
Speech-language pathologists
Home health aides
Homemakers
Pharmacists
Other team members, depending on the hospice's unique mission and population served

Depending on the size of the hospice, some team members may have more than one role, and not all hospices may have easy access to these specialists and services. The hospice team works in collaboration with the patient and family to define and plan care throughout the hospice patient's length of stay.

Administrative staff may include the following:

Administrators and managers
Secretaries and office support team members
Bereavement coordinators
Volunteer coordinators
Billing personnel
Other team members as the hospice organization's mission requires (e.g., massage, pet, and music therapists)

Hospice care is a team effort. To work effectively, meet patient needs and goals, and ensure smooth operation, hospice care depends on clear, open, and positive communications among team members. Team conferences or interdisciplinary group (IDG) meetings should occur on an ongoing basis and according to the hospice organization's policy. Figure 1-2 presents an example of an IDG form that shows communications and coordination among the team members.

Therapists, clinicians, volunteers, the physician, the aide or certified nursing assistant (CNA), and other personnel involved with a particular hospice patient all participate in developing the plan of care (POC). It goes without saying that hospice patients and their families or designated caregivers are the focus around which the other team members revolve. This ensures that hospice care is client centered and directed.

1

HOSPICE INTERDISCIPLINARY TEAM (IDT) MEETING NOTES

Primary Physician:_____ SOC Date:_____

	No Change	Continue Care Plan	Change or New Needs	Comments
Oxygen ___lpm PRN ___lpm continuous				
Equipment (circle applicable equipment)	Hospital bed, over bed table, bath bench, monitor, w/c, walker, commode, cane, other_____			
Medication				
PROBLEM (Only mark applicable ones) 1. Alteration in Pain/Comfort/Safety				
2. Potential/Actual Alteration in Cardiopulmonary Status				
3. Alteration in Nutrition				
4. Alteration in Elimination *URINARY:* Retention Dysuria Incontinence *BOWEL:* Diarrhea Constipation Incontinence				
5. Self Care Deficit/Mobility Bathing/Hygiene Dressing/ Grooming Feeding Toileting				
6. Ineffective Coping/Impaired Communication				
7. Grieving, Anticipatory				
8. Spiritual Distress				

IDT Meeting Date:_____ **DNR:** ☐ Yes ☐ No
Level of Care: ☐ Routine home care ☐ Respite ☐ Inpatient ☐ Continuous

Anticipated visit frequency next 2 weeks
SN _____ x   Aide _____ x wk.
SW _____ x wk.   Volunteer _____ x wk.
Chaplain _____ x   Dietitian _____ x wk.
Therapy (PT, OT or ST) _____ Other _____

IDT Signatures*:
RN _____ Medical Dir_____
MSW _____ Chaplain _____
Volunteer _____ Other _____
Therapist (PT, OT, ST, Music, Massage) _____
☐ *Discipline representative signatures on separate sheet.

PATIENT NAME - Last, First, Middle Initial   ID#

Form 3455P © BRIGGS, Des Moines, IA 50306 (800) 247-2343 www.BriggsCorp.com
1002   PRINTED IN U.S.A.   HOSPICE INTERDISCIPLINARY TEAM (IDT) MEETING NOTES

Figure 1-2 Hospice interdisciplinary team meeting notes form. (Courtesy Briggs Corporation, Des Moines, IA.)

All hospice team members providing care must maintain liaison with each other to ensure that their efforts are coordinated effectively and support the objectives outlined in the IDG and the patient's clinical record or minutes of care conferences. The documentation should establish that effective interchange, reporting, and coordination of patient care occur.

Roles of Hospice Team Members

The following are the members of the hospice care team:

1. **Clinicians**
   Health care must be provided by or under the supervision of an RN functioning within a medically approved plan of care. Just as (or even more than) in the hospital, physician orders are needed for all care or changes to the plan of care. Hospice clinicians should be experienced in the art and science of pain and symptom management and have well-developed physical assessment skills.

   Health care in hospice may be provided by clinicians and/or specialists. Some hospice clinicians may be master's prepared or have additional training and education and certification for their chosen areas of specialization. Certification is available through the National Board for Certification of Hospice and Palliative Nurses, an affiliate of the Hospice and Palliative Nurses Association (HPNA). (See the Resources in Part 8 for more information.)

   Services provided by the clinician are as varied as the hospice patient population. They may include the following:
   - Comforting an end-stage heart failure patient
   - Observing and assessing a patient through such data sources as weight, pedal edema, patient history and input, shortness of breath, and respirations
   - Administering medication and managing symptoms
   - Monitoring the patient's status and reporting to the physician
   - Teaching an elderly caregiver how to care for a loved one with end-stage disease

2. **Medical social workers**
   The medical social worker is an important member of the hospice team. Support, active listening, and resource identification are just some of the services that medical social workers provide to hospice patients and their family members. Problems addressed by social work in hospice include financial, housing, and caregiver status concerns. Most social workers in hospice are master's prepared and have clinical experience in addressing the counseling and other needs of terminally ill patients and their families.

3. **Physicians**
   The physician is a key member of the team and the interdisciplinary group and plays an important role in the care plan and the review of care.

1

Medicare and other medical health insurance plans cover or pay for "medically necessary" care. They require that the physician (1) certify that the patient needs the services and (2) sign the plan of care supporting the care. Some hospices have their own forms, and others use a facsimile of the form 485 from the Centers for Medicare and Medicaid Services (CMS—formerly the Health Care Financing Administration), also called the Home Health Certification and Plan of Care. Medicare law requires that payment for services can be made only if a physician certifies the need for services and establishes a plan of care. All care, changes in the plan of care, and changes in the patient's condition must be reported to the physician and documented in the patient's clinical record. It goes without saying that all verbal orders or any changes must be obtained, put in writing, and sent to the physician for signature. The organization will have policies relating to the forms and process for receiving and documenting verbal and other physician orders. From legal, quality, and standards of practice perspectives, it is very important that the hospice team members communicate and coordinate care with the patient's physician(s).

Many hospice organizations have a medical director or advisor. For Medicare-certified hospice this is a requirement of the Conditions of Participation (COPs). This is an important role and has numerous responsibilities, including acting as a resource to the organization's management and clinical team members and providing direction related to clinical services. Although specific roles, programs, and practices vary, the following are some of the important responsibilities of the hospice medical director:

- Providing guidance about the development of new or revised policies and procedures
- Serving on the hospice advisory committee or other boards or committees
- Collaborating and consulting with the managers and facilitating problem solving toward meeting the patient's needs
- Participating in team conferences
- Serving as the liaison between the hospice organization and physician members of the medical community
- Supporting the hospice organization through teaching, public relations endeavors, education of physicians about hospice and palliative care in the community (e.g., who is appropriate, needing MD orders, communications)
- Acting as a role model by making home visits if possible and attending scheduled team and other meetings and other activities that support the mission of the hospice organization

The physicians will look to the hospice clinicians for recommendations and solutions to care needs for their patients.

The physicians most involved with hospice are the hospice organization's medical director and the local community physicians who refer patients and families for specialized hospice care. The medical director's role varies among hospices but is always very important to the operations of the hospice and effective hospice and family care. The following are some of the multifaceted responsibilities of the medical director, as based on the unique needs of the hospice:

- Providing direction and acting as a resource to hospice team members on palliative care and practice
- Providing guidance about the development of medical and clinical policies relating to the provision of hospice
- Providing insight and feedback from a physician perspective about clinical and administrative areas
- Serving as a member of the hospice advisory board or performance improvement (PI) committees
- Collaborating with the hospice managers to facilitate problem solving toward meeting patient and family needs
- Participating in team or IDG meetings
- Consulting with other hospice team members
- Serving as the liaison between the hospice program and members of the medical community
- Supporting the tenets of hospice in the community through education and public relations endeavors
- Educating physicians and other health care professionals about hospice and the care of the terminally ill patient in the community
- Contacting new physicians who refer patients to hospice, assisting them through the process, answering their questions, and coordinating care
- Assisting in the resolution of difficulties that may arise between members of the team and physicians in the community
- Acting as a role model by making home visits if possible to hospice patients and their families

Counseling includes dietary counseling with respect to the care of the terminally ill individual and bereavement counseling with respect to the survivors' adjustment to death. Although Medicare hospice puts dietary counseling and bereavement counseling together under the heading "counseling," these important counseling services are very different.

4. **Dietitians/Dietary counselors**

Dietary counselors are very important for the provision of quality hospice care. Many hospice patients have symptoms and side effects that have an impact on their nutritional status. Anorexia, mouth sores and pain, swallowing disorders, diarrhea or constipation, and nausea are common symptoms and challenges in hospice. The nutritional status of the patient and the family/caregiver response to nutritional changes often are a source of conflict and uneasiness with the unit of care and among caregivers. The importance of educating patients and family members about nutritional and dietary changes cannot be overemphasized. Hospice dietary counseling is usually provided by a dietitian. Depending on the state and licensure requirements, the dietitian may be a licensed dietitian (LD) and/or registered dietitian (RD).

The role of the professional dietitian in hospice home care is expanding as more patients are cared for in the community setting or at home. One important part of the role of the dietitian is to make home visits to patients and families and provide consultative services to promote optimal comfort and nutrition to hospice patients. Another important part of the role of the dietitian is to be an inservice educator for the other hospice team members. The dietitian assists in the development of educational polices, procedures, and tools for use by clinicians and patients and families.

Many home care and hospice programs have dietitians available to make home visits and provide consultative services to promote optimal nutrition. To determine whether nutritional services or intervention is required, clinicians in hospice assess patients for being at risk for conditions such as cachexia by monitoring weight loss and checking that the refrigerator is stocked with an adequate supply of food. For accreditation, standards require that the patient's nutritional status be assessed, interdisciplinary nutritional care planning be performed, counseling or nutrition intervention be carried out, and appropriately qualified staff members be designated to coordinate services. Hospice has traditionally relied upon hospice nurses to identify, coordinate, and implement nutrition-related services. Hospice organizations may need the dietitian for diet modification and counseling and use of oral supplements. The dietitian may also make recommendations relating to enteral and parenteral nutrition therapies. Other services include teaching about complex diets, identifying educational materials for use with patient teaching, and acting as an inservice educator and resource on nutrition services. Resources relating to hospice nutritional services are listed in Part 9; Part 6 is a guide to planning and implementing hospice nutritional care.

5. **Bereavement counselors**

Bereavement counselors are important to comprehensive hospice care. The standards for bereavement counseling and care include that bereavement care be offered for 13 months after the patient's death to bereaved survivors. This counseling is based on an assessment performed when the patient is initially admitted to hospice. High-risk and other problematic areas are identified on admission and updated through the length of hospice care to best address the needs of the bereaved family members.

Bereavement counseling is a part of the hospice organization's planned intervention program for the survivors and is a key indicator of the quality of hospice services. Components of the bereavement program may include a standardized assessment tool to identify at-risk families or family members, organized support meetings, cards and letters, and counseling services. Services may be provided by specially trained bereavement volunteers under the direction of the hospice and by social workers, psychologists, or others with a background in counseling, grief, and loss. See Figures 1-3 and 1-4 for examples of a bereavement assessment tool and a follow-up tool.

BEREAVEMENT ASSESSMENT

Date of Contact _____/_____/_____

❏ Home Visit   ❏ Telephone Consult

1

GENERAL INFORMATION

Name of Bereaved: _____

Address: _____

City/State/ZIP: _____

Telephone No.: (_____) _____

Age: _____ Sex: ❏ Male   ❏ Female

Bereaved's Relationship to Deceased: _____

Length of Relationship: _____

Patient Address: _____

City/State/ZIP: _____

Date of Patient's Death: _____/_____/_____

Place of Patient's Death: _____

Circumstances of Death (Describe): _____

SUPPORT SYSTEMS

Person(s) Providing Support:

Spouse: _____

Family Member(s): _____

Friends: _____

Clergy: _____

Professionals: _____

Others: _____

Support Person(s) Available:

❏ Daily ❏ Several Times a Week ❏ Once a Week

❏ Other (Specify): _____

Meaningful Activities (Describe):

_____

Important Dates:

Birthdays: Patient _____ Bereaved _____

Other (Specify): _____

EMPLOYMENT

Employment Situation (Describe): _____

PHYSICAL STATUS

Sleep Patterns:	❏ Unchanged	❏ Changed	Comments _____
Appetite:	❏ Unchanged	❏ Changed	Comments _____
Appearance:	❏ Neat	❏ Unkempt	❏ Not Observed
Recent Illnesses:	❏ None	❏ Present	❏ Describe _____
Weight:	❏ Gain	❏ Loss	❏ Unchanged

Additional Comments: _____

BEHAVIOR OBSERVED/FEELINGS EXPRESSED

Behavior Observed: ❏ Depressed ❏ Guilty ❏ Angry ❏ Withdrawn ❏ Denial ❏ Tearful ❏ Restless ❏ Talkative

Other (Specify): _____

Comments: _____

Suicide Considered: ❏ No   ❏ Yes   Comments: _____

Alcohol Intake: ❏ None   ❏ Occasional   ❏ 2 or more times a week   ❏ Daily

Comments: _____

Drug Intake: ❏ None   ❏ Occasional   ❏ 2 or more times a week   ❏ Daily

Comments: _____

PATIENT NAME–Last, First, Middle Initial   ID#

Form 3451P © 1995 Briggs Corporation, Des Moines, IA 50306
To order, phone 1-800-247-2343 www.BriggsCorp.com PRINTED IN U.S.A.   **BEREAVEMENT ASSESSMENT**

Figure 1-3 Bereavement assessment tool. (Courtesy Briggs Corporation, Des Moines, IA.)   *Continued*

6. **Spiritual counselors/Chaplains**

Spiritual counseling is a core component of quality hospice. A spiritual assessment should be part of the comprehensive assessment that is performed upon evaluation and admission to hospice. The spiritual care services provided should be consistent with the belief systems of the patients and family. Many hospices have a network of community clergy who provide support and spiritual care to patients according to their own

BEREAVEMENT ASSESSMENT

PSYCHOSOCIAL	
History of Ability to Cope: ❑ Poor ❑ Fair ❑ Good ❑ Excellent	
Comments: _____	
Assessment of Coping Ability: _____	

OTHER STRESS SOURCE

Additional Recent Losses: _____

Finances: ❑ Unchanged   ❑ Changed   ❑ Sufficient   ❑ Insufficient
Comments _____

Living Situation: ❑ Unchanged   ❑ Changed   ❑ Stable   ❑ Uncertain
Comments _____

Health: ❑ Unchanged   ❑ Changed   ❑ Improved   ❑ Deteriorated
Comments _____

PROBLEMS

Major Problems: _____

BEREAVEMENT FOLLOW-UP

Is Bereaved Interested in Follow-Up?   ❑ Yes   ❑ No
Does Bereaved Feel a Need For Immediate Support?   ❑ Yes   ❑ No
Others Needing/Desiring Follow-Up (Indicate name and relationship):
_____ Phone _____
_____ Phone _____

PLAN/INTERVENTION

Plan/Intervention: _____

COMMENTS

_____

Signature and Title of Assessor _____ Date ___/___/___

BEREAVEMENT ASSESSMENT

Figure 1-3, cont'd Bereavement assessment tool. (Courtesy Briggs Corporation, Des Moines, IA.)

beliefs or the religious community. Other hospices have their own chaplain team, which works with the local community spiritual representatives.

Hospice spiritual services are varied. For purposes of clarity only, the term *chaplain* will be used, though a rabbi, minister, or priest also could fill this important role. The chaplain (or other spiritual counselor) serves a population that spans the life continuum from infancy through death.

Figure 1-4 Bereavement follow-up tool. (Courtesy Briggs Corporation, Des Moines, IA.)

The chaplain, like other hospice team members, interfaces with patients and their family members during some of the most difficult times of their lives. This struggle with the meaning of life, a common experience among patients who have significant health concerns, is the work of the chaplain, regardless of any formal religious beliefs the patient may have. The chaplain's role varies depending on the patient and family and their

SPIRITUAL ASSESSMENT

Information Obtained By: ❑ Phone ❑ Visit

GENERAL INFORMATION

	Patient	Primary Caregiver	Family
Faith/Denomination			
Church Affiliation			
Name of Pastor/Priest/Rabbi			
Phone No.	( )	( )	( )
Contact Requested	❑ Yes ❑ No	❑ Yes ❑ No	❑ Yes ❑ No
Hospice Chaplain Referral Requested	❑ Yes ❑ No	❑ Yes ❑ No	❑ Yes ❑ No
Importance of Religion in Life: (Great, Moderate, Unimportant, Unknown)			

PATIENT ASSESSMENT

Current Support Systems:

❑ Family ❑ Friends ❑ Community Groups ❑ Religious Groups
❑ Prayer/Meditation ❑ Worship Services ❑ Religious Rituals (sacraments, etc.)
❑ Other (Specify)__________

Patient is satisfied with current spiritual support: ❑ Yes ❑ No (Explain)__________

INDICATORS OF SPIRITUAL STRENGTH (Check all that apply) Patient demonstrates/expresses:	**INDICATORS OF SPIRITUAL DISTRESS (Check all that apply)** Patient demonstrates/expresses:
Acceptance of Reality	Depression
Eternal Life Beliefs	Anxiety
Spiritual Discipline	Guilt
Serenity/Peace	Shame
Life Meaning/Purpose	Anger
Hope	Hopelessness/Despair
Forgiveness	Powerlessness
Reconciliation	Meaninglessness
Acceptance of Limits	Grief
Self Worth	Denial of Reality/Pain
Unknown at This Time	Withdrawal/Isolation
Other (specify)	Self Pity
	Suicidal Thoughts
	Fear of (specify)
	Other (specify)

Overall patient demonstrates: ❑ Spiritual Connection ❑ Spiritual Distress ❑ Uncertain
Further spiritual follow-up desired: ❑ Patient ❑ Primary Caregiver ❑ Family
Specify type of follow-up desired:__________

Comments/Counseling/Care plan implementation:__________

Signature and Title of Assessor__________ Date ___/___/___

PATIENT NAME–Last, First, Middle Initial | ID#

Form 3468P © 1995 Briggs Corporation, Des Moines, IA 50306 To order, phone 1-800-247-2343 PRINTED IN U.S.A. SPIRITUAL ASSESSMENT

Figure 1-5 Spiritual assessment tool. (Courtesy Briggs Corporation, Des Moines, IA.)

unique belief systems and needs. Responsibilities may include providing bereavement counseling, serving on ethics committees, supporting hospice staff and attending team meetings, performing the sacraments for the sick, and intervening in other ways. The chaplain facilitates patients' and families' movement toward their own resolution of life's questions. A spiritual assessment form is presented in Figure 1-5. It is completed initially by admitting team members and later reviewed and addressed/completed in detail by the chaplain.

1

7. Volunteers

Volunteers and their supportive care and services are a unique and valued part of hospice care. Conceptually the role of the specially trained hospice volunteer varies among hospices. Some hospices have volunteers who are dietitians, clinicians, and social workers providing some of the patient and family care and support. The primary role of these volunteers is to offer respite for the family. Other hospices have volunteers who are specialized in areas such as bereavement, spiritual support, and art or other therapies. Still other hospices "pair" volunteers, having them work together with an assigned hospice patient and family. Most try to match the hospice patient to the volunteer, depending on availability. An example is a hospice volunteer who is an engineer paired with a patient who shares the same profession and/or background. Hospice volunteers make an important difference in the quality of life for hospice patients and families. A frequent sentiment heard from families is, "I could not have done it without my volunteer(s)."

Hospice volunteers are special people who are specially trained in this poignant work. Activities that a volunteer might assist with include listening, reading, transportation, meal preparation, plant care, and numerous other tasks, depending on the patient's needs and the relationship forged.

New hospice team members, such as new clinicians, may be a part of the volunteer training program. Some hospices use this mechanism as a way for new team members to get to know the new hospice volunteers.

The team concept is at the core of all hospice care and is particularly important for relations between the hospice clinicians and volunteers because the volunteers must be comfortable reporting changes and generally updating and reporting on the patient's progress to the clinician. In addition to fulfilling their all-important role in patient care, other volunteers may participate in fund-raising, bereavement counseling, spiritual support, massage, and committee work. Examples of a volunteer care plan and an activity record are presented in Figures 1-6 and 1-7 for review.

Other services, depending on physician orders, the hospice, and the patient's and family's unique needs, may include the following:

8. Physical therapists

Physical therapists (PTs) are sometimes called *licensed physical therapists* (LPTs). Members of the rehabilitation team have very important roles in hospice. Physical therapy in hospice care is based on the patient's problems, and its goals are usually directed toward safety and comfort. An example is the patient who has a pathological hip fracture but refuses surgical intervention. The therapist in this case teaches the clinician aide, and other team members safe positioning, movement, and pain control. One of the primary skills of the PT in hospice is teaching the family or caregivers the home exercise program (HEP) to promote comfort and safe care at home. The PT, like other team members, provides input into the plan and any necessary revisions of the plan, prepares clinical documentation, and participates in inservice programs.

Figure 1-6 Volunteer assessment care plan. (Courtesy Briggs Corporation, Des Moines, IA.)

9. **Occupational therapists**

Occupational therapists (OTs) assist the hospice patient to attain the maximum level of physical and psychosocial independence. Areas of expertise generally include fine motor coordination, perceptual/motor skills, sensory testing, adaptive techniques, assistive devices, activities of daily living (ADLs), and specialized upper extremity/hand therapies. Problems frequently seen in hospice care that may require OT intervention include

VOLUNTEER ACTIVITY RECORD

	DAY→	SUN	MON	TUE	WED	THU	FRI	SAT	WEEK OF
	Date								/ /
	Time In								
	Time Out			·					THROUGH
	SITE OF SERVICE:								
	Home								/ /
	Nursing Home								
	Hospice Office								
	Other (Specify)								
PSYCHOSOCIAL SUPPORT	**PATIENT-RELATED ACTIVITIES**	SUN	MON	TUE	WED	THU	FRI	SAT	**COMMENTS** (All comments must be dated)
	Companionship–Patient								
	Respite–Primary Caregiver								
	Emotional Support:								
	Patient								
	Primary Caregiver								
	Bereavement:								
	Telephone Call								
	Support								
	Attend Funeral								
ACTIVITIES	Shopping								
	Meal Preparation								
	Light Housekeeping								
	Yard Work								
	Laundry								
	Other (Specify)								
HOSPICE	**ORGANIZATIONAL ACTIVITIES**	SUN	MON	TUE	WED	THU	FRI	SAT	
	Fund-raising Assistance								
	Answer Phone								
	Clerical Work								
	Other (Specify)								

VOLUNTEERS ASSIGNED		
INITIALS	**VOLUNTEER NAME**	**DATE**
		/ /
		/ /

PATIENT NAME–Last, First, Middle Initial	ID#

Form 3469P © 1995 Briggs Corporation, Des Moines, IA 50306
To order, phone 1-800-247-2343(800) 247-2343 PRINTED IN U.S.A.   **VOLUNTEER ACTIVITY RECORD**

Figure 1-7 Volunteer activity record. (Courtesy Briggs Corporation, Des Moines, IA.)

end-stage lung processes such as chronic obstructive pulmonary disease (COPD). OT can train patients in diaphragmatic breathing and relaxation techniques for comfort and energy conservation training. Safety assessments for hospice patients wishing to remain at home also are appropriate for the OT who specializes in safety measures relating to daily function.

10. **S-LP Speech-language pathologists**
    Speech-language pathology (S-LP) services are an important part of
    therapy for patients with various speech and swallowing problems.
    Patients who may need specialized S-LP services in hospice include
    those with cerebral vascular accidents (CVAs), tracheostomies, laryn-
    gectomies, or various neuromuscular diseases such as amyotrophic
    lateral sclerosis and multiple sclerosis. Like all the team members, the
    S-LP creates clinical documentation, provides input into the plan of
    care, and attends case conferences about the patient's status and
    progress on a regular basis for care coordination.

11. **Home health or hospice aides**
    Home health aides (HHAs), or certified nursing assistants (CNAs), as
    they are called in some states, provide what is probably the most impor-
    tant service for many patients. HHAs are truly the "eyes and ears" of the
    hospice organization. They are often the team members who visit the
    patient the most because they provide personal care and assistance in
    the activities of daily living to support the patient in maintaining com-
    fort at home. The HHA's role and functions are pivotal in the determi-
    nation of whether hospice patients can remain at home safely. Because
    the HHA usually spends more time with the patient and family than any
    other team member, the HHA's contribution is invaluable to both the
    team process and patient and family satisfaction. The Medicare stan-
    dards for home health aides require that they be specially trained. Home
    health aides are selected on the basis of such factors as a sympathetic
    attitude toward the care of the sick; the ability to read, write, and carry
    out directions; and the maturity and ability to deal effectively with the
    demands of the job. From a Medicare perspective, home health aides
    must be proficient or competent in 12 subject areas:
    1. Communication skills
    2. Observation, reporting, and documentation of patient status and
       the care or service furnished
    3. Reading and recording of temperature, pulse, and respiration
    4. Basic infection control procedures
    5. Basic elements of body functioning and changes in body
       function that must be reported to the aide's supervisor
    6. Maintenance of a clean, safe, and healthy environment
    7. Recognition of emergencies and knowledge of emergency
       procedures
    8. Physical, emotional, and developmental needs of hospice
       patients and families and ways to work with the populations
       served by the hospice, including respect for the patient and the
       patient's privacy and property
    9. Appropriate and safe techniques in personal hygiene and
       grooming, including:
           Bed bath
           Sponge, tub, or shower bath
           Shampoo, sink, tub, or bed

Nail and skin care
Oral hygiene
Toileting and elimination
10. Safe transfer techniques and ambulation
11. Normal range of motion and positioning
12. Adequate nutrition and fluid intake

HHAs should also be proficient in any other task that the organization may choose to have aides perform. HHAs are closely supervised by the RN or other team members to ensure their competence and comfort in providing the best hospice care to patients.

12. Homemakers

Homemakers maintain the patient care area in a manner acceptable to provide safe and effective hospice care. Some hospices define home-maker services as those services required to keep patient care areas maintained. Homemaker services may include housekeeping duties such as cleaning, vacuuming, and grocery shopping.

13. Pharmacists

The important role of the pharmacist is growing as the complexities of drug–drug, drug–disease, and drug–food adverse reactions increase. In hospice care, nurses are acutely aware that many patients are inappropriately medicated or overmedicated. Traditionally most hospice patients are elderly and have multiple risk factors for therapeutic misadventures secondary to drug therapy. They may have multiple pathologies, have different prescribers, and exhibit polypharmacy (both prescription and non-prescription medications), and they are at greater risk for adverse effects from medications because of altered physiology secondary to aging and disabilities (e.g., poor eyesight, impaired hearing, arthritic fingers).

The clinician in the community sees the whole picture, including the shoeboxes full of medications given to patients by multiple physicians. It is in this instance that the hospice clinician addresses safety concerns related to medications, acts as the patient's advocate to clarify medications and orders, and consults with the pharmacist, who can effectively evaluate the multiple medication regimens.

Traditionally the pharmacist has been considered simply the provider of a product, that is, drugs. Although this is certainly one of the pharmacist's roles, the pharmacist, as a medication expert, can offer many other services to the hospice care team, including the following:

- Providing the hospice care team with inservice education and information about medications
- Reviewing medication regimens and screening for interactions and incorrect doses or dosage forms
- Suggesting simplifying medication regimens by altering drug delivery systems or medication administration scheduling
- Monitoring and assessing the therapeutic or toxic effect of drugs
- Participating in case conferences, hospice rounds, and IDG meetings

- Perhaps most importantly, acting as a resource for pain and other symptom control for hospice patients, their families, and the hospice team

14. **Other services**

Other services may be available, such as music or art therapy or massage, depending on the hospice organization's mission and specialty programs.

Although the entire team is very much involved with the patient's care, hospice clinicians make most visits in the community. Safety is an important issue in hospice home care, as it is in all our communities. Information for the entire team about home care safety follows.

DEFINING HOSPICE NURSING

Whatever the organizational structure of the hospice, the hospice clinician plays a key role on the team. Hospice health care practice is the provision of palliative health care for the terminally ill and their families, with the emphasis on their physical, psychosocial, emotional, and spiritual needs.[5] Hospice health care is a synthesis of special skills that are used to create the environment for the best outcomes for hospice patients and their families.

The hospice clinician's role is often that of case or care manager as the nurse coordinates the implementation of the plan of care. Whatever the role defined by the organization, the following are key aspects of the hospice home care specialty that must be learned, nurtured, and improved through continued education and experience. Experienced clinicians new to hospice may be paired with an experienced hospice clinician as a preceptor through the new clinician's orientation. It goes without saying that, as with any specialty, home health care clinicians without additional orientation, education, and experience cannot successfully make the transition to hospice. Hospice is very different from home health care practice, even though some of the care interventions appear similar, and the care site—the patient's home—may be the same place.

HALLMARKS OF EFFECTIVE HOSPICE AND PALLIATIVE CARE

The following are some of the areas in which hospice team members must be proficient when caring for hospice patients and their families.

1. **Pain and symptom management skills**

This is a specialty area in hospice. Because of the teamwork in hospice, this is often an interdisciplinary effort with input from the hospice clinician, the physician, the pharmacist, and other team members, such as a social worker and a spiritual counselor. Because the focus of care is palliative and supportive, it is imperative that hospice clinicians be competent in pain assessment, intervention, and evaluation. The fifth vital sign, pain, should be assessed during every patient encounter. Modalities for pain relief and optimal comfort range from pharmaceutical agents to acupuncture, imagery, massage, and other care interventions. Most patients receive a complement of pain solutions (e.g., massage and analgesics). Readers are referred to the Agency for Health Care Policy and Research's *Clinical Practice Guidelines Number 9: Management of Cancer Pain,* which is free and can be obtained by calling 1-800-358-9295. This fact-filled text of over 200 pages has numerous recommendations and pain assessment models, resources, and tools to improve pain control and patient comfort. Examples of pain assessment tools are included in Part 7. Please refer to the "Pain" care guideline for an in-depth discussion on pain.

2. **Knowledge of concepts related to death and dying**
   Hospice integrates the dying process as a part of life. Team members' philosophies and belief systems should be congruent with the basic tenets of hospice care. Dr. Elisabeth Kübler-Ross's research on the stages of dying and other studies may be incorporated into patient care and care planning. The theoretical framework in Kübler-Ross's work provides the rationale for intervention and identification of resolutions to challenges that patients and families face.

3. **Stress management skills**
   Hospice clinicians and colleagues have varied mechanisms for providing support to themselves and each other. Hospice care may be stressful for clinicians and other hospice workers. Hospices provide staff support mechanisms to assist in the resolution of problems and for review of care and feelings raised through hospice care. Staff support may be structured, such as scheduled meetings with a trained facilitator, or may be volunteer-initiated, with varying models. It is important that all hospice team members take care of themselves and find activities and events that promote emotional well-being, nurture, and support. Whatever model staff support takes, it is a means for sharing, caring, team building, validating, and processing the important work of hospice.

4. **Sensitive communication skills**
   Communication skills are essential for effective hospice team members. There is untold intimacy and poignancy in hospice. A clinician walks into the homes of patients who may have been battling cancer for years and are now ready to change the focus from fighting the disease to enjoying their last days in their chosen way. The patient's sole priority while beginning growth work through hospice may seem to be the care of their pets or the maintenance of a garden. These values also become the hospice team's priority to support care and respect the patient's wishes. The psychosocial and spiritual components of hospice are very important to quality of life and patient and family satisfaction. Hospice staff can facilitate closure or the mending of difficult relationships. Figure 1-8 presents an example of an initial psychosocial assessment tool.

Text continued on p. 28

INITIAL PSYCHOSOCIAL ASSESSMENT

PRIMARY CAREGIVER INFORMATION

Name ——————————————

Address ——————————————

City/State/ZIP ——————————————

Phone No. (——) ——————————————

Age ———— ❏ Male ❏ Female

Relationship to Patient ——————————————

Health Status ——————————————

SOCIAL HISTORY ASSESSMENT

Family System Background (General History) ——————————————

Family Stability ——————————————

Caregivers and Supporters (in Addition to Primary Caregiver) ——————————————

Members of Immediate Family/Significant Others Living with Patient

Members of Immediate Family/Significant Others NOT Living with Patient

Patient s Most Significant Relationship ——————————————

Length of Relationship ——————————————

Patient s Educational History (Indicate Number of Years Completed)

Elementary———— Jr. High/Middle School———— High School———— College———— Vocational————

Patient s Occupational History ——————————————

Ethnic and Cultural Considerations ——————————————

Significant Losses/Crises Experienced with Family or Other Significant Others ——————————————

PATIENT NAME—LastFirst, Middle Initial | ID#

Form 3457P · 1995 Briggs Corporation, Des Moines, IA 50306
R1102   To order, phone 1-800-247-2343 www.BriggsCorp.com PRINTED IN U.S.A.

INITIAL PSYCHOSOCIAL ASSESSMENT

Page 1 of 4

Figure 1-8 Initial psychosocial assessment tool. (Courtesy Briggs Corporation, Des Moines, IA.)

SUPPORT SYSTEM ASSESSMENT

Discuss the questions listed below with the patient and family. Summarize their responses in the space provided.

What has this experience been like for you? Do(es) family/patient talk about illness with you? How is that for you?

Patient: _____

_____

_____

Family: _____

_____

_____

Have there been changes in the roles of members of your family? Changes in family plans/routines?

Patient: _____

_____

_____

Family: _____

_____

_____

What are the reactions to increased dependency?

Patient: _____

_____

Family: _____

_____

Who/what in your community can you count on in hard times?

_____

_____

RISK ASSESSMENT						
Check the appropriate response for each question below. A "yes" response indicates a risk potential.						
	PATIENT			PRIMARY CAREGIVER		
	YES	NO	Uncertain	YES	NO	Uncertain
Are there children/adolescents in immediate family?						
Are there dependent family members (handicapped, elderly, sick)?						
Is a parent still alive?						
Will death result in loss of financial provision?						
Will death mean loss of constant companion/emotional support?						
Will death mean loss of home (feared or actual)?						
Does the family have difficulty making decisions?						
Is family unable to share feelings?						
Is there reluctance to face facts of illness?						
Is there marital or family discord?						
Are there communication difficulties in the family?						
Is there a concurrent life crisis?						
Has there been difficulty in dealing with previous losses?						
Is the family inflexible?						
Has the patient or family members had excessive or prolonged emotional problems/mental illness?						
Is there a lack of community support?						

INITIAL PSYCHOSOCIAL ASSESSMENT

Page 2 of 4

Figure 1-8, cont'd Initial psychosocial assessment tool. (Courtesy Briggs Corporation, Des Moines, IA.)

Continued

INITIAL PSYCHOSOCIAL ASSESSMENT

PHYSICAL RESOURCE ASSESSMENT

Environmental Factors —

Source and Adequacy of Income —

Other Financial Factors —

SERVICE NEEDS

Does the patient need assistance in any of the areas listed below?

	YES	NO	TYPE OF ASSISTANCE/REFERRAL NEEDED
Budget Counseling			
Other Financial Need			
Social Services			
Funeral Arrangements			
Legal Will Preparation			

EMOTIONAL ASSESSMENT

Is the patient exhibiting or experiencing the following?

	YES	NO		YES	NO			YES	NO
Memory Problems			Withdrawal			Feelings of:	Loneliness		
Changes in Sleep Patterns			Hostility				Isolation		
Anxiety			Anger				Guilt		
Alertness			Irritability			Moodiness			
Lethargy			Depression			Hallucinations			

Does the patient have impaired comprehension, judgment, or reasoning?   ❏ Yes (If yes, explain)   ❏ No

COMMENTS ON PATIENT/FAMILY RISK POTENTIAL AND EMOTIONAL STATUS (Discuss risk potential of patient/family and the primary problems observed. Include family dynamics, present and anticipated coping, support systems, etc. Also include grief potential within the family and any factors that would influence the intensity or level of grief.)

Figure 1-8, cont'd Initial psychosocial assessment tool. (Courtesy Briggs Corporation, Des Moines, IA.)

ASSESSMENT SUMMARY AND PLAN

Signature and Title
of Assessor _____   Date ____ / ____ / ____

INITIAL PSYCHOSOCIAL ASSESSMENT   Page 4 of 4

Figure 1-8, cont'd Initial psychosocial assessment tool. (Courtesy Briggs Corporation, Des Moines, IA.)

Communication skills include active listening, realizing the work of "getting things in order," presence as an intervention, and being sensitively cued to what the patient and family are saying (and sometimes asking for). An example is Sarah, a 39-year-old woman with an aggressive, recurrent breast cancer. At a nursing visit, Sarah said to the hospice clinician, "Anne, I want to renew my vows with my husband before I die." Anne said that she would talk to her later about that because she was doing her dressing change. However, this discussion did not occur, and Sarah later expressed the same wish to the HHA, who reported it at the patient care conference. Because of this team effort, Sarah did renew her vows before her death. Especially in hospice, because of the limited time factor, patient and family needs must be addressed in a timely manner and followed up. In addition, this example shows an important component of hospice, spiritual care.

Patient and family needs, both those clearly articulated and those that are more veiled, should be identified to ensure that the hospice team is meeting them. These spiritual and other psychosocial needs are a key component in the provision and evaluation of high-quality hospice nursing.

Another challenge is family members asking, "When is he/she going to die?" Box 1-1 provides a useful list of some of the signs that family members may expect to see with the approach of death.

5. **A sense of humor**
   It is only in the past few years that the healing power of laughter has finally come to be recognized. A kind sense of humor helps the entire team and patients and their families on particularly rough days or in meeting unique challenges.

6. **Flexibility**
   Patients and families in hospice control their care and care planning. Because the days shared with the hospice team are the patient's last months or weeks, the patient calls the shots. This includes scheduling, visit times, length of visits, and a myriad of other decisions. Respect for and acceptance of the patient's choices and decisions are part of effective daily operations in hospice and are required by law through patient self-determination acts.

7. **Hospice and palliative care knowledge**
   It is very important that the hospice clinician have a strong base of knowledge grounded in hospice care and practice. A body of literature is emerging related to hospice, and all team members must keep current.

IDENTIFIED DIFFERENCES BETWEEN HOME CARE AND HOSPICE NURSING

Because of the growth of hospice and the bulk of care being provided in the patient's home, it is important to note that many patients may be in home

BOX 1-1

APPROACHING DEATH
Signs and Symptoms

The following are some of the signs and symptoms as death approaches. It is important to note that not all of these symptoms may ever appear, nor will they appear at the same time. Some of the most common symptoms are as follows:

1. *Cooling of the extremities* means that the patient's hands, arms, or feet are cool to the touch, and mottling or a purplish coloring may appear. Sometimes the skin also darkens with the decrease in circulation as death approaches. Interventions are related to keeping the patient warm, but electric blankets should not be used for safety reasons.

2. *Breathing slows and becomes irregular.* Cheyne-Stokes breathing may occur as the cerebrum, the control center for respirations, begins to fail. This breathing is usually characterized by irregularity and apnea, sometimes with long periods between breaths.

3. *The patient sleeps almost all the time.* This occurs as the slow but progressive failure of body systems occurs and metabolic needs decrease proportionately toward death.

4. *Fluids begin to build up in some patients.* This may appear as increased secretions in the throat or create a sound like a "rattle." The body can no longer absorb the secretions, and the fluid is heard as a result. The rattle, which can be distressing to family members, can sometimes be controlled with medication. The patient may also be suctioned or repositioned for comfort in some instances.

5. *The patient may appear confused or restless.* Confusion states are a common part of the death process and may be very upsetting to family members. Caregiver and family members may want to reassure the patient or provide presence to the patient. It is important that the restlessness be assessed as being caused by the lack of oxygenation and not from pain or other discomfort.

6. No matter what the symptoms or signs of approaching death, it is important that family members support the patient through this changing period with their presence and support. *Patients can still hear* even if their eyes appear glassy and unresponsive.

care health care or home health care oncology program and have been receiving home visits. Patients and clinicians seeking to make the transition to hospice commonly want clarification of the major differences. The following information seeks to address some of the many differences. It is important to note that the dimensions of scope, depth, and breadth of quality hospice care extend well beyond those of the standard medically directed and focused home health care program.

1

1. *In home care:* The patient is the unit or focus of care. Patient care is usually directed toward health and ultimately self-care. Care is the traditional medical model, as Medicare, a medical insurance program, pays for medically necessary care. Care in home care is usually related to illness and therapeutic, curative, interventions.

   In hospice: The patient, partner, family, and/or identified caregivers are a single unit and are the recipients of care. Hospice is what all clinicians learned in health care school; here the patient and family are an inseparable unit of care, and the patient is an equal partner in determining that care and making choices related to care and care planning.

2. *In home care:* Much of the care is medically focused on curative interventions and outcomes. Care and programs are structured for reimbursement and regulatory reasons.

   In hospice: The care and outcomes are focused on comfort and relief of suffering, pain management, and other palliative or symptom-control interventions. Because of this, hospice clinicians and their hospice teammates are often experts in symptom management and care planning. Because hospices have historically grown out of grassroots initiatives to provide special supportive care in a local community, they have a flexibility and creativity unknown to most traditional health care models. This means that there are unique programs to support patients, their families, and surviving loved ones. Creative programs offered by hospices include specialized bereavement camps for children, music therapy programs, art therapy interventions, and others. In fact, some hospices continue to be community- and volunteer-based, are not Medicare certified, and do not provide "insurance-covered" care, with its attendant rules and structures.

3. *In home care:* In the best organizations, home care is a team effort.

   In hospice: In hospice, care and care planning are truly a team effort. A standard in all hospice programs is that the patient and family care is planned and provided by an interdisciplinary team.

4. *In home care:* Medicare has traditionally been a cost-based reimbursement system that sometimes reinforced unneeded or medically unnecessary visits. As home care becomes a prospective payment system, the need for efficiencies becomes paramount.

   In hospice: The Medicare hospice benefit is a managed care system of reimbursement. An in-depth discussion about Medicare hospice can be found under the heading *Medicare Hospice 101*. The Medicare/Medicaid certified hospice program is reimbursed on a daily capitated rate (amount per day) to provide palliative care related to the terminal illness. This is also called a *per diem* rate ("daily" in Latin).

5. *In home care:* In home care, it can be frustrating when a patient chooses not to have hospice when the clinician has determined that the patient and family (and the care team) would have additional support and that needed care cannot be provided under the auspices of regular home care. For this reason, some programs have a "bridge," or "pre-hospice," program.

In hospice: Volunteer support, staff support mechanisms, and the true team concept all assist and support the team members through the patient's death and beyond. Continuity and closure are also offered through bereavement services for the patient's survivors with trained bereavement counselors for 13 months after death. The supportive and nurturing nature of the team encourages members to support each other, avoiding the "I'm out there alone" feeling.

6. *In home care:* Productivity and other parameters of effectiveness are designated by time frames (e.g., 6–7 visits per day, or 25–30 visits per week both, on average).

In hospice: Time frames may be more difficult to project in hospice because of lengthy or extended visits. The initial hospice visit may take more than one visit and may be over 2 hours. Hospice clinicians may make only three to four visits a day, depending on the patient/family needs and status. Although there may be productivity standards, the hospice team visits as long as reasonably needed to meet patient/family needs.

Not only is there much information to provide on admission; it must be provided in a sensitive manner with the patient and family usually setting the pace. Some hospices have both a clinician and a social worker admit the patient for the first or initial admitting visit. If the hospice is Medicare certified and the patient is admitted under the hospice benefit, the rules must be explained, multiple forms, such as a hospice consent, must be signed, and clinical and physical assessment data must be gathered. All this is labor intensive. It is only with experience that admission and subsequent visits become more efficient and effective.

MEDICARE HOSPICE 101

Many insurers now cover or reimburse hospice programs for hospice services. How hospice services are defined may vary, as may the specific coverage and documentation requirements. Medicare has a Medicare hospice benefit (MHB), which many state Medicaid programs mirror. The hospice team is expert on communicating coverage and other information to patients and families in the advocacy role. It is for this reason that hospice team members should know the fundamentals of the Medicare hospice program.

Congress enacted the benefit in 1983 and made it a permanent program in 1986. The following five requirements must be met for a patient to be eligible for the Medicare hospice benefit:

1. The patient is eligible for Medicare Hospital Insurance (Part A).
2. The patient is certified by an attending physician and the hospice medical director to have a limited life expectancy with a poor prognosis (usually 6 months or less if the disease runs its expected course).
3. The patient resides in a geographic area where there is a Medicare-certified hospice program.
4. A written plan of care is established and regularly reviewed
5. The patient elects the Medicare hospice benefit. See form entitled "Election of Medicare Hospice Benefit" (Figure. 1-9).

ELECTION OF MEDICARE HOSPICE BENEFIT

I, ______________________ (Social Security # ______________________), choose and
NAME—First, MI, Last

consent to have ______________________ Hospice provide for my care under

the Medicare Hospice Benefit, effective ___/___/___
(Month/Day/Year)

I understand that the Medicare Hospice Benefit takes the place of Medicare Part A or my Medicare HMO plan for treatment of my terminal illness. *Medicare Part B or my Medicare HMO plan remains responsible for physician services as long as I pay my premium.* I will be evaluated at the end of each benefit period (90 days, 90 days, and an unlimited number of subsequent 60 day periods) for my continued eligibility.

I understand that by choosing the Medicare Hospice Benefit, I will be entitled to the following services if certified necessary by my doctor and the Hospice Team:

1. Intermittent visits by nursing personnel, a homemaker, home health aide, social worker, chaplain, volunteers and other professionals as defined on the Informed Consent Form.
2. Intermittent visits and/or consultation by auxilliary team members providing dietary, physical, occupational and speech therapies.
3. Extended hours of care in the home in times of medical crisis, as determined by the Hospice Team and defined by the Medicare Hospice Benefit. Hospice is on call twenty-four (24) hours a day, seven (7) days a week.
4. Medical supplies, equipment and prescription medications (less deductible, if applicable) that are related to my terminal diagnosis.
5. Hospital care for acute pain and symptom management that cannot be achieved at home. Short-term inpatient care is provided only as arranged by Hospice.
6. Respite care to relieve the family/caregiver for up to five (5) days per stay per period.

I understand that I may revoke this Benefit anytime and re-elect in the next certification period. I may transfer to another Medicare Certified Hospice Program without reducing the benefits to which I am entitled. I consent for Medicare to reimburse this hospice organization directly for service. I will be informed of any costs Medicare does not cover and if I agree to these services, I will be responsible for this cost.

Date ___/___/___ ______________________
Month/Day/Year — Signature of Patient or Responsible Person (if Patient Is Unable to Sign)

Date ___/___/___ ______________________
Month/Day/Year — Signature of Primary Contact Person or Family/Caregiver Member

Date ___/___/___ ______________________
Month/Day/Year — Signature of Hospice Representative

PART 1 —Hospice PART 2 —Patient

PATIENT NAME —Last, First, Middle Initial	ID#

Form 3466/2P © 1995 Briggs, Des Moines, IA 50306 PRINTED IN U.S.A. (R203)

DON'T BREAK THE LAW MAKE THE CALL Save 13%* 1-800-247-2343 www.BriggsCorp.com

*savings on buying vs. copying

ELECTION OF MEDICARE HOSPICE BENEFIT

Figure 1-9 Election of Medicare hospice benefit form. (Courtesy Briggs Corporation, Des Moines, IA.)

Simply put, the patient who elects the hospice benefit "gives up," or "waives," regular Medicare benefits for the admitting disease or diagnosis. This is usually not a problem unless the patient wants more care than can be delivered through hospice. Patients who elect the benefit receive palliative and noncurative care and support for certain benefit periods. These periods are for two initial 90-day benefit periods, followed by an unlimited number of subsequent 60-day periods. The benefit periods may be used consecutively

HOSPICE BENEFIT CERTIFICATION

CERTIFICATION STATEMENT

I certify/recertify that it is my professional judgment, based on the medical information available to me, that_____
(First Name of Patient)

_____, who elected the Medicare or Medicaid Hospice Benefit for_____
(Last Name of Patient)   (Circle One)   (Diagnosis)
is terminally ill with a life expectancy of six months or less if the terminal illness runs its normal course.

INITIAL 90-DAY CERTIFICATION (PERIOD I)

Start Date ____ / ____ / ____   End Date ____ / ____ / ____

Verbal order to certify from Primary Physician received by:_____ Date ____ / ____ / ____
(Signature and Title)

Verbal order to certify from Hospice Physician received by: _____ Date ____ / ____ / ____
(Signature and Title)

* Primary Physician's Signature _____ Certification Date ____ / ____ / ____

* Hospice Physician's Signature _____ Certification Date ____ / ____ / ____
* Physician signature also serves as counter signature for verbal order

RECERTIFICATION: 90 DAYS (PERIOD II)

Start Date ____ / ____ / ____   End Date ____ / ____ / ____   I ❑ Do ❑ Do Not recertify at this time.

Verbal order to certify from Hospice Physician received by: _____ Date ____ / ____ / ____
(Signature and Title)

* Hospice Physician's Signature _____ Date ____ / ____ / ____

* Remainder of benefit period revoked/transferred as of Date ____ / ____ / ____* Physician signature also serves as counter signature for verbal order.

RECERTIFICATION: SUBSEQUENT 60 DAYS (PERIOD III)

Start Date ____ / ____ / ____   End Date ____ / ____ / ____   I ❑ Do ❑ Do Not recertify at this time.

Verbal order to certify from Hospice Physician received by: _____ Date ____ / ____ / ____
(Signature and Title)

* Hospice Physician's Signature _____ Date ____ / ____ / ____

* Remainder of benefit period revoked/transferred as of Date ____ / ____ / ____* Physician signature also serves as counter signature for verbal order.

RECERTIFICATION: SUBSEQUENT 60 DAYS (PERIOD IV)

Start Date ____ / ____ / ____   End Date ____ / ____ / ____   I ❑ Do ❑ Do Not recertify at this time.

Verbal order to certify from Hospice Physician received by: _____ Date ____ / ____ / ____
(Signature and Title)

* Hospice Physician's Signature _____ Date ____ / ____ / ____

* Remainder of benefit period revoked/transferred as of Date ____ / ____ / ____* Physician signature also serves as counter signature for verbal order.

RECERTIFICATION: SUBSEQUENT 60 DAYS (PERIOD V)

Start Date ____ / ____ / ____   End Date ____ / ____ / ____   I ❑ Do ❑ Do Not recertify at this time.

Verbal order to certify from Hospice Physician received by: _____ Date ____ / ____ / ____
(Signature and Title)

* Hospice Physician's Signature _____ Date ____ / ____ / ____

* Remainder of benefit period revoked/transferred as of Date ____ / ____ / ____* Physician signature also serves as counter signature for verbal order.

RECERTIFICATION: SUBSEQUENT 60 DAYS (PERIOD VI)

Start Date ____ / ____ / ____   End Date ____ / ____ / ____   I ❑ Do ❑ Do Not recertify at this time.

Verbal order to certify from Hospice Physician received by: _____ Date ____ / ____ / ____
(Signature and Title)

* Hospice Physician's Signature _____ Date ____ / ____ / ____

* Remainder of benefit period revoked/transferred as of Date ____ / ____ / ____* Physician signature also serves as counter signature for verbal order.

Part 1 – Clinical Record   Part 2 – Physician

PATIENT NAME–Last, First, Middle Initial | ID#

Form 3463/2P © 1995 Briggs Corporation, Des Moines, IA 50306
To order, phone 1-800-247-2343 www.BriggsCorp.com PRINTED IN U.S.A.

Figure 1-10 Hospice benefit certification form. (Courtesy Briggs Corporation, Des Moines, IA.)

or at intervals. Regardless of whether patients use the benefit periods consecutively or at different times, they must be certified each time (by the physician) as terminally ill. Patients can "revoke" the benefit should they wish to withdraw from the hospice program and revert to standard Medicare coverage. A hospice benefit certification form and revocation form are presented in Figures 1-10 and 1-11. Note that if a patient revokes in the

STATEMENT OF REVOCATION

Medicare Number_____

Effective_____/_____/_____, I, _____ , choose to revoke
         Date of Revocation   Patient s Name
election for Medicare coverage under the Hospice Medicare Benefit.

   1. I understand that I am revoking Hospice Medicare Benefit for the remainder of
      the current benefit period for the following reason: _____

      _____

   2. I understand that if I am in the first, second or subsequent benefit periods, as
      listed below, I can at any time in the future elect Hospice Medicare coverage
      for the remaining benefit period(s). I am, however, forfeiting Hospice Medicare
      coverage for the days remaining in the current benefit period.

      The benefit periods are as follows:

               First Benefit Period —90 Days
             Second Benefit Period —90 Days
        Subsequent Benefit Periods —Unlimited 60 Day Periods

   3. I understand that the Medicare health care benefits I waived to receive Hospice
      Medicare coverage will be resumed after the effective date of this revocation.

Signature of Patient
or Legal Representative _____ Date _____/_____/_____

Signature of Witness _____ Date _____/_____/_____

Signature of Witness _____ Date _____/_____/_____

PART 1 —Clinical Record	**PART 2 —Physician**	**PART 3 —Patient/Representative**
PATIENT NAME—LastFirst, Middle Initial		ID#

Form 3456/3P   1995 Briggs Corporation, Des Moines, IA 50306 www.BriggsCorp.com
        To order, phone 1-800-247-2343 PRINTED IN U.S.A.

HOSPICE MEDICARE BENEFIT REVOCATION

Figure 1-11 Hospice Medicare benefit revocation form. (Courtesy Briggs
Corporation, Des Moines, IA.)

middle of a benefit period, the remaining days in that benefit period are lost.
In addition, some of the requirements of regular Medicare home care are
waived for these patients. For example, the patient does not have to be
homebound or meet skilled care requirements as skilled care is defined in
the Medicare home health benefit.

    The strength of the Medicare hospice program is that it is a comprehen-
sive managed care program where all services and care are coordinated

through one entity—the hospice organization. Coverage for services related to the terminal illness generally includes physician services, health care, medical supplies and equipment, short-term inpatient care (including respite care), home health aide services, physical therapy, speech-language pathology services, and medical social services and counseling, including dietary counseling. Patients have limited cost-sharing for drugs and inpatient respite care. The hospice program is the expert on the rules related to the Medicare hospice program. Although the Medicare hospice program is a needed and viable program for some Medicare beneficiaries seeking hospice, it may not be appropriate for all patients, some of whom may desire curative care or treatment through death.

SKILLS AND KNOWLEDGE NEEDED IN HOSPICE CARE

1. **A knowledge of the core care standards and rules for hospice care**
   These consist of both administrative and clinical information and are important to being an effective team member. For Medicare-certified hospices or hospices that are also home health agencies (HHAs), knowledge of the following is required:
   - The Medicare Conditions of Participation for hospice (and home care if dually certified)
   - The Medicare Hospice Manual provisions about hospice coverage
   - If dually-certified, the section of the home health agency manual that addresses the correct completion of the OASIS and other forms
   - National Patient Safety Goals (NPSGs)

   Other important core care standards are the NHPCO's *Standards of a Hospice Program of Care* and relevant accreditation standards related to hospice, such as those issued by the Joint Commission on Accreditation of Healthcare Organizations (JCAHO) or Community Health Accreditation Program (CHAP).

   Because Medicare sets many standards, it is important to be familiar and up to date with these rules. Some other insurers also use Medicare's criteria for qualifying and/or coverage. In addition, many insurers, such as state Medicaid programs or private insurers, use facsimiles of the HCFA form 485 as the POC and provide hospice services that mirror the Medicare coverage. In hospice the HCFA form 485 is not mandated, but a plan of care is.

2. **A repertoire of service-driven and patient-oriented interpersonal skills**
   Community liaison and public relations activities are a part of the hospice home care clinician's busy day. To those we meet, such as the community pharmacist or a family member of a patient, we represent hospice. Make those impressions positive!

1

3. **The ability to pay incredible attention to detail**

   This is true both in addressing complex patient and family care needs and in documentation. Both are equally important, and they go hand in hand in the provision of high-quality hospice care.

4. **The possession of multifaceted skills accompanied by flexibility**

   It is the hospice clinician who must "bend" or renegotiate to meet patient and family needs and achieve patient-centered outcomes. This flexibility usually includes visiting times and scheduling but can also include aspects that center on accommodating patient and family/caregiver needs.

5. **The possession of a reliable car and safe, effective driving skills**

   The hospice clinician in the community must like, or at least not mind, driving (even in inclement weather), have a good sense of direction (or a map!).

6. **The ability to assume responsibility for the patient and family's care and the patient's POC**

   Holistic care is a reality in quality hospice care. From the initial hospice assessment through the identification of patient and family needs and challenges, the hospice clinician assumes the planning and follow-through for care. Sometimes only a limited number of core hospice team members are involved in the care, depending on the patient and family needs. Because of these factors, the hospice clinician in the community setting can directly affect the care and see the results of that planned and continually evaluated care. Close communication is required between the hospice clinician and the other team members and any case managers involved with the care. This patient-management function, with its associated prioritizing and sometimes complex decision making, makes hospice practice unique. It is from this aspect that hospice team members often receive personal satisfaction and positive feedback from patients and their families, friends, and caregivers.

7. **Strong clinical skills and the ability to function as both a specialist and a generalist clinician**

   Hospice patients may be of all age-groups, from infants to the elderly. In addition, the diagnoses and care needs of patients may vary from day to day. Within the hospice organization, a wide range of clinical problems and nursing diagnoses may exist. Developing an area of expertise and acting as a resource for clinicians new to hospice care are important assets for the individual clinician or manager's own professional growth.

8. **Self-direction and the ability to function autonomously in a nonstructured atmosphere**

   Self-direction means having well-developed and effective time-management skills to address the many aspects of care, including visits scheduled, documentation, and detail-oriented administrative duties (e.g., completing and updating plans of care, returning a phone call in a timely way).

1

9. **The desire to continue learning and being open to new information and clinical skills**

   This is particularly important given the many new kinds of technologies being used in the home setting. Dobutamine management, new pain- and symptom-management methods, and ethical dilemmas may be some of the care problems competent clinicians and managers address daily. For this reason, "resources for care and practice" are listed in each care guideline, and journal articles, books, and other resources that may assist in the goal of ongoing lifelong education and learning are listed in Part 6.

10. **A sincere appreciation of people**

    This includes interacting positively with and being empathetic to all patients, families, and caregivers, who are often in the midst of crises. Because many family caregivers continue to work outside the home, hospice team members use their observation, assessment, teaching, and training skills to maintain patient safety in the home. This teaching or consulting role brings job satisfaction as well as comfort and security to the families.

11. **The ability to be open and sincerely accepting of people's unique and chosen lifestyles and of the effects that these lifestyles have on their health**

    Being accepting is easier said than done! We have all cared for patients with end-stage COPD who continue to smoke two to three packs a day and do not adhere to the safety instructions they have been taught regarding oxygen. These ethical dilemmas of safety versus self-determination are a part of professional hospice practice.

12. **The awareness and acceptance that a constant balance must be maintained between clinical and administrative demands**

    In addition, the clinician must know that both demands are equally important, but in different ways and for different reasons.

13. **The knowledge that change can be difficult**

    The hospice home care culture is very different from the "down the hall" camaraderie, supervision, and peer consultation available in the inpatient hospice setting.

14. **The possession of a kind sense of humor that can help patients, families, and peers get through the rough times**

    This sense of humor is finally being recognized for its healing power when used appropriately.

15. **Knowledge of the economics of health care and the larger environment that is affecting home care health and hospice specifically**

    A basic knowledge of reimbursement, including differences among payer sources, utilization, and payment mechanisms and what this means to hospice patients and their families, is very useful in the clinician's role as admission and insurance specialist on the initial visits.

16. **Time-management skills to be able to prioritize and manage diverse and sometimes equally important tasks and responsibilities**
The best clinicians in hospice home care are very well organized and use their organizational skills in their daily routines. They create and keep detailed schedules, document at the patient's home (unless there are safety concerns), and generally seek to do things right the first time. Day scheduling calendars, cellular phones, voice mail, and other technological tools also assist these important aspects of communication and care.

17. **The practical wisdom of hospice care and practice**
Practical wisdom is information that comes with reading and practice. It may be called "the best way to do things." Much of this knowledge base comes from watching and learning from experienced hospice clinicians. It includes such practical tips as always having two supplies with you (the Noah's Ark approach) because the time you don't will be the time you'll need that second catheter or other item. Other areas where experience helps include organizing paperwork, setting up your schedule, and tracking physician orders. Try to impart to others the information you needed when you began and have now.

THE HOSPICE ORIENTATION

All new hospice team members need an appropriate orientation period. A high-quality orientation is important to being successful and feeling comfortable in the hospice team member role. No matter how understaffed the program may be, prospective team members should, when possible, try to define or address their orientation (including time span and content) before accepting the position. The following list addresses some of the information that an orientation should include. Obviously, if the clinician or manager has been in hospice home care for some time, it may not be appropriate or necessary to review all this information; however, it is important that all team members have an understanding of these hallmarks of hospice.

- The organization's orientation manual
- The Medicare COPs for Hospice (and/or Home Health Care if the organization is a dually Medicare-certified program)
- The schedule of hospice team and staff support meetings
- The Medicare hospice and/or HHA manual (the coverage of services sections) if the organization provides hospice services as a Medicare-certified hospice and/or HHA
- The hospice clinical and administrative policy and procedure manual(s)
- An overview of the organization's clinical records, documentation system, and required forms, including where the paperwork goes and when it must be completed and submitted

- Guidelines for hospice home visits and what they entail, including verbal orders, the referral process, and scheduling
- The opportunity to "buddy" with an experienced hospice clinician from the organization
- The hospice's required forms, including the Health Insurance Portability and Accountability Act (HIPAA) rules of privacy and security
- Hospice coverage and documentation requirements, including confidentiality and the timeliness of physician orders
- Administrative details and processes (e.g., payroll, on-call scheduling, mileage reports)
- Equipment and supply acquisition (e.g., venipuncture supplies, personal protective equipment [PPE], lab forms, and drop-off locations)
- The specific automated clinical documentation system, where applicable
- Performance improvement (PI) activities and processes and the clinician's role in identifying and reporting information (e.g., patient infection, falls, missed visits, adverse drug reactions)
- Benefits, employee handbook, mileage, on-call process and pay, lab pick-up schedules, and other miscellaneous information unique to the program
- Occupational Safety and Health Administration (OSHA) requirements, including (1) hepatitis B virus vaccination, (2) the HHA-related policies and supplies for bloodborne pathogens and tuberculosis, (3) standard precautions supplies with appropriate barriers and related disposal of supplies, and (4) record-keeping activities
- Completion of a skills checklist or proficiency testing and ongoing educational plan
- Information related to compliance with laws and regulations (e.g., home health aide supervisory visit frequency, timeliness for obtaining physician orders)
- Pain- and symptom-management skills
- An orientation to the hospice's response and plans for the NPSGs
- On-call strategies and skills
- The roles of the other team members of the hospice IDG

A more in-depth narrative discussion about hospice orientation follows.

Hospice Orientation Considerations

Hospice orientation varies in scope, depth, and time span, depending on the organization and the new team member's experience. Remember that you are not alone in making the transition to a new area of care or practice and that orientation and education continue long after the formal orientation period. In fact, the best hospice clinicians and managers truly make learning a lifelong endeavor. There is always more to know!

Everyone knows how exciting and difficult it can be to leave what is known and familiar and move on to learn new skills in a foreign environment. The challenge is well worth the work. *It goes without saying that no clinician new to home health care or hospice should care for patients without an effective orientation.* The *Webster's Collegiate Dictionary* definition of *orient* is "to acquaint with the existing situation or environment." The

American Nurses Association (ANA) defines *orientation* as "the means by which new staff members are introduced to the philosophy, goals, policies, procedures, role expectation, physical facilities and special services in a specific work setting." The information in this section provides a framework for review and reference during this transition.

Orientation is perhaps the most important period in the role transformation to hospice, and the initial information presented may set the stage for future growth, professional development, and the clinician's satisfaction in the role and the organization. The orientation period is the time designated for honing clinical skills, taking the time to find answers, and developing new relationships with peers and managers. It has been said that excellence "is in the details," and this is very true in hospice care. During orientation, information will be provided about documentation, detailed assessments, thoughtful data analysis, and the importance of clear communications to other hospice team members. These are the kinds of details that contribute to effective and quality hospice care. Perhaps most important, orientation is the time to be detail oriented and acquire the knowledge that constitutes the "practical wisdom" of hospice.

Defining the Hospice Orientation

Many important aspects of hospice care must be covered in the limited "official" orientation period. Overall behavioral outcomes or goals for the transitioning clinician include:

- Completing the orientation within the time allocated
- Identifying key staff members and customers (defined by the organization)
- Describing and explaining new patient assignment processes
- Demonstrating clinical competence in the home hospice setting
- Adhering to policies and procedures as observed/monitored
- Knowing where to go for questions or challenges related to practice and operations
- Other goals defined as policies and procedures by the individual hospice organization

Competency Assessment and Validation

Employees new to hospice can expect their new or existing employer to check their references and request completion of a self-assessment tool or checklist. These checklists identify specific skills or areas of knowledge and education, including areas where the clinician may need to review or be observed. They are also a way to validate competency, which is a hallmark of quality in hospice practice. The process of identifying educational and orientation needs is a way for the organization to ensure competency by hiring qualified team members.

It is important to note that some organizations identify their own list of high-risk, low-volume skills and may have all nurses demonstrate competency in these skills. Examples include tracheostomy care and specialty assessments. A preceptor may accompany the new clinician in the field to observe certain skills and thereby ensure safe and effective patient care and standardization of care and care processes among team members and across the organization.

Organizational Orientation Topics

The topics that may be addressed by the organization's orientation program cover a broad range of content. The information under these topics is prioritized in this section to emphasize the regulatory aspects interfacing with clinical patient care that must be understood to function safely in hospice. This section then lists topics and areas that should be addressed for quality, safety, practice, and accreditation reasons.

Although this looks like a voluminous amount of information, it all will make sense over the months to come (see Box 1-2 for orientation tips). In fact, colleagues who have successfully made the transition are likely to say that "about 6 months into this, it all came together and made sense." This information is presented in a functional format to make sense to clinicians making this important transition. There are numerous policies in hospice, but those listed below and their associated processes/outcomes provide a practical overview of the hospice specialty. This list is by no means all-inclusive but identifies those areas with the most direct impact on hospice clinicians.

BOX 1-2

ABSORBING IT ALL
Five Tips for Orientees

1. Complete assessment questions (or weekly evaluation forms, etc.) completely and accurately. This assists you and your manager/instructor/preceptor in goal revision.
2. Take notes. Orientation presents voluminous and important information, and it is sometimes difficult at the beginning to see the bigger picture. These notes can refresh your memory.
3. Ask questions. Others may have the same questions and not ask them. As well as addressing any confusing issues, your questions may inspire additional explanations that will help you remember certain information.
4. Listen actively. The depth and breadth of information demand this level of participation.
5. Provide feedback at the conclusion or after a defined time period. When the evaluation process occurs, complete evaluation forms and provide comments to assist the organization in its ongoing efforts to improve the orientation program and related processes.

Adapted from Marrelli: *The Nurse Manager's Survival Guide: Practice Answers to Everyday Problems*, ed. 3, 2004, Mosby.

1

Orientation may include, in addition to clinicians, other new hospice team members, such as therapists, social workers, pharmacists, spiritual counselors, volunteers, home health aides or certified health care assistants, intake coordinators, and clinical managers or educators. This is a great way to meet new colleagues and team members in a new hospice organization. From the beginning, you will see that the best hospice care is truly a team effort and that "everyone works from the same page."

As health care moves to the standardization of care and care processes for quality purposes, much of the same information must be provided to all the team members. Some organizations provide an orientation that is standardized for all new employees at the beginning and then, as the information becomes more specific, such as for nursing, the orientation continues with only the nurses.

1. **Mission, vision, values, philosophy**

   Hospice organizations have their own unique mission. Simply put, the mission is the bottom line of what the organization does and why it exists. The mission statement can be one sentence or a few sentences long if it articulates the vision and values to which the organization ascribes. Examples of mission statements include the following: "XYZ Hospice provides the best palliative care with the most competent staff"; "St. Elsewhere Home Care follows the mission of St. Elsewhere Hospital into the community, where we provide comprehensive and high-quality health care services, including hospice, in the community."

   Process/outcome: The orientee may receive a copy of the mission statement in the orientation packet with the history of the hospice organization. Sometimes the mission statement is written on the back or front of the identification/name badge, on business cards and letterhead of the organization, or on the agency's brochures. All team members in hospice must work together, and the mission can help in this quest. The new orientee should be able to restate the hospice mission statement and goals on completion of the orientation.

2. **Hospice brochure**

   The organization's brochure contains important information about the services provided. This is the information shared with patients, discharge planners, and other customers who may be interested in hospice services. This brochure indicates whether the organization is state licensed or Medicare-certified and/or accredited; how patients reach the organization; the on-call system and how to access care after regular business hours; the specific services their organization provides through its program; and any specialty programs or other information. Usually the brochure is provided during or before the application process. However, it may be given during the formal orientation as part of the packet of materials for new team members. The geographical areas covered by the hospice also may be listed in the brochure or provided as a policy.

   Process/outcome: This information is also provided initially and is explained by the nurse during the admitting visit and reinforced on subsequent visits. The new orientee should be able to list and describe the services and other information in the brochure about the hospice organization.

3. **Organizational chart**
   The new employee's position in relation to the hospice organization is very important for reporting, operational, and communication reasons. The organizational chart or table of organization clearly shows the lines of communications and the manager to whom the new hospice team member will report. Keep in mind that in some larger hospice organizations, new clinicians may spend more time with the preceptor or instructor than with their immediate supervisor, particularly during orientation, depending on the size and organizational structure of the hospice.

   Process/outcome: The hospice clinician in orientation should be able to identify managers, peer interdisciplinary patient care providers, where he/she is located in the chain of command, who to go to with questions, and their voice in organizational operations.

4. **Office information**
   Office information includes the business hours of hospice operations (i.e., when the office itself is open), time card and payroll processes, beeper or pager acquisition, car phone and/or allowance, equipment and supply closet/acquisition process, mileage reimbursement, nurse bag sign-out or purchase procedure, schedule of staff meetings, and other processes and details.

   Process/outcome: The new team member should be able to obtain needed supplies or equipment for hospice patients and families using the standard process provided in the orientation and should know whom to call with a question or for assistance related to these important processes.

5. **Personnel or human resource (HR) information**
   The personnel staff can be very important to making a successful transition. Physical exams, any required lab tests, TB testing, hepatitis B vaccine acceptance or declination statement, benefit information, CPR training, license verification, professional liability policy, dress code, safety training, standards of conduct, the organizational grievance process, and other areas may all be under the purview of HR. HR may also request background checks, car insurance, and a valid driver's license. Many of these requirements or standards are based on compliance requirements under individual state laws, organizational policies, accreditation entities, and others (e.g., CDC, CHAP, JCAHO, OSHA).

6. **Position description**
   Orientees usually receive and may sign a copy of their position description and contract, if applicable.

   Process/outcome: An evaluation tool may be included with or as a part of the position description for the hospice team members at the organization. The new team member should identify the values of the

1

organization and work toward achieving high scores on the behaviors and skills listed on the performance appraisal tool.

7. **Important policies and procedures**
The orientee will review and may be asked to sign numerous but important policies and procedures. In addition, the new hospice clinician may be given an orientation manual that contains the specific applicable clinical and administrative policies. It is very important that the new orientee thoroughly review this information and demonstrate an ability to describe and adhere to these policies from accreditation, state survey, and risk management perspectives. Some of these policies follow.

- *Patient Rights and Responsibilities*
  The Patient Rights and Responsibilities policy is listed first because it is an important requirement of the Medicare COPs. This information is usually explained to the patient and family or other responsible person and read aloud if the patient needs assistance or has visual problems. This policy provides the patient and family with written notice of the patient's rights.

  An example of a patient rights and responsibility form is found in Figure 1-12. The five components of the bill of rights that may be the most important are as follows: (1) the patient and family are given a signed copy of their notice of rights; (2) the rights explain the respect that the organization will have for patients, their belongings, and their property; (3) patients should be notified of their right to confidentiality of medical record information, a policy that is upheld by hospice team members; (4) patients must be kept apprised of financial arrangements related to care and coverage, and changes must be communicated to patients per the rights and responsibility document; and (5) if the hospice is home health agency based, patients and caregivers must be made aware of the home health hotline, a 1-800 phone number in each state that patients can use for complaints related to home care and/or advance directives and for questions about local home health agencies.

  Process/outcome: The intent of this process is to ensure that at all times patients understand their rights and team members respect patient choices and decisions. Attitude is essential. Clinicians must know that they enter the home as guests, with services to offer that patients are free to accept or reject. Team members should be able to describe the intent and the process at the hospice organization for explaining patient rights and responsibilities.

- *HIPAA and Notice of Privacy Practice (NPP)*
  With the provisions of the Privacy Rule of HIPAA, all patients must now receive an NPP upon admission to hospice services. Patients must sign it as an acknowledgment.

- *Patient consent for hospice care*
  A written consent must be obtained for patients admitted to hospice. It is very important that the patient and family understand hospice, including the intent of the services, the hours of care available

As a home care patient, you have the right to be informed of your rights and responsibilities before the initiation of care/service. If/When a patient has been judged incompetent, the patient's family or guardian may exercise these rights as described below. As they relate to:

PATIENT RIGHTS, you have the right:

1. To receive services appropriate to your needs and expect the home care organization to provide safe, professional care at the level of intensity needed, without unlawful restriction by reason of age, sex, race, creed, color, national origin, religion or disability.
2. To have access to necessary professional services 24 hours a day, 7 days a week.
3. To have your pain management needs recognized and addressed as appropriate.
4. To be informed of services available.
5. To be informed of the ownership and control of the organization.
6. To be told on request if the organization's liability insurance will cover injuries to employees when they are in your home, and if it will cover theft or property damage that occurs while you are being treated.

PATIENT CARE, you have the right:

1. To be involved in your care planning, including education of the same, from admission to discharge, and to be informed in a reasonable time of anticipated termination and/or transfer of service.
2. To receive reasonable continuity of care.
3. To be informed of your rights and responsibilities in advance concerning care and treatment you will receive, including any changes, the frequency of care/service and by whom (disciplines) services will be provided.
4. To be informed of the nature and purpose of any technical procedure that will be performed, including information about the potential benefits and burdens as well as who will perform the procedure.
5. To receive care/service from staff who are qualified through education and/or experience to carry out the duties for which they are assigned.
6. To be referred to other agencies and/or organizations when appropriate and be informed of any financial benefit to the referring agency.

RESPECT AND CONFIDENTIALITY, you have the right:

1. To be treated with consideration, respect, and dignity, including the provision of privacy during care.
2. To have your property treated with respect.
3. To have staff communicate in a language or form you can reasonably be expected to understand and when possible, the organization assists with or may provide special devices, interpreters, or other aids to facilitate communication.
4. To maintain confidentiality of your clinical records in accordance with legal requirements and to anticipate the organization will release information only with your authorization or as required by law.
5. To be informed of the organization's policies and procedures for disclosure of your clinical record.

FINANCIAL ASPECTS OF CARE, you have the right:

1. To be informed of the extent to which payment for the home care services may be expected from Medicare, Medicaid or any other payer.
2. To be informed of charges not covered by Medicare and/or responsibility for any payment(s) that you may have to make.
3. To receive this information orally and in writing before care is initiated and within 30 calendar days of the date the organization becomes aware of any changes.

Form 3531   © 1994 Briggs Corporation, Des Moines, IA 50306
R1002   To order, phone 1-800-247-2343   www.BriggsCorp.com   PRINTED IN U.S.A.   **RIGHTS AND RESPONSIBILITIES**

Figure 1-12 Example of a patient rights and responsibilities form. (Courtesy Briggs Corporation, Des Moines, IA.)   *Continued*

(as opposed to regular organizational office hours), and the roles of the hospice in the care of the patient and family. An example of a patient consent for care form is given in Figure 1-13.

   Process/outcome: The information on the consent form should be reviewed with the patient or family before the provision of hospice care, the form should be signed by the hospice patient, and the patient or the patient's representative should be given a copy.

SELF-DETERMINATION, you have the right:

1. To refuse all or part of your care/treatment to the extent permitted by law and to be informed of the expected consequences of said action.
2. To be informed in writing of rights under state law to formulate advance directives.
3. To have the organization comply with advance directives as permitted by state law and state requirements.
4. To be informed of the organization's policies and procedures for implementing advance directives.
5. To receive care whether or not you have an advance directive(s) in place, as well as not to be discriminated against whether or not you have executed an advance directive(s).
6. To be informed regarding the organization's policies for withholding of resuscitative services and the withdrawal of life-sustaining treatment, as appropriate.
7. To not participate in research or not receive experimental treatment unless you give documented, voluntary informed consent.
8. To be informed of what to do in an emergency.
9. To participate in consideration of ethical issues that may arise in your care.

COMPLAINTS, you have the right:

1. To voice complaints/grievances about treatment or care that is (or fails to be) furnished, or regarding lack of respect for property without reprisal or discrimination for same and be informed of the procedure to voice complaints/grievances with the home care organization. Complaints or questions may be registered with

   _____
   Define individual(s)
   by phone, in person or in writing. The address and phone are _____

   _____.

   The organization investigates the complaint and resolution of same.

2. To be informed of the State Hotline. The _____ also has a State Hotline for complaints
   Define entity
   or questions about local home care agencies as well as to voice concerns regarding advance directives.

   The State Hotline number is ___**1-800-**_____

   and the days/hours of operation are _____

   _____.

PATIENT RESPONSIBILITIES

As a home care patient, you have the responsibility:

1. To provide complete and accurate information about illness, hospitalizations, medications, pain and other matters pertinent to your health; any changes in address, phone or insurance/payment information; and changes made to advance directives.
2. To inform the organization when you will not be able to keep your home care appointment.
3. To treat the staff with respect and consideration.
4. To participate in and follow your plan of care.
5. To provide a safe environment for care to be given.
6. To cooperate with staff and ask questions if you do not understand instruction or information given to you.
7. To assist the organization with billing and/or payment issues to help with processing third party payment.
8. To inform the organization of any problems (including issues with following the plan of care), dissatisfaction with services or recommendations for improvement.

RIGHTS AND RESPONSIBILITIES

Figure 1-12, cont'd Example of a patient rights and responsibilities form. (Courtesy Briggs Corporation, Des Moines, IA.)

- *Infection control*
  There are very specific infection control processes unique to caring for patients in the home environment. OSHA is the government department responsible for defining occupational safety for workers. Universal/standard precautions are the method used for infection control, and these protection and prevention guidelines related to bloodborne pathogens are also outlined by OSHA. Various policies addressing the

PATIENT CONSENT FOR CARE

I, _____, hereby consent to admission to and care by
Patient's Name

_____ Hospice. I understand that:

1. Hospice's goal is not to cure my terminal illness. The goal of hospice is to maintain quality of life through the management of pain and other symptoms when no further curative measures are planned. Hospice staff will also provide emotional and spiritual support (when requested) to me and my family and/or primary caregiver.

2. _____ will be considered my
Name
my "primary caregiver." This means he/she will be the person mainly responsible for overseeing my care at home.

3. Hospice services are provided by a team of staff specially trained in hospice care. Services may include medical, nursing, social work, homemaker/health aide, dietary, pastoral/spiritual and volunteer. The role of each hospice team member has been explained to me.

4. Care will be provided by scheduled appointment, but assistance is available 24 hours a day, 7 days a week. I can reach Hospice by calling (_____) _____.

5. While I am enrolled in this hospice program, a hospice team of caregivers will manage my care whether I'm being cared for in my home or in a hospital or nursing home.

6. The hospice medical record will contain information about me, my family and/or my primary caregiver. Every effort will be made to keep this information confidential. However, I authorize the organization to disclose and release information contained in my clinical record to the health care providers involved in my care, third party payers, utilization review and professional standard review organizations, regulatory review and accreditation entities and any other organizations, companies, community resources, etc. that may/will assist me to meet my hospice care and/or health needs. Information about me will be exchanged with my family.

7. This consent may be withdrawn at any time.

8. Hospice does not take the place of the caregiver, but rather, supports the caregiver.

In summary, I have been advised of my rights and responsibilities. All services have been explained to me and I have had ample opportunity to ask questions.

Signature of Patient
or Legal Representative   _____   Date_____/_____/_____

Signature of Witness   _____   Date_____/_____/_____

Part 1 – Clinical Record	Part 2 – Patient/Family
PATIENT NAME–Last, First, Middle Initial	ID#

Form 3460/2P © 1995 Briggs Corporation, Des Moines, IA 50306
B902   To order, phone 1-800-247-2343 www.BriggsCorp.com PRINTED IN U.S.A.

PATIENT CONSENT FOR CARE

Figure 1-13 Patient consent for care form. (Courtesy Briggs Corporation, Des Moines, IA.)

identification, handling, and disposal of biohazardous wastes in the home setting will be provided to new clinicians. Other policies and activities are education related to infections, sharps disposal, prevention, reporting, identification and tracking of infections in hospice patients, a tuberculosis exposure control plan, disinfection of supplies, and other aspects of infection control.

Process/outcome: The organization should have proper PPE available to hospice team members. This equipment includes disposable latex and non-latex gloves, masks, aprons, goggles, and other coverings; mouth-pieces for CPR; and other equipment as necessary. CPR masks should be kept on the clinician's person (e.g., not in the car parked in front of the patient's home). Infection control related to the home visit bag and equipment must be maintained. The contents and equipment must be protected from contamination, particularly because they can be sources of cross-contamination. The organizational policies related to the cleaning of supplies and the frequency of these cleanings should be reviewed. Some organizations have designated "bag check" days when an inventory of the contents is made and the process for retrieval and storage of equipment is reviewed.

Effective and regular handwashing is critical to the provision of high-quality care. Organizations provide paper towels and soap or alcohol-based soap ("waterless wash"). Team members should use the paper towels instead of the patient's cloth towels (unless they are known to be clean) and liquid soap instead of the bar of soap in the patient's home. Infection control and adherence to related policies are standards heavily weighted by accreditation (e.g., CHAP, JCAHO, ACHC) surveyors as well as important indicators of quality. On completion of the orientation the orientee should be able to describe infection control practices as specified by the hospice (Box 1-3) and verbalize and correctly demonstrate bag technique.

- *Self-Determination/Advance Directives*
  The Federal Patient Self-Determination Act of 1990 was designed to enable patients to decide in advance what health care decisions are to be made should the patient lose the capacity to do so. A goal of hospice is that the patient's self-determined choices be upheld and implemented in the framework of quality care. All Medicare-participating entities, such as hospices and HHAs, must comply with the advance directive provisions of the Omnibus Budget Reconciliation Act (OBRA) law. This policy is usually distributed to new team members during orientation.

  Most hospices have the admitting clinician or other hospice team member provide this information to the patient. The law requires that the hospice or HHA inform patients in writing of its policies regarding the implementation of advance directives and educate staff and the community on issues concerning advance directives.

  Process/outcome: Many times, patients who have come out of the hospital are well aware of advance directives and may have thought about and/or discussed them with their family members or physician. The admitting clinician's role is usually to provide an informational flyer identifying resources should the patient wish more information. Upon completion of orientation the orientee should be able to describe the intent of the self-determination law and the hospice team member's role in implementing and complying with this requirement.

- *Community resources*
  A listing of available community resources may be provided during orientation. This list should provide linkage to services in the community and may include such educational and/or financial support resources as

BOX 1-3

1

NINE TIPS FOR INFECTION CONTROL

When the hospice patient is cared for at home, one hallmark of quality care is infection control and related practices. The following nine tips may contribute to improved practice and patient care while supporting accreditation and other standards.

1. Although it is well known that handwashing is the most effective way to prevent the spread of infection, numerous studies show that it is not always performed or is not performed enough.

    Tip: Wash hands, apply clean gloves, provide care, discard gloves, and wash hands. Always wash hands (and change gloves) between patient contact, even between tasks or procedures on the same patient to prevent cross-contamination. If there is no running water or paper towels, use foam or waterless soap/cleansing agents and paper towels from your bag. Do not use bar soap. Do not use the patient's towel unless you know it is clean (e.g., right out of the washer and dryer).

2. Urinary tract, wound, infusion site, or strep infections may appear to be isolated cases until looked at from a trending perspective.

    Tip: Report patient or staff infections to your manager for data collection, analysis, and trending within the organization.

3. Every patient cared for is automatically cared for using Standard Precautions.

    Tip: Use Standard Precautions at all times, and always carry your PPE in your bag.

4. Equipment may be a source of cross-contamination in households and among patients.

    Tip: Clean thermometers and scissors after each use. When possible, have the patient keep his or her own thermometer and scissors for use in home care. Follow your organization's policies on the cleaning of blood pressure cuffs, stethoscopes, and the clinical bag.

5. Hazardous waste management is an important part of infection control and risk management. The most common and problematic area is needles and other sharps.

    Tip: Never recap needles! Use the biohazardous sharps container provided by the hospice. These containers are usually hard plastic and should be leak resistant and puncture proof for safety. It goes without saying that overfilling these containers is to be avoided.

6. The clinician's bag is usually divided into clean and dirty sides for infection control purposes. It may be a challenge to know where to place the bag once inside the home.

Continued

BOX 1-3

NINE TIPS FOR INFECTION CONTROL — cont'd

Tip: Try to identify a clean surface in the home for the bag and needed supplies. A barrier should be placed under the bag, such as a chux, a piece of plastic, or a newspaper. If there is no clean spot or there are many roaches or other obvious infestations, the bag may be hung on a doorknob or only what is needed may be brought into the home in a clean plastic bag.

7. There is much discussion in conference rooms and in medical literature about aseptic versus sterile techniques in wound care at home. For this reason specific orders are needed from the physician for the patient's care.

    Tip: Obtain specific orders from the physician about dressing changes, including whether to use sterile or aseptic techniques. Consider speaking with your manager about working with a wound, ostomy, continence nurse (WOCN) about problematic wounds in hospice patients and possible inservice education about the many options for wound care supplies and products now available.

8. In caring for patients with various cancers and other illnesses necessitating immunosuppression, it is important to be aware of terms such as *pathogens* (i.e., disease-producing microorganisms), *contamination* (i.e., introducing harmful or infectious material), and *cross-contamination* or *cross-infection* (i.e., moving or transferring pathogens from one site or source to another).

    Tip: There is clearly a higher risk of cross-contamination when the infection is especially virulent. There recently has been much information disseminated about infections resistant to certain antibiotics. With this in mind, try to schedule immunosuppressed patient care before visiting and caring for patients with infected or difficult wounds or other sources of known infection.

9. Caring for challenging hospice patients and their families can be difficult on certain days. Infection control is an important component for both patients and clinicians.

    Tip: Take care of yourself by eating properly, exercising regularly, getting plenty of sleep, practicing effective infection control on and off the job, and taking time for yourself to rejuvenate.

the local cancer or other societies, community loan closets, and area offices on aging.

Process/outcome: The hospice clinician in the case manager role coordinates care for the patient across health care settings and notifies patients of services available. Linkage and rapport with available community resources assist in ensuring effective communications and assisting patients and families in accessing needed services. Upon completion the orientee should be able to reference and identify possible resources based on examples or patient cases discussed during orientation.

- *Emergency preparedness*
  The hospice organization should have a process prepared in case an emergency occurs where the normal operations of the organization or office are shut down. Examples include fire, floods, hurricanes, ice storms and blizzards, activities related to homeland security, power outages that affect local phone service, and earthquakes. The process has a plan that is practiced should such an event occur.

  Process/outcome: Patient care will continue as far as possible, patients will be prioritized based on their needs, and hospice team members will know their roles and activities in the process. Cellular phones, telephone trees for communications, a listing of the patients with an assigned priority number in the on-call book, and mock fire drills or other drills should all be part of an emergency preparedness and safety plan that works should an unforeseen event occur.

  Many other policies may be provided to the orientee for review. Some organizations may also have a scavenger hunt to test team members' ability to locate and identify these policies, procedures, supplies, or equipment.

SAFETY IN HOSPICE

Personal safety is an appropriate concern in community-based practice when making home visits to hospice patients and families. It is particularly important to team members entering unfamiliar geographical areas and/or at unusual hours.

The clinician should review any protocols the hospice organization has related to staff safety and home visits. Organizational procedures such as calling in a schedule to coordinators may assist in staff safety, as may beepers, pagers, and car phones. Some organizations have local law enforcement persons who provide training and education about home visiting and safety. The information shared is valuable to team members both as clinicians and as members of a community.

Personal safety starts with awareness of the surroundings (see Box 1-4 for a list of personal safety tips). Use those well-honed skills of observation and assessment wherever you are!

BOX 1-4

PERSONAL SAFETY TIPS

When going anywhere for the first time, get specific, detailed, and correct directions to the patient's home and have them validated by the patient or caregiver.

If you are unsure of a neighborhood or have heard about problems, talk with your supervisor, who may contact the local police. The police know the communities and the problems best and can be very helpful in identifying problem areas and working with the care team on solutions.

Organizations may have contracts with security staff. Your supervisor will know of such arrangements and the process for their use.

Know the community. As you are driving, always be aware of your surroundings.

You may want to call patients and families before leaving so they can be watching for you. Ask about parking too.

Lock the car doors and keep any valuables, such as purse, supplies, and any patient information, out of sight.

Wear a seatbelt while driving.

When nearing the home, look for the landmarks described and address numbers on houses.

Keep maps out of sight where possible and try to avoid looking as though you are unfamiliar with the area.

Try to park in well-lit areas and in front of the home or as close as possible. Lock the car and identify your route to the front door.

Be cautious when boarding elevators.

Have your needed supplies in an accessible area so you are not searching in the trunk for a given supply.

When making evening or night visits, let your family know where you are going and when you expect to return.

When walking to your car, have your keys out, ready to unlock the car. Many of the newer car models have "keyless entry," which works with a computer chip and unlocks the door when the mechanism is pointed toward the car and pressed.

Before getting back in the car, check the back seat and floor areas.

If you feel unsafe, you probably are. Trust your feelings and intuition and call your supervisor from a safe spot.

Speak with your supervisor about your organization's unique policies relating to home visiting safety.

BOX 1-5

CAR SAFETY TIPS

Car safety is also very important. It begins with a knowledge of the strengths and weaknesses of your car. Successful and safe home visiting team members have good driving records and reliable cars that are usually not gas guzzlers. A small car can make it easier to find a parking spot on snowy streets or downtown in metropolitan areas. Always make sure you have enough gas. Some hospice clinicians make it a habit never to let the gas tank get below one half full. Do not make visits running on empty!

Carry 1 gallon of water, a blanket, and a first aid kit. A candle in a coffee can help heat your car in cold weather, but be careful! Lock all car doors when entering or leaving the car.

Store sand, rug mats, or kitty litter in your trunk to assist you out of ice and snow.

If your organization gives you a sign that identifies you as a health care worker, use it per program policies. Sometimes these signs help you obtain and keep a parking spot in front of the hospital or lab.

Consider obtaining gas credit cards and joining an automobile club for assistance in emergencies such as towing, running out of gasoline or fuel, and/or dead batteries.

Take good care of your car, winterize it if you live where the weather is cold, and maintain it well.

Have the oil and fluid levels checked regularly.

Make sure that your spare tire is in good condition and inflated and that you have the tools and knowledge and ability to change a flat tire.

MAP READING: UPDATE OF AN IMPORTANT SKILL

All team members making home visits need the skill of map reading. Many organizations cover a large and diverse geographical catchment area that may cover urban, suburban, and rural areas. With this in mind, you cannot know every side street or bridge in a given area. Experienced clinicians and managers have found the ability to navigate and read maps sorely tested. In communities where there is rapid growth, sometimes the newer roads and access routes may not even be on the map. For that reason the large county book maps that are updated fairly frequently seem to work well. When taking directions from patients or their family members or caregivers, write down landmarks such as schools, playgrounds, trash dumps, marinas, shopping centers, or other identifying information that will confirm that you are on the right track.

Personal safety is enhanced by the ability to get from one patient and family's home to the next easily (see Box 1-5 for car safety tips).

Supervisors or experienced colleagues will know the nuances of any community that can plague a planned day. These include when and where streets are cleaned, making parking almost impossible; snow emergency routes where cars seemingly are towed when the first snowflake falls; or streets that change direction during rush hours to accommodate the traffic so that "you can't get there from here." These challenges can tax the most experienced visiting staff. Be prepared!

SUMMARY

The kinds of patients and families cared for through hospice have grown and changed. Historically hospice has provided care primarily to patients with cancer. Patients and families of patients with Alzheimer's, amyotrophic lateral sclerosis, and end-stage heart disease and other organ failures are now also finding support and care through hospice. All kinds of patients of varying ages and problems who are seeking comfort and care with a limited life expectancy are turning to hospice. Hospice care is limited by the prognosis, not the disease.

The special qualities, skills, and characteristics of caring people go into making up the hospice team. Clinicians may have the unique role of case manager at many hospices. As such, the clinician coordinates and clarifies the desires of patients and their families or partners. Expertise in symptom control, the desire for continued learning about pain and its relief, flexibility, and a sense of humor are all assets for clinicians wishing to make the transition to a practice setting where hospice team members make an important difference in care and life or throughout the dying process for patients and their families. Whatever the individual role of the clinician or other team member at an individual hospice, the focus is always centered on the patient and caregiver and their unique, individualized choices and journeys.

Orientation is an important period in a new hospice team member's tenure. It is the time when the organization's standards and other information are provided. Orientation varies among organizations, and the orientation may set the precedent for and establish the value of the care and education that the organization espouses. Everyone comes with different skills and competencies, so orientation is the time to identify areas for improvement and provide needed education and information. Welcome to hospice!

REVIEW EXERCISES

1. List six of the services offered by hospices.
2. Describe the basic tenets of hospice.
3. Identify the reason that documentation is an important component in hospice care.
4. List three reasons for the growth in hospice.
5. Define hospice and hospice health care.
6. Describe the different kinds of hospice organizations.
7. Identify four of the differences between home care and hospice health care.
8. What is the focus of hospice?
9. Who is the unit of care in hospice?
10. What kinds of patients and families are cared for through hospice?

References

1. National Hospice and Palliative Care Organization: *NHPCO Facts and Figures*. Alexandria, VA, 2003, The Organization.
2. Carney K, Burns N: Economics of hospice care, *Oncology Nursing Forum,* 18:761-786, 1991.
3. NHPCO: *Standards of Practice for Hospice Programs*. Alexandria, VA, 2000, NHPCO.
4. APNA. *Statement on the Scope and Standards of Hospice and Palliative Nursing Practice.* Dubuque, IA, Kendall/Hunt, 2000.
5. HPNA, ANA. *Scope and Standards of Hospice and Palliative Nursing Practice*. Washington, DC, ANA, 2002.

PART TWO

AN OVERVIEW OF HOSPICE DOCUMENTATION

Part 2 seeks to assist both new and experienced hospice nurses in meeting various requirements and documenting the specific information required by any payer, illustrating the patient's condition and responses to interventions, and accurately chronicling the patient's care and course.

HOSPICE DOCUMENTATION

Hospice team members and their clinical practice are described every day to surveyors, peers, and managers through the review of clinical records. Visit records, notes, and other information that appear in the record reflect the standard of hospice care as well as the particular care provided to a specific patient. Hospice clinicians must be able to integrate knowledge of regulatory criteria, care coordination, and practice into effective documentation that supports coverage while demonstrating quality to any reviewer. Today, numerous third-party payers make quality and reimbursement decisions based on the care the patient received as evidenced in the hospice clinical record.

The clinician's entries in the patient's clinical record are recognized as a significant contribution that documents the standard of care provided to a patient. As the practice of hospice has become more complex, so too have the factors that influence documentation. These factors include requirements of regulatory agencies and accreditation bodies (e.g., Joint Commission on Accreditation of Healthcare Organizations [JCAHO], Community Health Accreditation Program [CHAP], state licensure departments, government entities), consumers of health care, and legal entities. Hospice clinicians must try to satisfy these various requirements all at once, often with little time in which to accomplish the important task of documentation. Fortunately, many organizations have integrated these requirements, where possible, into the organization's policy and/or procedure manuals and documentation forms. Clinicians must remember that the written clinical record is their best defense against malpractice or negligence litigation.

The increased specialization of practice and the complexity of patient problems contribute to the provision of multiple and varied services to patients. The clinical record is the only source of written communication—and sometimes the only source of any communication—for all team members. The team members not only contribute their unique and individual assessment findings, interventions, and outcomes, but also may actually base their subsequent actions on the events documented by another hospice team member.

A hospice chart audit tool is a way to assist in evaluation of the overall clinical record (see Figure 2-1). This review may be useful as a way to identify areas that may need improvement, such as care coordination, pain and medication management, and spiritual and psychosocial support.

Why Is the Clinical Record So Important?

The clinical record is a legal document, and it is the only document that chronicles a patient's stay from start of care through discharge. As such, it

HOSPICE CHART AUDIT TOOL

Date of Review _____
Reviewer _____
Team _____

Patient Name _____ Medical Record # _____
SOC Date _____ D/C Date _____
Primary Dx _____ Secondary Dx _____

Hospice Admission and Benefit Election	Yes	No	N/A	Comments (describe any missing components, opportunities for improvement)
Attending MD and medical director certification of terminal condition (certification obtained within state licensure and federal guideline requirements)				
Informed consent for hospice				
Election statement with date				
Evidence that rights and responsibilities were reviewed				
Documentation of terminal diagnosis and prognosis				
Assessment of advance directive (e.g., DNR, Living Will, etc.)				
If patient has advance directive, copy or written documentation of content				
Team Assessments and Care Planning				
Complete nursing assessment, including comprehensive pain and symptom assessment and assessment of HHA need				
Home environment and safety assessment				
Assessment and appropriate ordering of DME				
Assessments comprehensive and timely (evidence of contact within ____ days from SOC)				
Spiritual assessment				
Assessment for volunteer need				

Figure 2-1 Hospice chart audit tool. (Courtesy Anne L. Rooney, RN, MS, MPH.)

should be completed as soon as possible per rules, regulations, standards of practice, and organizational policy. This includes beginning and completing the physician's orders, plan of care, or other required forms and the daily visit record or notes as soon as possible. It is recommended that the documentation be completed at the time the care is provided. In the inpatient setting, it would have been unheard of not to complete the documentation as care and plans for care were developed for the patients.

Other assessments when ordered (e.g., dietary, physical therapy, occupational therapy, speech therapy)				
Interdisciplinary team care plan, including clear and measurable goals, signed by MD				
Evidence of patient/family involvement in care planning				
Signed and dated verbal orders when needed for changes in frequencies, medications, treatments, etc.				
Care plan revised when necessary				
Current HHA or HCA plan of care, if applicable				
Do progress notes for all team services reflect implementation of the plan of care as written? Are interventions appropriate to the assessed needs? **Note:** Address visit frequencies, planned follow-up interventions. Note discrepancies under comment section.				
Care Coordination				
Ongoing care conference notes that reflect updates to plan of care				
Progress notes that reflect ongoing interdisciplinary communication				
Communication with the MD for significant changes or concerns				
Evidence that hospice team assumes professional management responsibility for care, regardless of setting				
Evidence of care coordination with other involved organizations (e.g., SNFs, case managers from other agencies)				
Evidence of communication with receiving organization when patient transfers between settings (e.g., transfer summary)				

Figure 2-1, cont'd Hospice chart audit tool. (Courtesy Anne L. Rooney, RN, MS, MPH.)
Continued

Important facets of hospice documentation include the patient's condition, the status (e.g., psychosocial, spiritual) of the family or other caregivers, the environment of care, a description of the specific care provided, the patient's pain and symptom presentation and associated interventions and evaluations, communications with the physician or other team members, and the observed or verbal patient/family response(s) to interventions and care.

Pain and Symptom Management and Medication Monitoring				
Current medication profile that matches MD orders **Note:** Check travel chart for current profile				
Allergies noted				
Progress notes that reflect ongoing assessment of pain and other symptoms (e.g., pain scale, usage of breakthrough pain medication, monitoring of bowel status)				
Progress notes that reflect evidence of education on medications, management of side effects, etc.				
Documentation of all medications administered by hospice staff				
Reassessment and Recertification				
Evidence of ongoing interdisciplinary assessments				
Documentation that reflects assessment of continued appropriateness of hospice care (e.g., according to NHO guidelines, especially for noncancer diagnoses)				
Communication with attending MD and medical director before recertification				
Bereavement Care				
Risk assessment completed for at least PCG and other at-risk survivors (e.g., children)				
Bereavement plan of care appropriate to assessed survivor risk and needs				
Documentation of bereavement care as described in bereavement plan of care				
Appropriate intervention when complicated grief identified (e.g., suicidal ideation)				
General Issues				
HHA supervision documented every 2 weeks				

Figure 2-1, cont'd Hospice chart audit tool. (Courtesy Anne L. Rooney, RN, MS, MPH.)

Factors Contributing to More Emphasis on Documentation

The following discussion addresses five specific areas that have increased the importance of clinical documentation.

1. **The current economics of our health care system and the emphasis on utilization management**

   Patients continue to be discharged sooner or stay home while they are considerably ill. In response to spiraling health care costs, third-party payers, such as government, commercial, and business self-insurers,

Documentation legible, dated, authenticated by signatures				
Errors corrected according to policy (e.g., no correction fluid; item should be crossed through with "error" written above)				
Other technical documentation issues				
Revocation form signed and dated, if applicable. Does documentation reflect reason for revocation?				
In reviewer's opinion, were the patient's/family's needs addressed and coordinated?				
In reviewer's opinion, were the utilization of hospice services and level of care appropriate?				
General comments/suggestions				

Figure 2-1, cont'd Hospice chart audit tool. (Courtesy Anne L. Rooney, RN, MS, MPH.)

have increased their scrutiny and control of limited resources. Initially these programs, called *utilization review* or *utilization management,* were influential in decreasing hospital lengths of stay. This review of care then moved into the outpatient, home care, and hospice arenas.

The phrase often heard to describe this phenomenon is "quicker and sicker." In general, the decreased length of hospital stays has increased the disease acuity levels of patients at home. This often translates into increased care needs, as is evidenced by the increase in the number of visits or hours patients are seen. In addition, some managed-care programs are decreasing their number of home visits while also limiting the patient's inpatient stay, which places stress on team members as they continue to provide needed care and, many times, "negotiate" for the patient so that the appropriate levels of safe, effective care are provided. Third-party payers often need substantiating evidence and documentation clearly showing that appropriate care was provided.

The information in the clinical record is one of the sources with which third-party payers make payment or denial decisions. It is important to note that Medicare, by law, can pay only for covered care. It is primarily the clinical documentation that is the objective basis for payment determinations. These notes reflect the care (admission, visit notes, discharge, and ordered services) provided to hospice patients at home.

2. **The emphasis on performance improvement**
   As quality initiatives in all health care settings evolve, patient outcomes are being recognized as valid indicators of care. Hospice care is concerned with patients and families having and retaining self-determined courses of care and death with comfort and dignity at home. Clinical documentation is the written record demonstrating the care provided, based on the hospice interdisciplinary plan of care, and movement toward achieving patient-centered, quantifiable

goals of care. The documentation must reflect the patient's condition and, in essence, paint a clear picture for any reviewer assessing for coverage and quality reasons. Because the reviewer has not seen the patient, it is important to express objectively the way the patient "looks" throughout the clinical documentation.

The interdisciplinary focus on quality efforts creates an incentive for the entire hospice team to work together to achieve these outcomes for hospice patients and their loved ones. The clinical documentation in the written record demonstrates care coordination, and this collaboration is in the format of interdisciplinary group or team meetings, conferences, or other team activities and communications.

Performance improvement (PI) is based on date measurement and assessment. PI addresses what is actually done and how well it is accomplished and focuses on the design (or redesign) of processes or functions within the hospice organization. Examples of PI activities include revamping the patient education tools, the documentation system, the hospice admission process and referral form, the comprehensive orientation program or redesigning the physician order retrieval process to improve the timely returns of hospice physician orders.

3. **The emphasis on standardization of care, policies and procedures, and processes**

All patients are entitled to a certain level or standard of hospice care. Operationally this means that regardless of which clinician is assigned, the patient receives the same level of care and the same interventions in the same order as designated by our organizations and managers. This ensures standardization of care and related processes across the organization. This standardization ensures that the same "brand" of hospice care is provided in a community by all team members. In fact, the use of a text such as this by all clinicians in a given organization contributes to standardization of patient care.

As patients and their families become more proactive consumers in their purchases of health services, patient satisfaction with the care provided becomes key to any organization's reputation and ultimate survival. More patients are demanding care in their own homes. Because of their healing skills and other areas of professional proficiency, hospice clinicians are pivotal in fostering patient satisfaction. Further, the roles of patient advocate, listener,and teacher has become widely accepted in recent years. In general, it also is known that satisfied patients are less likely to sue. A hospice satisfaction questionnaire is provided for review in Figure 2-2.

4. **The recognition and empowerment of the nursing profession with the nursing shortage**

Although more nurses are in the work force than ever before, qualified professional hospice nurses continue to be needed and are projected to be in ever more demand in the future.

The nurse's notes can become the factor by which documented quality becomes demonstrated quality. All health care professions,

HOSPICE SATISFACTION SURVEY

DATE _____/_____/_____

Thank you for allowing us to provide hospice services to your family. We are interested in your ideas or opinions about our program. Please take a moment to answer the following questions. Additional comments are welcome and can be recorded on the back of this form. If you need assistance in completing this form, please feel free to contact our office.

For questions 1 - 10, please circle the appropriate number that best describes your opinion.
1-Strongly Agree   2-Agree   3-Disagree   4-Strongly Disagree   5-No Opinion or N/A

1. We were satisfied with the care provided by the hospice staff.	1 2 3 4 5
2. Medication/Supplies were delivered on time.	1 2 3 4 5
3. Equipment was delivered on time.	1 2 3 4 5
4. We were involved in decision making regarding the plan of care for our family.	1 2 3 4 5
5. Staff treated our family, our home and belongings with respect.	1 2 3 4 5
6. Staff explained care, services, rights and responsibilities, and other procedures related to the care provided.	1 2 3 4 5
7. We were able to reach hospice staff in a timely manner whenever necessary.	1 2 3 4 5
8. We would recommend this hospice to friends and relatives.	1 2 3 4 5
9. Staff provided emotional support during our hospice experience.	1 2 3 4 5
10. Staff assisted with managing our loved one/family member's pain and symptom control.	1 2 3 4 5

11. Suggestions for improvements/additional comments: _____
_____
_____

12. What most impressed us about the hospice care/services was: _____
_____
_____

How long did you receive hospice services: ❏ less than 1 month ❏ 1-3 months ❏ 3-6 months ❏ 6-9 months ❏ 9-12 months ❏ greater than 12 months	❏ We would ❏ would not like to discuss our responses further. Please return the completed survey in the enclosed, self-addressed stamped envelope.
Thank you for your valuable feedback. This confidential information will be used only in efforts to improve care/services. Sincerely, _____ *Director/Administrator*	_____ *Optional Signature* _____/_____/_____ *Date*

2

Form 3471 © 1995 Briggs Corporation, Des Moines, IA 50306
To order, phone 1-800-247-2343 www.BriggsCorp.com PRINTED IN U.S.A.

HOSPICE SATISFACTION SURVEY

Figure 2-2 Hospice satisfaction survey. (Courtesy Briggs Corporation, Des Moines, IA.)

including nursing, have recognized standards of care. As society becomes more litigious, the hospice nurse must become aware of state practice and other accepted standards of care. Standards of care represent the minimum level that any patient can expect in similar circumstances. Other standards include policies and procedures, state or federal regulations, and the published standards of professional nursing organizations. These standards necessitate keeping current with and informed of the standards of practice through affiliation with specialty groups or other professional groups. Readers are referred to the resources section entitled "nursing resources."

An example of a hospice organization's standards of care is as follows: Every patient and family shall have an assessment that is comprehensive, on a standardized form that is completed in the same way, addresses specific patient needs, is performed by a registered nurse on admission, and is documented in the clinical record by a set time line. Through complete, effective documentation the hospice clinicians demonstrate that the standard of care has been maintained.

5. **The emphasis on effectiveness and efficiency in all settings in health care, particularly community-based care**
   As organizations continue to streamline their operations, administrative tasks historically performed by clinicians are being reconsidered for their effectiveness. Repetition or duplication of documentation has been an area of appropriate concern to clinicians and their managers. Some organizations have moved toward automation to help prevent the duplication of much clinical and administrative information needed for effective daily operations. Quality, not quantity, is now emphasized with regard to documentation. Effective documentation may not need to be lengthy or wordy; it needs only to support appropriate and covered care.

All the previously discussed factors have created an environment in which hospice clinicians must meet increased responsibilities, often in less time.

Importance of the Hospice Record

The importance of documentation in the clinical record relates to the fact that this record has the following characteristics:

- It is the only written source for reference and communication among members of the hospice care team
- It is the primary source (written or verbal) for reference and communication among the members of the hospice team
- It is the text that supports insurance coverage or denial
- It is the evidence of the basis on which patient care decisions were made
- It is the only legal record
- It is the primary foundation for the evaluation of the care provided
- It is the basis for staff education or other study
- It is the objective source for the organization's licensing (where applicable), certification, accreditation, and state surveyor review

The Centers for Medicare and Medicaid Services (CMS), previously called the Health Care Financing Administration (HCFA), which manages Medicare programs, instructs the fiscal intermediaries on the administration of the Medicare hospice program. These instructions have implications for hospice clinicians who provide care to patients covered under the Medicare hospice benefit. Regional Home Health Intermediaries (RHHIs) are specialized fiscal intermediaries that contact the CMS to process and make payment determinations on all hospice (and home care) claims from across the country.

The RHHIs can pay only for hospice care under Medicare provisions that are covered by law. They look to the hospice's clinical documentation in the medical record to decide whether to support covered care.

Because of the high volume of claims, the RHHIs cannot look at each hospice claim individually. The RHHIs direct their medical review efforts toward areas and claims where the risk of inappropriate payment is greatest. Hospice claims are subject to more reviews based on the RHHIs initiatives and findings identified in claims processing. Usually, these reviews entail the screening of claims with the greatest risk of overutilization of program payment. This happens through database analysis and referrals. Through various initiatives, the government has increased its scrutiny of hospice and other Medicare services and claims. Because of this heightened review, it is more important than ever that hospices effectively document and manage clinical records. All government or Medicare reviewers hold Medicare-participating hospice organizations to the Medicare Conditions of Participation (COPs) for hospice.

Documentation: The Key to Coverage, Compliance, and Quality

Documentation is critical to the positive outcome of any review process. Paint a picture with your documentation from the onset of care through continuation of hospice services. Distinguish clearly in your documentation between the chronic and terminal phases of a disease, especially if it is long and chronic in nature. Specify any patient periods of exacerbation, stabilization, and further deterioration. Document the way treatments and medication play a palliative role in the plan of care (POC). Remember that notes from all caregivers are usually reviewed, and documentation in all notes should complete the picture of the terminally ill patient. Remember that what is "normal" and "stable" to a hospice team member may still indicate a clearly terminal patient if the details are provided in the documentation. Avoid generalizations such as "no change" or "as tolerated"; insurers need to pay for covered care, and all documentation plays an important role.

Because home health care and hospice clinicians often need to meet these documentation requirements simultaneously, they are appropriately concerned about their ability to do so. Clinicians in practice today can meet these needs and produce clear, effective documentation. The tips in Box 2-1 and Table 2-1 can assist in this goal.

HOSPICE DOCUMENTATION 101

Medicare, like any medical insurance program, has both covered services and exclusions. For payers, documentation is the only paper trail of the care provided and the patient's response to that care.

Text continued on p. 71

BOX 2-1

DOCUMENTATION TIPS

- Write legibly or print neatly. The record must be readable.
- Use permanent ink, preferably black or blue.
- For every entry identify the time and date; sign the entry and include your title.
- Describe care or interventions provided or mark appropriate box on flow sheet and the patient's response to care.
- Write objectively when describing findings (e.g., behaviors).
- Document in consecutive and chronological order with no skipped areas.
- Document or data-enter information either at the patient's home (if safe and appropriate) or as soon as possible after care is provided.
- Be factual and specific.
- Use patient, family, or caregiver quotes.
- Use the patient's name (e.g., "Mr. Smith").
- Document patient complaints or needs and their resolutions. (Remember to discuss the complaint with your manager, who may also document it in the complaint log and note the resolution or follow-up actions taken and any trends.)
- Make sure the patient's name is listed correctly on the visit record, daily note, or other form.
- Be accurate, complete, and thorough.
- Write out what you are saying if anything is questionable. (Avoid potentially confusing abbreviations.)
- Chart only the care that you provided.
- Promptly document any change in the patient's condition and the actions taken based on such a change.
- Document the patient's, family's, or caregiver's response to teaching or any other care intervention.
- To correct an error: (1) draw a line through the erroneous entry, (2) briefly describe the error (e.g., wrong date, spilled coffee on visit record), and (3) add your signature, the date, and the time (or as per organizational policy).

Try to Avoid the Following:
- Relying on memory.
- Whiting out or erasing any entries.
- Crossing out words beyond recognition.
- Making assumptions, drawing conclusions, and blaming.
- Leaving blank spaces between entries and your signature.
- Waiting too long to record entries.
- Leaving gaps in documentation.
- Using abbreviations except where they are clear and appear on the organization's list of approved, acceptable abbreviations.
- Using terms or abbreviations that have been identified as dangerous and/or ambiguous (see Table 2-1).

TABLE 2-1

DO *NOT* USE THESE DANGEROUS ABBREVIATIONS OR DOSE DESIGNATIONS

Abbreviation/ Dose Expression	Intended Meaning	Misinterpretation	Correction
Apothecary symbols	Dram Minim	Misunderstood or misread (symbol for dram misread for "3" and minim misread as "mL").	Use the metric system.
AU	Aurio uterque (each ear) or left or right ear	Mistaken for OU (oculo uterque—each eye).	Don't use this abbreviation. "left ear", "right ear" or "both ears"
D/C	Discharge Discontinue	Premature discontinuation of medications when D/C (intended to mean "discharge") has been misinterpreted as "discontinued" when followed by a list of drugs.	Use "discharge" and "discontinue."
Drug Names			**Use the complete spelling for drug names**
ARA°A	Vidarabine	Cytarabine ARA°C	
AZT	Zidovudine (Retrovir)	Azathioprine	
CPZ	Compazine (Prochlorperazine)	Chlorpromazine	
DPT	Demerol- Phenergan-Thorazine	Diphtheria-pertussis-tetanus (vaccine)	

Modified from Institute for Safe Medication Practices, 2003 (www.ismp.org).
For a list of additional abbreviations refer to the ISMP List of Error-Prone Abbreviations, Symbols, and Dose Designations, 2004, JCAHO.

Continued

2

TABLE 2-1

DO *NOT* USE THESE DANGEROUS ABBREVIATIONS OR DOSE DESIGNATIONS—cont'd

Abbreviation/ Dose Expression	Intended Meaning	Misinterpretation	Correction
HCl	Hydrochloric acid	Potassium chloride (The "H" is misinterpreted as "K")	
HCT	Hydrocortisone	Hydrochlorothiazide	
HCTZ	Hydrochlorothiazide	Hydrocortisone (seen as HCT 250 mg)	
$MgSO_4$	Magnesium sulfate	Morphine sulfate	
MSO_4	Morphine sulfate	Magnesium sulfate	
MTX	Methotrexate	Mitoxantrone	
TAC	Triamcinolone	Tetracaine, ADRENALIN, cocaine	
$ZnSO_4$	Zinc sulfate	Morphine sulfate	
Stemmed Names			
"Nitro" drip	Nitroglycerin infusion	Sodium nitroprusside infusion	
"Norflox"	Norfloxacin	Norflex	
mg	Microgram	Mistaken for "mg" when handwritten.	Use "mcg."
o.d. or OD	Once daily	Misinterpreted as "right eye" (OD—oculus dexter) and administration of oral medications in the eye.	Use "daily."
TIW or tiw	Three times a week	Mistaken as "three times a day."	Don't use this abbreviation.
Per os	Orally	The "os" can be mistaken for "left eye."	Use "PO," "by mouth," or "orally."

Abbreviation	Intended Meaning	Misinterpretation	Correction
q.d. or QD	Every day	Mistaken as q.i.d., especially if the period after the "q" or the tail of the "q" is misunderstood as an "i."	Use "daily" or "every day."
qn	Nightly or at bedtime	Misinterpreted as "qh" (every hour).	Use "nightly."
qhs	Nightly at bedtime	Misread as every hour.	Use "nightly."
h.s.	Half-strength	Mistaken for "hour of sleep"	Write out "half strength"
q6 PM, etc.	Every evening at 6 PM	Misread as every 6 hours.	Use 6 PM "nightly."
q.o.d. or QOD	Every other day	Misinterpreted as "q.d." (daily) or "q.i.d." (four times daily) if the "o" is poorly written.	Use "every other day."
sub q	Subcutaneous	The "q" has been mistaken for "every" (e.g., one heparin dose ordered "sub q 2 hours before surgery" misunderstood as every 2 hours before surgery).	Use "subcut." or write "subsubcutaneous."
SC	Subcutaneous	Mistaken for SL (sublingual).	Use "subcut." or write "subcutaneous."
U or u	Unit	Read as a zero (0) or a four (4), causing a 10-fold overdose or greater (4U seen as "40" or 4u seen as 44").	"Unit" has no acceptable abbreviation. Use "unit."
IU	International unit	Misread as IV (intravenous).	Use "units."
cc	Cubic centimeters	Misread as "U" (units).	Use "mL."
x3d	For 3 days	Mistaken for "three doses."	Use "for 3 days."
BT	Bedtime	Mistaken as "BID" (twice daily).	Use "hs."
ss	Sliding scale (insulin) or ½ (apothecary)	Mistaken for "55."	Spell out "sliding scale." Use "one-half" or use "½."

Continued

Modified from Institute for Safe Medication Practices, 2003 (www.ismp.org).
For additional abbreviations, please refer to the ISMP List of Error-Prone Abbreviations, Symbols, and Dose Designations, 2004, JCAHO.

TABLE 2-1

DO *NOT* USE THESE DANGEROUS ABBREVIATIONS OR DOSE DESIGNATIONS—cont'd

Abbreviation/ Dose Expression	Intended Meaning	Misinterpretation	Correction
> and <	Greater than and less than	Mistakenly used opposite of intended. Use "greater than" or "less than."	
/ (*slash mark*)	Separates two doses or indicates "per"	Misunderstood as the number 1 ("25 units/10 units" read as "110" units.)	Do not use a slash mark to separate doses. Use "per."
Name letters and dose numbers run together (e.g., *Inderal 40 mg*)	Inderal 40 mg	Misread as Inderal 140 mg.	Always use space between drug name, dose, and unit of measure.
Zero after decimal point (1.0)	1 mg	Misread as 10 mg if the decimal point is not seen.	Do not use terminal zeros for doses expressed in whole numbers.
No zero before decimal dose (.5 mg)	0.5 mg	Misread as 5 mg.	Always use zero before a decimal when the dose is less than a whole unit.

Modified from Institute for Safe Medication Practices, 2003 (www.ismp.org).
For additional abbreviations, please refer to the ISMP List of Error-Prone Abbreviations, Symbols, and Dose Designations, 2004, JCAHO.

2

To qualify for the Medicare hospice benefit, a patient must have Medicare and be terminally ill, the physician must certify that the patient is terminally ill, the patient must choose to receive hospice care instead of the standard Medicare benefits for the illness, and the care must be provided by a Medicare-participating hospice program.

For documentation purposes, the patient is considered terminally ill under the Medicare guidelines if one of the following conditions applies:

- The medical documentation meets the criteria in the National Hospice and Palliative Care Organization (NHPCO) prognosticating guidelines and supports that the patient is terminally ill (i.e., there is no conflicting or inconsistent information in the record to suggest that the patient is not terminally ill even though the guidelines are met).
- The medical documentation in the record supports that the patient is terminally ill even though criteria in the NHPCO guidelines are not met or the patient's condition is not covered by the NHPCO guidelines.
- The patient dies from the illness for which he or she elected the hospice benefit.
- Medical documentation is insufficient to make a decision, but the hospice medical director or attending physician provides clinical documentation to support the certification of terminal illness. The documentation should be clear and in the records.

Documentation may include results of tests or narrative descriptions of the clinical indicators or progression of disease.

The patient must have a prognosis of 6 months or less for most hospice programs, including those under Medicare. If on admission the family member states, "Grandma's been like this for 3 years," the admission nurse must identify the changes that now make this patient appropriate for hospice. Remember that the recertification process confirms the patient's projected length of care or time limits related to the prognosis.

Always try to review the documentation objectively after completion. Remember that the clinical documentation and the record must support that the patient under care has an illness of a terminal nature and the progress and other notes must describe the condition.

The RHHIs, when reviewing Medicare hospice claims, look to the following items, at a minimum, to support covered hospice services:

- Hospice admission history and physical (including the assessment)
- Election form with designated effective date
- Certification of the terminal illness with clinical indicator(s) supporting justification
- Visit, prognosis, and other notes describing the patient's condition
- Recertification(s)

Some hospice organizations also provide a written summary that shows the hospice benefit is appropriate for the patient's condition. *Remember that by law the RHHIs can pay only for covered care and the documentation is the source that supports the covered hospice care.* When summaries are written, the following may be included:

- Patient diagnoses, including any illness affecting the terminal diagnoses
- Any co-morbidity that affects the prognosis

- History and progression of the illness
- Physical baseline (e.g., weight and weight changes, vital signs, heart rhythms, rales, edema sites and amount)
- Objective change, such as "clothes are looser" or "baggy," as reported by family caregivers, etc.
- Physician's prognosis stating rationale for life expectancy of 6 months or less

Medicare Hospice Documentation: A Checklist Approach

✔ Are the physician's certification, assessments, and recertification(s) of terminal illness complete and included?

✔ Are all discipline visits notes and/or telephone calls signed, dated, legible, and descriptive of the course of care related to the patient, family, and caregivers?

✔ Has the physician provided written material that chronicles the patient's course of illness and care to date?

✔ Are all the laboratory or other test results included?

✔ Is the hospice election form signed and dated by the hospice provider and the patient/family or other responsible party?

✔ Is the effective date for the care clearly marked?

✔ Has the hospital or physician provided a discharge summary, history, and results of a physical?

✔ Is the POC established, updated, and being followed?

✔ Has a copy of the election form been left with the patient, family, or other responsible party?

✔ If and when different levels of care are used, is there documentation of the date, time, and reason for the change in the level of care and services?

✔ Does the documentation support that the patient is terminally ill?

✔ Is the certification obtained on a timely basis?

✔ Do patient assessments paint a clear picture of the patient's status, including the following core aspects of hospice care: functional, spiritual, nutritional, clinical, emotional, psychological, and physical assessments and plans?

Effective Hospice Documentation: A Checklist Approach

✔ Are handwritten notes or other entries legible to team members or others who may require the information?

✔ Are data elements or areas requiring completion addressed in an understandable manner? For example, is a legend or a list of acceptable abbreviations included in instances where abbreviations occur?

✔ Does the care plan reflect the problems identified during the comprehensive assessment?

✔ Are new team members oriented to forms and provided with accurately completed examples?

✔ Does the clinical record paint a clear picture of the hospice patient and family, interventions, responses, and outcomes (or quantifiable goals of care)?

✔ Do the hospice record and the documentation overall pass the test of effective care planning and coordination? Could another colleague, in your absence, review the record and be able to continue effectively with the hospice plan of care?

✔ Does the clinical documentation support the level of service provided (e.g., continuous care, inpatient care)?

✔ Does documentation show the active and ongoing management and reassessment of pain and symptoms?

✔ Are the prevention and treatment or interventions related to secondary symptoms such as constipation carried out and documented in the clinical notes?

✔ Are the psychosocial and spiritual concerns of the patient and family receiving acknowledgment and follow-up?

✔ Are initial and ongoing assessments of the dying patient clearly identified in the clinical record?

✔ Are interventions based on the patient's/family's needs as documented in the comprehensive assessment and the subsequent entries throughout the patient's care?

✔ Does the documentation emphasize the reasons that the patient/family needs or continues to need hospice services?

✔ Does the documentation support covered care as defined by Medicare, the case manager, or payer?

✔ Are the clinical records reviewed on an ongoing and timely basis for quality, completion, and identification that the patient either (1) has met predetermined goals or (2) needs continued care with possible changes to the plan based on the ongoing assessment findings and response to interventions? This includes dates, communications, and physician order follow-up procedures.

✔ If a surveyor, payer, patient, or accreditation entity were to review your record, would the clinical documentation reflect the provision of safe, quality, and effective hospice patient care?

✔ Does the documentation simultaneously do the following:
1. Demonstrate the care provided and the patient's response to that care?
2. Show that the current standards of care are maintained?
3. Meet documentation requirements for Medicare and other payers?

✔ Are the clinical record and entries legible, neat, and organized consistently? How the clinical record looks may be seen as an indicator in assessing care and the organization.

✔ Are telephone calls and other communications with physicians, community agencies, and other team members documented? Do they explain what occurred with the patient, what actions were ordered, modified, and implemented, and what the patient's/family's response was to these interventions?

✔ Is the care planning process demonstrated in the record? Look for problem identification, assessment, implementation of ordered interventions and actions, movement toward patient-centered goals, assessment of the patient's response, and continued evaluation.

✔ Are goal achievement and/or progress toward goals and outcomes documented? Are the goals realistic, quantifiable, and centered on patient and family?

✔ Are family/caregiver teaching and their responses/demonstration of behavior and learning documented?

✔ Is the patient's response to care interventions documented?

✔ Are the interventions modified based on the patient's response, where appropriate?

✔ Is evidence of interdisciplinary team conferences and discussions documented?

✔ Are continuity of care planning goals and consistent movement toward outcomes/goal achievement by all members of the team shown?

✔ Does the record tell the story of the patient's care, needs, and progress while the patient/family was receiving hospice services?

✔ Is compliance with organizational, regulatory, licensure, and quality standards demonstrated?

Clinical Path Considerations

As hospice and home care organizations seek to become more efficient, new models of care and documentation are emerging. Clinical paths, or care pathways, are one way to ensure that all team members are on the same page as they work together to achieve patient goals. More paths are emerging in hospice and becoming available to all the staff involved in the plan of care and the patient and family. Clarifying the expectations for care, integrating standards of care into the path, and identifying quantifiable patient goals at the onset create an environment for improved communications and care. The NHPCO has a path specifically designed for hospice.

Clinical paths are one way of defining a clinical budget or the amount of resources needed to care for a particular patient or group of patients. The reason clinical paths are initiated is to improve quality of care; the main focus must be on the patient.

Defining Clinical Paths

Clinical paths are tools that organize, sequence, and time the major interventions of clinicians for a particular case type, medical condition, diagnostic category, or functional diagnosis. They identify and standardize tools and information, interventions, and processes for achieving predetermined outcomes (quantifiable goals of care). The development and implementation of clinical paths are similar to project management, wherein certain key processes that are mapped out schematically can be used to monitor the effectiveness of the plan and determine progress through a process of quality improvement to positively impact and improve patient care.[1]

Clinical paths demand the standardization of care and care processes. For example, goals are clearly defined, and all care to be provided is specifically explained, laid out in a linear design, and based on the organization's historical data. Your organization may have paths for certain groups of patients or diagnoses as a way to ensure quality care for patients with those particular problems. Not all patient problems will have a path; the course of some medical problems cannot be easily projected.

Automation: Effectively Integrating Care and Documentation

There is no question that we need to be more effective in health care; automation or computerization is one method to increase efficiency while enabling team members to provide more detailed and accurate documentation. However, computers are not the answers to all care planning and scheduling issues in hospice. Data, whether documented on paper or keyed into a computer, must be correct for the entire process to flow toward billing and discharge.

To be able to compare "apples to apples," everyone must collect the same information in the same format and manner while using the same glossary in communications. Benchmarking with peers, performance improvement activities, and data management and collection will only become more important in the coming years. Dr. Deming,[2] the guru of quality, has been credited with saying, "In God we trust; all others must have data." Only through standardized data collection tools, methods, and definitions are valid comparisons for cost and care efficiencies possible. These data will help direct our collective efforts to improve hospice care for patients and their loved ones.

SUMMARY

The hospice clinician plays an important role in supporting coverage of hospice through the generation and maintenance of effective documentation. Hospice documentation should reflect that the patient clearly has a terminal illness with a limited life expectancy of less than 6 months. The hospice documentation should emphasize the patient's prognosis, whatever the diagnosis; this is the reason for hospice.

Hospice team members practicing in the community must be service oriented, flexible, strong clinically, and able to document effectively. Payers and insurers must continue to address spiraling health care costs. The customary way to do this has been to decrease authorized visits and services and add additional review levels. The emphasis on the collection of data quantifying the impact of care will only increase in the coming years.

The professional can validate the need for skillful hospice care and back it up with effective documentation. Clinicians must know the coverage criteria for specific insurers, such as Medicare, and the documentation needed to support covered care. The documentation and related coverage criteria go hand in hand, and their importance cannot be overstated. They assist in meeting patients' needs, marketing services, safeguarding team members and the organization against alleged Medicare fraud or abuse claims, and ensuring reimbursement for services. They also provide the baseline for community education related to hospice services and a benchmark for reviewing visit or care utilization.

Clinical documentation continues to be an important indicator of the quality of care provided. In community-based hospice home care, in which a reviewer or surveyor cannot walk down inpatient halls and see patients receiving care, the clinical record and its format, organization, and timeliness of filing become important as the link to the quality of the care provided. From this perspective, with the spiraling costs of health care, the clinical record reflects the organization and their belief that "excellence is in the details." In hospice care the details of clinical documentation are a driving force toward payment and certification; more important, they help ensure that patients and families receive quality hospice care.

REVIEW EXERCISES

1. Explain the following statement: "Hospice and clinical practice are described every day through review of patient records."
2. List three reasons for the importance of clinical documentation and the record.
3. Who are the Regional Home Health Intermediaries (RHHIs), and what important role do they plan in hospice?
4. Explain the following statement: "The RHHIs can pay only for hospice care under Medicare that is covered by law."
5. List the hallmarks of effective hospice documentation.
6. Describe the hospice documentation needed to support covered care.
7. What is the test of effective care planning and care coordination?
8. Define a clinical path and the role it plays in effectively managing a patient's care across the care continuum.
9. Explain the rationale that supports the standardization of care and care processes.
10. Describe the clinician's role in compliance related to Medicare and documentation requirements.

References

1. Marrelli T, Hilliard L: *Home care and clinical paths. Effective care planning across the continuum,* St Louis, 1996, Mosby.
2. Deming WE: *Out of the crisis,* Cambridge, Mass, 1986, Massachusetts Institute of Technology Center for Advanced Engineering Studies.

PART THREE

PLANNING AND MANAGING
CARE IN HOSPICE

PLANNING AND MANAGING CARE IN HOSPICE

Frequency of visits and length of service are usually based on the hospice team's assessment and ongoing evaluation of the patient and family status and the patient's biopsychosocial and unique family system needs. The current health care environment and the increasing emphasis on quality initiatives demonstrated by positive patient outcomes identify the need for research and evaluation regarding the frequency and length of time the patient needs to be under care. The following is a discussion of the process and knowledge that may assist in determining frequency and length of service. Throughout this discussion, remember that all visits require orders by the physician, and the nurse must maintain compliance with the Medicare Conditions of Participation, state licensure, surveyor directives, and other regulations or laws.

Much has been written about the appropriate time to admit patients to hospice. In addition, Medicare-participating hospices and government initiatives have been developed to save the Medicare Trust Fund from alleged overutilization, fraud, and abuse. These efforts have heightened awareness of the types of patients and their problems and histories when admitted to hospice.

A number of considerations help in determining the appropriate frequency and length of hospice visits. This discussion provides a framework to assist hospice clinicians in making these decisions appropriately; however, it is not meant to take the place of ongoing meetings with the hospice manager or interdisciplinary group (IDC) to determine patients' unique frequency and duration needs. Rather, this discussion is designed to help hospice clinicians become aware of the many factors that go into making this determination.

The introduction of diagnosis-related groups (DRGs) and other prospective payment systems (PPSs) in inpatient settings has increased the scrutiny of admission to and frequency and duration of home health and hospice services. Nurses practicing in the community are acutely aware of the decreased lengths of stay in hospitals and the increased patient acuity in both the hospital and the home setting. The increasing complexity of patient needs is demonstrated in the changing case mix of the clinician's caseload.

Experienced hospice and community health clinicians know that they are in an important position for identifying the patient's specific service and visit frequency needs. The objective findings in comprehensive hospice assessments are the basis for the recommendations that are made by the team member and communicated to the physician. Some patients may be seen infrequently by their physician after discharge because they lack adequate transportation to the physician's office or, in some instances, the physician does not or will not make needed home visits. The professional nurse's judgment skills can help in making these important visit frequency decisions. Box 3-1 lists some factors that are considered in determining frequency and duration of care.

The clinician's rationale, experience, and sometimes intuition contribute to the decision-making process related to frequency and length of stay. Home health and hospice are two settings in which experienced clinicians

3

BOX 3-1

PATIENT-RELATED CONSIDERATIONS

The following is a list of the most common patient-related considerations that the clinician evaluates when formulating plans and beginning
care. This alphabetical list is not all-inclusive; other considerations may
apply, such as the hospice patient caseload and availability of services
or other resources. In addition, many of these factors are interrelated.

Absence of caregiver
Activities of daily living (ADLs) limitations
Adaptive or assistive devices
Affect (e.g., depression)
Behavioral or mental disorders
Belief systems
Caregiver support
Chemical or drug problems (e.g., alcoholism)
Chronic illness(es)
Clinician assessment and reassessment findings
Clinician diagnoses
Cognitive function
Communication
Competency (patient/family)
Compliance/Noncompliance
Coping skills
Cultural status
Directives
Disabilities
Discharge plan
Drug considerations (e.g., number, type, interactions)
Educational level/barriers
Environment
Family
Fatigue
Fire safety
Functional limitations
Goals/expected outcomes
Handicaps
History
Home medical equipment
Home setting
Independence
Instrumental activities of daily living (IADLs)
Knowledge of emergency procedures
Language
Learning needs
Loneliness

BOX 3-1

PATIENT-RELATED CONSIDERATIONS—cont'd

Loss of significant other(s)
Medical equipment or supply needs
Medications
Mobility
Motivation
Nutritional status
Orthotic needs
Other considerations, based on patient's/family's unique needs
Pain
Parenting
Pathology
Physical assessment findings
Physical setting for care
Polypharmacy
Probability of further complications
Prognosis
Psychopathology
Psychosocial needs
Reason for prior hospitalization, for referral to hospice
Rehabilitative needs
Resources (e.g., financial, human)
Rights
Risk factors
Safety
Self-care status
Skin integrity
Social factors
Social supports
Socioeconomic condition
Spiritual needs
Stability
Support systems
Swallowing
Values
Voice

use their broad knowledge base to make effective patient care decisions, such as those determining frequency and level of stay, that can have a direct impact on patient and family outcomes. The clinician also can look to the manager for specific information, feedback, and standards of the hospice organization or program.

Health care reform is primarily addressing three of the greatest problems within the U.S. health care system—access, cost, and quality. Cost is the issue that hospice programs address daily when a case management company questions or limits needed visits, services, or hours of care. As hospice experts, clinicians, managers, and administrators must articulate to a case manager or third-party payer the objective rationale and plan for projected care. Clinicians must be able to communicate objectively the skills used during care and explain why those visits may vary even though patients may have the same general diagnoses or problems. Clinicians and other hospice clinicians can do their jobs because of their education and experience.

Payment is for the professional clinician's judgment and observational and other skills. Only clinicians can compare one wound with others seen in their practice experience, make a judgment regarding healing or infection, identify dehiscence, evaluate the wound in relation to other pathological conditions, obtain a baseline assessment, teach the patient and caregivers, and apply a myriad of other skills to patients daily in homes. The role and responsibility of home care and hospice professionals are to educate others, including case managers, payers, consumers, and families, about the cost effectiveness, quality, and demonstrated positive outcomes experienced by the patients. As performance improvement focuses on the consumer of services, the industry must move toward standardizing processes, continually looking at methods to improve results (positive patient outcomes) and objectively measuring performance and demonstrated outcomes.

Research-based practice guidelines, outcome measures, and standards of care are important because of the increased emphasis on cost-effective high-quality care. These practice parameters assist clinicians in determining patient needs and care frequency and better projecting length of service.

Standardized care plans are based on North American Nursing Diagnosis Association (NANDA International) health care diagnoses and clinician's experience with particular patient problems. Other organizations have developed or purchased automated systems that help them track and define objective findings and demonstrate outcome achievement based on outcome criteria. Clinicians in practice are aware of the ongoing concern regarding provision of adequate patient care in a climate of tighter reimbursement, more limited resources, frequent ethical dilemmas, and heightened emphasis on both quality and effectiveness. This cost/quality equation must balance out for the maintenance of patient and family satisfaction and success, productivity, viability of organizations, and clinician satisfaction in their ability to meet patient and family needs.

Managers and clinicians need to be adept in articulating and quantifying patient care needs based on objective evidence and supporting documentation. As clinicians identify the need to streamline and more effectively provide and demonstrate care, use of such systems will help in creating and maintaining cost- and time-effective operations and quality improvement. The use of standardized care plans as the basis for individualizing hospice care helps clinicians as they teach patients and family members to prioritize new or multiple health needs.

HOSPICE CARE EXAMPLES

The following are examples of some patients and patient problems seen in hospice. They are just examples, and the hospice clinician's professional judgment, recognized standards of care, and information gathered from all aspects of the assessment process are still the basis for identifying patient and family services, visit frequency, and service duration needs. All hospice documentation must clearly show the disease progression of the terminally ill patient.

The answers to the following questions may help the hospice clinician determine the frequency and intensity of hospice services. Determinations must be based on the patient's and family's unique findings, situation, and supports. Generally, hospice patients may have more intensive needs toward the end of care than at the beginning. This situation is the opposite of the typical home health care scenario, in which the patient is working toward independence and the team pulls back toward discharge. Keep in mind, however, that some patients are admitted to hospice appropriately for intensive services at the onset for hospice's specialty skills of support and pain and symptom management.

- What symptoms or clinical information supports the need for hospice?
- What is the patient's current activity level, how has it changed, and how rapidly has it changed?
- What information has the doctor, patient, or others provided that supports the contention that the patient has a limited life expectancy?
- What are the expectations related to hospice care and support, and how can we best meet them?
- If this is a new diagnosis, what services are identified during the assessment and how do these services support fulfillment of the patient and family needs?
- What are the special skills and services that hospice will bring to this patient and family?
- If the patient has Alzheimer's disease, cardiac, or lung disease, or another illness that may have long-term or chronic disease implications, what occurrences or symptoms lead the physician and clinicians to believe that the patient is dying?
- Are symptoms or side effects from therapy emerging in the history and physical assessment?
- Why were the patient and family referred to hospice? Can hospice meet their unique needs?
- What are the patient and family expressing/identifying as their needs?

1. The patient is 82 and was recently diagnosed with cancer of the prostate. He moved into his daughter's home after his last hospitalization, hoping to return to his own home "after he was stronger." The patient had a suprapubic catheter and complained of lower back pain. After several weeks of care, it is apparent that he will not get any stronger, and he continually asks his daughter to let him go home—especially if he is dying. Understandably upset, his

daughter has had multiple discussions with the physician, and hospice was called for an assessment. Because of her work schedule, the daughter frequently is not home.

In an effort to address the patient's stated desire to return to his home, the hospice admitting clinician assesses the patient at his daughter's home. The patient clearly states that the next visit will be at his home, mentioning that he thinks his niece will move in with him if necessary. Because the patient is a widower who lives alone, the hospice team initially focuses efforts on the need for a primary caregiver. The effective use of care conferencing assists the patient and his daughter in the decision-making process and assessment of the appropriate time to make the transition to hospice and for the patient to return home.

This patient does return to his own home, with his daughter (when available) and niece as his primary caregivers. The IDT's support contributes to the patient's ability to return home. His death occurs some 3 weeks later, and bereavement support assists his daughter and niece (who was identified as at risk for a difficult bereavement) during the period following his death.

Visit frequency for this patient was daily, at the onset, as the patient experienced continued discomfort with the catheter and was concerned about possible dislodgment. The certified nursing assistant (CNA) assisted with personal care, activities of daily living, and meal preparation. The CNA noted increasing discomfort on standing or turning in certain positions and reported this to the hospice nurse, who reassessed the patient and called the physician for a change in the medication regimen and plan of care. The niece, who at another time had moved in with and assisted another family member who had later died, was very concerned about the patient's dying at home and her being alone. The social worker visited once a week and discussed a system of communication with her to try to decrease this possibility and her anxiety. Because of this history, all team members were very clear in their communications with the niece when she daily asked, "Is he near?" or "Is it close?" The catheter was finally removed, which made the patient more comfortable and mobile. The patient died at home pain-free, and the niece was not alone; both the patient's daughter and the hospice nurse were there, and the niece and daughter had uncomplicated bereavement periods.

2. The patient is a 46-year-old woman with an aggressive metastatic breast cancer and a history of bilateral mastectomies, chemotherapy, radiation, and alternative therapies over a span of 6 years. She was initially referred to hospice by her physician for pain control and support to the patient, her husband, and their three children, who are 6, 8, and 14 years old. On admission, the hospice clinician notes that her pain was assessed as a 2 on a scale of 1-10, and the patient notes that it worsens with movement or any activity. The hospice team contacts the physician and the pharmacist, and changes are made in her medication regimen that cause the pain to decrease to 0 with

activity. Massage therapy, which the patient identifies as most effectively assisting her comfort level, is integrated into her plan of care.

Hospice volunteers assist with support for the family, and the patient dies at home, according to her request, with her symptoms fairly well controlled. At the bereavement visits, her husband verbalizes the importance of the care and support they all received from hospice. In this example the frequency of visits is intense on admission for pain assessments and reassessment and management, stabilizes as the patient's symptoms are controlled, and then increases significantly as the patient and family needs increase just before death.

3. The patient is a 47-year-old woman with cancer of the liver who is admitted for hospice care. The hospice clinical specialist who admits the patient and family to the program explains the hospice philosophy and proposes a care regimen based on the needs identified. Health care, home health aide care, and other components of the hospice team are explained, and care is scheduled to begin. The frequency issue is sometimes more complex in patients with clearly shortened life spans.

Depending on the patient's and family's unique needs, it can be appropriate for the same amount of care to be provided throughout the hospice admission. Keep in mind that many patients are admitted to hospice at the end stages of their disease after high-technology interventions and cure-oriented therapies have been exhausted. As the focus changes from cure to palliation, the hospice takes a holistic approach to care, with the frequency determined solely by patient and family needs. For such a patient, services could consist of 3-times-weekly RN visits with home care aides and volunteer support or any combination of services provided by the hospice IDT. The goals/outcomes identified in this case are symptom-controlled death at home with hospice support and family presence.

SUMMARY

Clinicians working in hospice must be flexible and able to explain objective reasons for frequency related to the plan of care. These and other decisions and the underlying rationale must be communicated clearly to the manager or third-party payer representatives who are responsible for tracking, approving, or denying vists or care. We must be able to articulate the clinical and other needs of the patient. This advocacy role will ensure quality care while the patient remains at home. Those who can explain needs based on objective information and patient findings to numerous reimbursement gatekeepers will be successful as advocates for patients and families who elect hospice care. The increasing complexity of caring for patients sent home with limited resourced and coverage demands these skills for safe, effective patient care.

REVIEW EXERCISES

1. List five factors that are taken into account when projecting care needs for hospice patients and families.
2. Describe a hospice patient example and the rationale that supports the frequency and the interventions planned.
3. Explain three reasons that support a patient's admission to hospice (assume, of course, that the patient and family desire hospice).
4. Support the following statement: "We should use standardized care plans as the basis for individualizing patient/family hospice care."

3

PART FOUR

MEDICAL-SURGICAL CARE GUIDELINES
Special Patients and Families

OUTLINE FOR CARE GUIDELINES

1. **General Considerations**

2. **Needs for Visit**

3. **Safety Considerations**

4. **Potential Diagnoses and Codes**

5. **Skills and Services Identified**
   - Hospice Nursing
     a. Comfort and Symptom Control
     b. Safety and Mobility Considerations
     c. Emotional/Spiritual Considerations
     d. Skin Care
     e. Elimination Considerations
     f. Hydration/Nutrition
     g. Therapeutic/Medication Regimens
     h. Other Considerations
   - Home Health Aide or Certified Nursing Assistant
   - Social Worker
   - Volunteer(s)
   - Spiritual Counselor
   - Dietitian/Nutritional Counseling
   - Occupational Therapist
   - Physical Therapist
   - Speech-Language Pathologist
   - Bereavement Counselor
   - Pharmacist (for some diagnoses)
   - Music, Massage, Art, or Other Therapies or Services

6. **Outcomes for Care**

7. **Patient, Family, and Caregiver Educational Needs**

8. **Specific Tips for Quality and Reimbursement**

9. **Queries for Quality**

10. **Resources for Hospice Care and Practice**

ACQUIRED IMMUNE DEFICIENCY SYNDROME (AIDS) CARE

1. General considerations

Every year, an estimated 40,000 new HIV infections are reported. Of the approximately 850,000 to 950,000 Americans living with HIV, a fourth don't know they are infected.

Home continues to be the care setting for most patients with acquired immune deficiency syndrome (AIDS). Care is directed toward palliation of opportunistic infections and other HIV-related conditions and prevention of further problems. *Pneumocystis carinii* pneumonia continues to be one of the most serious processes in the adult patient with AIDS. The provision of comfort, support, education, and palliative care to patients and their caregivers is key to effective hospice care in the community.

Please refer to "Cancer Care," "Pain Care," "Infusion Care," and "Bedbound Care" should these sections also pertain to your hospice patient.

2. Needs for visit

Physician order for hospice care, specific to the hospice program's admission criteria and policies
Standard precautions supplies
Vital signs equipment for baseline assessment
Other supplies or equipment, based on physician orders

3. Safety considerations

Infection control/standard precautions
Night-light
Extra caution on slippery surfaces
Removal of scatter rugs
Tub rail, grab bars for bathroom safety
Supportive and nonskid shoes
Handrail on stairs
Fall precautions
Protective skin measures
Identification and report of any skin problems
Smoke detector and fire evacuation plan
Assistance with ambulation
Municipal water source/safety
Pet care (e.g., mobility, infection control)
Others, based on the patient's unique condition and environment

4

4. Potential diagnoses and codes

AIDS (general)	042
Anemia	042 and 285.29
Anorexia	042 and 783.0
Bacterial infections, recurrent	042 and 041.9
Burkitt's lymphoma	042 and 200.20
Cancer, cervical	042 and 180.9

Candidiasis	042 and 112.9
Candidiasis, esophageal	042 and 112.84
Candidiasis, oral	042 and 112.0
Candidiasis, vaginal	042 and 112.1
Cervical cancer	042 and 180.9
Chorioretinitis	042 and 363.20
Colitis	042 and 558.9
Cryptococcus	042 and 117.5
Cytomegalovirus	042 and 078.5
Cytomegalovirus retinitis	042 and 078.5, 363.20
Dementia	042 and 294.10
Diarrhea	042 and 008.69
Encephalitis	042 and 323.0
Encephalopathy, AIDS	042 and 348.39
Endocarditis	042 and 424.90
Esophagitis	042 and 530.10
Failure to thrive, adult	783.7
Herpes simplex	042 and 054.9
Herpes zoster	042 and 053.9
Histoplasmosis	042 and 115.90
HTLV III	042
Hyperalimentation (procedure)	99.15
Kaposi's sarcoma	042 and 176.9
Lymphocytic interstitial pneumonia	042 and 516.8
Lymphoma	042 and 202.80
Lymphoma, non-Hodgkin's	042 and 202.80
Lymphoma of the brain	042 and 202.81
Malaise and fatigue	780.79
Meningitis	042 and 047.8
Mycobacterium avium intracellulare	042 and 031.0
Mycobacterium tuberculosis	042 and 011.90
Myocarditis, acute or subacute	042 and 422.99
Neuropathy, peripheral	042 and 357.4
Neutropenia	042 and 288.0
Paraplegia	042 and 344.1
Pelvic inflammatory disease (PID) (acute)	042 and 614.3
Pelvic inflammatory disease (PID) (chronic)	042 and 614.4
Peripheral neuropathy	042 and 357.4
Pneumocystis carinii pneumonia	042 and 136.3
Pneumonia (bacterial)	042 and 482.9
Pneumonia (NOS)	042 and 486
Pneumonia (viral)	042 and 480.9
Polymyositis	042 and 710.4
Polyradiculoneuropathy	042 and 357.10
Protein-caloric malnutrition	042 and 263.9
Quadriplegia	042 and 344.00
Retinal detachment	042 and 361.9
Retinal hemorrhage	042 and 362.81

4

Salmonella	042 and 003.9
Salmonella septicemia	042 and 003.1
Seizures	042 and 780.39
Septicemia	042 and 038.9
Shigella	042 and 004.9
Shigella dysentery	042 and 004.9
Thrombocytopenia	042 and 287.5
Total parenteral nutrition (TPN) (procedure)	9.15
Toxoplasmosis	042 and 130.9
Tuberculosis (pulmonary)	042 and 011.90
Varicella	042 and 052.9
Wasting syndrome	042 and 799.4
Zoster virus	042 and 053.9

5. Skills and services identified

• *Hospice nursing*

a. *Comfort and symptom control*

Complete initial assessment of all systems of patient with AIDS admitted to hospice for _____ (specify problem necessitating care)

Presentation of hospice philosophy and services

Explain patient rights and responsibilities

Assess patient, family, and caregiver wishes and expectations regarding care

Assess patient, family, and caregiver resources available for care

Teach family or caregiver physical care of patient

Provision of volunteer support to patient and family

Assess pain and other symptoms, including site, duration, characteristics, and relief measures

Assess patient q visit for change (increase) in levels of fatigue, weakness, or malaise

Assess and observe all systems and symptoms q visit, and report changes and new symptoms to physician

Instruct patient and caregiver to notify RN or physician for new symptoms, including fever, vomiting, diarrhea, cough, and other changes

Teach pain and symptom management regimen to caregiver

RN to instruct in pain control measures and medications

Teach caregiver or family about care of weak, terminally ill patient

Instruct in the need for elevation of edematous extremities and elevation of head of bed for comfort

Evaluate pain in relation to other symptoms, such as fatigue, confusion, diarrhea, nausea and vomiting, depression, and shortness of breath

RN to assess patient's pain or other symptoms q visit to identify need for change, addition or other plan, or dose adjustment

Measure vital signs, including pain, q visit

Assess cardiovascular, pulmonary, and respiratory status

Teach caregivers symptom control and relief measures

Oxygen at _____ liters per _____ (specific physician orders)

4

Identify and monitor pain, symptom, and relief measures

Implement nonpharmacological interventions for pain, such as
   progressive muscle relaxation, imagery, positive visualization,
   music, and humor therapy of patient's choice

Comfort measures of backrub and hand or other therapeutic massage

RN to provide and teach effective oral care and comfort measures

Teach patient and family about realistic expectations of disease process

Teach care of dying and signs/symptoms of impending death

Presence and support

Other interventions, based on patient/family needs

b. *Safety and mobility considerations*

Provide patient with home safety information and instruction related to
   _____ and documented in the clinical record

Instruct patient regarding pet care and avoidance of cross
   contamination, and check with physician about certain types of pets

Teach patient and caregiver care needed for safe, effective management
   at home

Teach caregivers care of the bedridden patient

Instruct patient and family regarding safety and standard precautions in
   the home

Teach patient and family regarding planning and pacing activities

Teach patient and family regarding energy conservation techniques

Instruct caregiver regarding need to maintain activity as tolerated, range
   of motion (ROM) exercises to prevent loss or decrease in mobility,
   and need to report changes to physician

Other interventions, based on patient/family needs

c. *Emotional/Spiritual considerations*

Psychosocial assessment of patient and family regarding disease and
   prognosis

Discuss need for guardianship or power of attorney

Discuss concepts of "living will," other advance directives, status
   regarding resuscitation, other medical/technical interventions, and
   patient's wishes

Assist with funeral plans, if appropriate

Inform patient/family/caregiver of available volunteer support

Assess patient's spiritual needs and address plan

Assess patient and caregiver coping skills

Provide emotional support to patient/family with chronic and/or
   terminal illness and associated implications

Assess patient for mental status and sleep disturbance problems or changes

Assist with emotional support concerning care of children and
   children's future

RN to provide emotional support to patient and family

Other interventions, based on patient/family needs

d. *Skin care*

Teach patient and caregiver all aspects of wound care, including safe
   disposal of dressing supplies

4

Care for and assess Kaposi lesions, cleanse with_____
(specify according to physician orders)
Teach caregiver regarding patient's skin care needs, including the need
for frequent position changes, appropriate pressure pads and
mattresses, and the prevention of breakdown
Assess skin integrity
Observation and evaluation of wound and surrounding skin
Evaluate patient's need for equipment, supplies to decrease pressure,
alternating pressure mattress, gel foam seat cushion, and heel and
elbow protectors
Teach family to perform dressing changes between RN visits, _____
(specify)
Teach patient, family, or caregiver about proper body alignment and
positioning in bed to prevent skin tears from shearing skin
Observe and apply skilled assessment of areas for possible breakdown,
including heels, hips, elbows, and ankles
RN to teach patient regarding care of irradiated skin sites
Assess patient's skin and mucous membranes for problems, including
bacterial infection, thrush, rashes, and other changes
Other interventions, based on patient/family needs

e. *Elimination considerations*
Assess bowel regimen, and implement program as needed
Instruct patient and caregiver to report increase in diarrhea (frequency,
amount) to physician
RN to teach caregiver daily catheter care
RN to evaluate the patient's bowel patterns, need for stool softeners,
laxatives, and dietary adjustments and develop bowel management plan
Check for and remove impaction as needed
Condom catheter or indwelling catheter as indicated
Teach catheter care to caregiver
Assess amount and frequency of urinary output
Observation and complete systems assessment of the patient with an
indwelling catheter
Other interventions, based on patient/family needs

f. *Hydration/Nutrition*
Instruct patient about specified diet _____ (specify according
to physician orders)
Teach food preparation and handling techniques, particularly hand
washing, handling of uncooked foods, and the need to cook all eggs,
meat, fish, and poultry products
Weigh patient q visit and review food intake diary and use of herbs,
vitamins/mineral supplements, and alternative nutrition therapies
Encourage patient to eat small, more frequent meals of choice
Closely monitor parenteral feeding catheter and IV therapy site for
infection or other problems/complications
Monitor patient on enteral nutrition therapy
Nutrition/hydration to be maintained by offering patient high-protein
diet and foods of choice as tolerated

4

Assess nutrition and hydration status
Counsel patient with anorexia about diet and nutrition
Teach feeding-tube care to family
Encourage use of commercially prepared nutrition supplements
(e.g., Ensure)
Teach patient and family to expect decreased nutritional and fluid
intake as disease progresses
Other interventions based on patient/family needs

g. *Therapeutic/Medication regimens*
Monitor patient for side effects of drugs and food/drug and drug/drug
interactions
Teach site care of Hickman catheter or other venous access device
Obtain blood samples as ordered for necessary monitoring
Implement nonpharmacological interventions with medication schedule,
possibly including massage, distraction, imagery, progressive muscle
relaxation, humor, biofeedback, and music therapies
Medication management of patient on complex and numerous drug
therapies
Teach regarding antiretroviral therapy medication
Teach patient and caregiver all aspects of medications, including routes,
schedules, functions, and side effects
Teach new pain and symptom control medication regimen
Assess weight as ordered
Measure abdominal girth for ascites and edema; document sites, amount
Obtain venipuncture as ordered q _____ (specify ordered frequency)
Teach new medications and effects
Assess for electrolyte imbalance
Teach new medications and effects
Teach patient and caregiver use of patient-controlled anesthesia (PCA)
pump
Observe for side effects of palliative chemotherapy, including
constipation, anemia, and fatigue, and teach patient relief measures
Venipuncture _____ (specify ordered frequency) for
monitoring platelet count, other values
Demonstrate and teach use of multiple medications to caregiver
Monitor patient's level of anemia and other lab values
Assess the patient's unique response to treatments or interventions, and
instruct patient/family to report changes or unfavorable responses or
reactions to the physician
Other interventions, based on patient/family needs

h. *Other considerations*
Instruct patient and caregivers in all aspects of effective handwashing
techniques and proper care of bodily fluids and excretions
Address sexuality concerns and implications for safer sexual
expression, including the use of latex condoms, abstinence, the use
of dental dams during oral sex, and other information
Assess progression of disease process

RN to assess the patient's response to treatments and interventions and to report to the physician any changes, unfavorable responses, and reactions

Teach patient and caregiver about waterborne infections

Other interventions, based on patient/family needs

- *Home health aide or certified nursing assistant*
  Effective and safe personal care
  Activities of daily living (ADL) assistance and support and ambulation and transfer assist
  Observation and reporting
  Respite care and active listening skills
  Meal preparation
  Homemaker services
  Comfort care
  Other duties

- *Social worker*
  Psychosocial assessment of patient and family/caregiver, including adjustment to illness and its implications, and the need for care
  Identification of optimal coping strategies
  Financial assessment and counseling regarding food acquisition, ability to prepare, and costs of needed medications
  Intervention/support related to terminal illness and loss
  Identification of caregiver role strain necessitating respite/relief measures or support
  Emotional/spiritual support
  Facilitate communication among patient, family, and hospice team
  Referral/linkage to community services and resources as indicated
  Grief counseling and intervention/support related to illness/loss
  Patient/caregiver counseling and support
  For patients who live alone with no support system (e.g., able, available, willing caregiver[s]): obtain linkage with necessary community resources to allow patient to stay in the home
  Identification of illness-related psychiatric condition necessitating support and care/intervention
  Evaluation of situation related to patient's child(ren) and future wishes for child(ren)and pets
  Depression and fears assessed
  Funeral and burial planning assistance

- *Volunteer(s)*
  Support, friendship, companionship, and presence
  Comfort and dignity maintained/provided for patient and family
  Errands and transportation
  Other services, based on interdisciplinary team recommendations and patient/caregiver needs

- *Spiritual counselor*
  Spiritual assessment and care

4

Pray with or for the patient/family, using prayers familiar to patient's religious background (per their wishes)

Counseling, intervention, and support related to that dimension of life related to life's meaning (consistent with patient's/family's beliefs)

Support, listening, and presence

Participation in sacred or spiritual rituals or practices

Funeral and burial planning assistance

Other supportive care, based on the patient's/family's needs and belief systems

- *Dietitian/Nutritional counseling*
  Assessment of patient with decreased intake, weight loss, anorexia, diarrhea, nausea, and skin breakdown

  Assessment and recommendations for swallowing difficulties

  Support and care with food and nourishment as desired by patient

  Encourage patient to ingest nutritional supplements and snacks to increase protein and caloric intake

  Counsel and instruct family regarding patient's decreased appetite and possible inability to eat

  Food and dietary recommendations incorporating patient choice and wishes

  Teach proper food preparation and handling, especially handwashing, handling of uncooked foods, and need to cook eggs, meat, fish, poultry, and dairy products

  Assess and teach use of alternative nutrition therapies, such as herbs, vitamin/mineral supplements, and macrobiotic diets

- *Occupational therapist*
  Evaluation

  Energy conservation techniques

  Evaluation of ADL and functional mobility

  Assess for need for adaptive equipment and assistive devices

  Safety assessment of patient's environment and ADL

- *Physical therapist*
  Evaluation

  Assessment of patient's environment for safety

  Safe transfer training

  Strengthening exercises/program

  Assessment of gait safety

  Instruct/supervise caregiver and volunteers with regard to home exercise program for conditioning and strength

  Assistive, adaptive devices of equipment and teaching

- *Speech-language pathologist*
  Evaluation for swallowing problems

- *Bereavement counselor*
  Assessment of the needs of the bereaved family and friends

  Support and intervention, based on assessment and ongoing findings

Presence and counseling

Supportive visits and follow-up and other interventions (e.g., mailings, calls)

Other services related to bereavement work and support

- *Pharmacist*

  Evaluation of hospice patient on multiple medications for possible food/drug, drug/drug interactions

  Medication monitoring regarding therapeutic levels and dosages

  Pain consult and input into interdisciplinary plan of care related to pain control, palliation, and symptom management

- *Music, massage, art, or other therapies or services*

  Evaluation and intervention based on patient's and caregiver's unique wishes and needs that support care and death in the setting of the patient's choice

  Pet therapy (including patient's pet, if available) and therapeutic intervention

  Assessment plan to engage patient and support comfort, quality, enjoyment, and dignity

6. Outcomes for care

- *Hospice nursing*

  Patient and caregiver verbalize satisfaction with care

  Educational tools/plans incorporated in daily care, and patient/caregiver verbalizes understanding of safe, needed care

  Patient will decide on care, interventions, and evaluation

  Caregiver is effective in care management and knows whom to call for questions/concerns

  Patient will express satisfaction with hospice support received and will experience increased comfort

  Patient will be made comfortable at home through death in accordance with the patient's wishes

  Patient verbalizes the effectiveness of pain and symptom control

  Patient verbalizes understanding of and adheres to care and medication regimens

  Patient and caregiver are supported through patient's death

  Comfort maintained throughout course of care

  The patient and family receive hospice support and care, and family members and friends are able to spend quality time with the patient

  Caregiver able and verbalizes comfort with role and lists when to call hospice team members

  Patient supported through and receives the maximum benefit from palliative chemotherapy and radiation with minimal complications

  Patient/caregiver lists adverse reactions, potential complications, signs/symptoms of infection (e.g., sputum change, chest congestion)

  Comfort maintained through death with dignity

  Pain effectively managed, and patient verbalizes comfort at _____ on 0–10 scale

4

Patient has stable respiratory status with patent airway (e.g., no dyspnea, infection free)

Patient protected from injury, stable respiratory status, and compliant with medication, safety, and care regimens

Comfort and individualized intervention of patient with immobility/bed-bound status (e.g., skin, urinary, musculature, vascular)

Spiritual and psychosocial needs met (specify) as defined by patient and caregiver throughout course of care

Successful pain and symptom management as verbalized by patient/caregiver

Patient will demonstrate adequate breathing patterns as evidenced by a lack of respiratory distress symptoms

Patient will be comfortable through illness

Patient/caregiver will demonstrate _____ % compliance with instructions related to care

Patient and caregiver demonstrate and practice effective handwashing and other infection-control measures (specify: e.g., disposal of waste, cleaning of linens)

Adherence to plan of care (POC) by patient and caregivers, and able to demonstrate safe and supportive care

Planned and effective bowel program, as evidenced by regular bowel movements and patient/family report of comfort

Death with dignity, and symptoms controlled in setting of patient/family choice

Optimal comfort, support, and dignity provided throughout illness

Death with maximum comfort through effective symptom control with specialized hospice support

Patient and caregiver able to list adverse drug reactions/problems with medication regimen and whom to call for follow-up and resolution

Pain and symptoms managed/controlled in setting of patient/family choice (e.g., patient/family report ability to eat, sleep, speak more clearly with pacing, other intervention)

Patient's/family's privacy, independence, and choices supported with respect and maintained through death

Enhancement and support of quality of life

Effective symptom relief and control (e.g., a peaceful and comfortable death at home, some enjoyment of life)

Maximizing the patient's quality of life (e.g., alert and pain free, or as patient wishes)

Pharmacological and nonpharmacological interventions such as localized heat application, positioning, relaxation methods, and music

Patient cared for and family supported through death with physical, psychosocial, spiritual, and other concerns/needs acknowledged/addressed

Patient- and family-centered hospice care provided based on the patient's/family's unique situation and needs

Infection control and palliation through death

Grief/bereavement expression and support provided

Caregiver demonstrates ability to manage pain, where applicable

Patient maintains comfort and dignity throughout illness
Patient rates pain as _____ to _____ on pain 0–10 scale by next visit
Patient's catheter will remain patent and infection free
Patient and caregiver adhere to/demonstrate compliance with multiple
    medication regimens (e.g., times, storage, refrigeration)
Patient's and family's educational and support needs met as verbalized
    by caregiver and adherence to plan
Death with maximum comfort through effective symptom control and
    specialized hospice support
Symptoms controlled in setting of patient/family choice
Effective pain relief and control (e.g., a peaceful and comfortable death)
Patient cared for and family supported through death with physical,
    psychosocial, spiritual, and other needs acknowledged/addressed
Patient- and family-centered hospice care provided based on the
    patient/family's unique situation and needs
Infection control and palliation

- *Home health aide or certified nursing assistant*
  Effective and safe personal care and hygiene maintained
  Safe ADL assistance and ambulation
  Safe environment maintained
  Hygiene and comfort maintained
  Adequate nutritional support and sleep

- *Social worker*
  Patient/caregiver able to cope adaptively with illness and death
  Identification and addressing/resolution of problems impeding the
      successful implementation of the POC
  Adaptive adjustment to changed body and body image
  Psychosocial support and counseling offered/initiated to patient and
      caregivers experiencing grieving process
  Resources identified, communitylinkage to appropriate patient/family
  Funeral and burial planning assistance

- *Volunteer(s)*
  Comfort, companionship, and friendship extended to patient/family
  Patient and caregiver support provided as defined by needs of patient
      and caregiver
  Support and respite provided as defined by the patient/caregiver

- *Spiritual counselor*
  Spiritual support offered and provided to patient, family, and caregivers
  Patient and family express a relief of symptoms of spiritual suffering
  Provision of spiritual support and care as based on the assessed and
      ongoing needs of the patient and family
  Intervention and support provided related to that dimension of life
      related to life's meaning (consistent with patient's beliefs)
  Participation in sacred or spiritual rituals or practices
  Others, based on the patient's/family's unique beliefs and needs
  Pray with or for the patient/family, using prayers familiar to the
      patient's religious background (per their wishes)

4

- *Dietitian/Nutritional counseling*

  Caregiver integrating recommendations into daily meal planning and prepares safe meals

  Nutrition and hydration optimal for patient with difficulty eating and lack of smell contributing to anorexia

  Nutrition and hydration optimal for patient

  Patient eating foods and supplements of recommended consistency

  Patient and caregiver know whom to call for nutrition-related questions/concerns

  Patient and family verbalize comprehension of changing nutritional needs

- *Occupational therapist*

  ADL level maintained at patient's optimal level

  Optimal functional, safe mobility maintained

  Patient using adaptive devices

  Quality of life improved through assistive/adaptive devices and energy-conservation techniques

  Patient and caregiver demonstrate ADL program for maximum safety and independence

  Patient and caregiver apply principles of energy conservation to daily activities and mobility

  Patient and caregiver demonstrate safe and effective use of assistive devices to increase functioning

  Patient and caregiver demonstrate effective use of energy conservation

  Verbalization/demonstration of improved functional activity level and enhanced quality of life

  Patient and caregiver demonstrate effective use of diaphragmatic breathing to reduce shortness of breath and relaxation techniques to help in pain/symptom management

- *Physical therapist*

  Patient performs home exercise regimen taught and has _____ % increase in mobility/function/strength

  Maintenance of balance, mobility, and endurance as verbalized and demonstrated by patient

  Prevention of complications

  Safety in mobility and transfers

- *Speech-language pathologist*

  Safe swallowing and functional communication

  Swallowing improved as verbalized by patient or caregiver

  Recommended food textures list for safety and patient choice

- *Bereavement counselor*

  Support services related to grief provided to patient and family

  Well-being and resolution process of grief initiated and followed through bereavement services

- *Pharmacist*

  Multiple medication regimens reviewed for food/drug and drug/drug interactions and problems

  Infusion medications and blood-level lab reports reviewed for therapeutic dosage and safe, effective patient response and reported to physician

  Stability and safety in complex multiple medication regimens

  Effective pain control and symptom management as reported by patient or caregiver

- *Music, massage, art, or other therapies or other services*

  Therapeutic massage/touch effective for patient as self-reported or observed by caregivers/family

  Improve muscle tone, relaxation, and/or sleep

  Patient comfortable and relaxed (e.g., sleeping) after therapy

  Music therapy intervention based on assessment to decrease pain perception, provide emotional expression and support

  Maintenance of comfort and physical, psychosocial, and spiritual health

  Holistic health maintained and comfort achieved through _____ (specify modality)

  Patient has pet's presence as desired—in all care sites, when possible

7. **Patient, family, and caregiver educational needs**

   Educational needs are the care regimens that contribute to safe and effective care at home between the hospice team's visits. These include the following:

   The basic tenets of hospice and the availability of support 24 hours a day, 7 days a week

   Home safety assessment and counseling

   The patient's medication regimen

   Safe and proper body mechanics to promote patient comfort and prevent caregiver safety problems

   Other teaching specific to the patient's and family's unique needs

   Support groups available to patient's family, such as the hospice program's "Caregiver Support Group" meetings for family members and friends of the patient

   Anticipated disease progression

   Symptom management

   The importance of optimal nutrition and hydration

   Standard precautions protocol

   Home safety concerns, issues, and teaching

   The avoidance of infection, whenever possible

   The importance of medical follow-up

   Support groups in the community available to the patient, caregiver, and family

   Other information based on the patient's/family's unique needs

4

8. Specific tips for quality and reimbursement

Unless the patient is in a hospice insurance program, some insurers will not pay for a skilled nurse visit that is made at death if the patient is dead when the nurse arrives at the home. From a Medicare hospice care perspective, the visit at the time of death may be covered when the orders and clinical record document assessment of the patient's status and signs of death/life or state law allows pronouncement of death by an RN.

Document any variances to expected outcomes.

The Medicare hospice benefit does not require that the patient be homebound or have identified skilled needs. For further information on this benefit, please refer to CMS Hospice Manual 21.

Should the patient's status deteriorate and necessitate increased personal care, obtain a telephone order for the increased service, noting frequency and estimating the duration.

Obtain a telephone order for all medication and treatment changes of the medical regimen and document these in the clinical record.

Document patient deterioration

Document dehydration, dehydrating

Document patient change or instability

Document pain, other symptoms not controlled

Document status after acute episode of _____ (specify)

Document positive urine, sputum, etc. culture; patient started on (specify ordered antibiotic therapy)

Document patient impacted; impaction removed manually

Document RN in frequent communication with physician regarding (specify)

Document febrile at _____, pulse change at _____, irr., irr.

Document change noted in _____

Document bony prominences red, opening

Document that RN contacted physician regarding _____ (specify)

Document marked shortness of breath (SOB), dyspnea

Document alteration in mental status

Document medications being adjusted, regulated, or monitored

Document unable to perform ADL, maintain personal care

Document all interdisciplinary team meetings and communications in the POC and progress notes of the clinical record

All team members involved should have input into the hospice POC and document their interventions and goals

Document in the clinical notes the clear progression and symptoms and interventions that demonstrate caring for a patient with terminal illness

Document when/if the patient has respiratory changes, SOB exacerbation of conditions, dysphagia, pain, and other symptoms and that they are identified and resolved

Remember that the clinical documentation is key to measuring ongoing compliance for quality and reimbursement purposes. Care coordination, timely verbal and initial physician orders, and assessment and addressing of spiritual and psychosocial needs should be clearly documented in the patient's clinical record

The documentation should support that all hospice care supports comfort and dignity while meeting patient/family needs

The documentation should include the ongoing assessment and management of pain and other symptoms and the anticipation and prevention of secondary symptoms such as constipation

It is important to note that all team members, including nurses and social workers, should assess, identify, and "hear" spiritual needs that the patient/family want to be addressed. These spiritual issues are key to the provision of high-quality hospice care and cannot be addressed effectively and promptly by the spiritual counselor only

Document clearly symptoms, clinical changes, and assessment findings that support the end stage of the disease process

Document patient changes, symptoms, and clinical information identified from visits and team conferences that supports hospice care and a limited life expectancy

Clearly support in the documentation the rationale that supports or explains the progression of the illness from the chronic to terminal stages

Document mentation, behavioral, and cognitive changes

Document dysphagia, weight loss, increased shortness of breath, dyspnea, infection, sepsis, new or changed medications, etc.

Document any skin changes (e.g., inflamed, painful, weeping skin sites)

Document when the patient is actively dying, deteriorating, or progressing toward death

Remember that the "litmus test" of care coordination rests on the quality of the clinical documentation completed by all team members. Review one of your patient's clinical records, and ask yourself the following: "If I was unable to give a verbal report/update on this patient, would a peer be able to pick up and provide the same level of care and know (from the documentation) the current orders, including specific medications and other details that contribute to effective hospice care?"

Document/report any variance to expected outcomes

Obtain a telephone order for any change in the POC, including changes in the frequency of the visits, medications, services provided, and concurrence of other team members

Document your care and the patient's response to your care interventions

Document the patient's problems or changes in status, especially an exacerbation of symptoms

Document increased sputum production, coughing, SOB, pain, diarrhea, or any change in the patient's mental status

Document patient deterioration and improvements

Document blood results, cultures, and treatments

Consider patient for case management or clinical path protocol

4

Consider AIDS/clinician or clinical specialist for consultation and
review of POC

Document any increase in temperature or other objective signs that
could signal a pending infection

Document the specific teaching provided and response to teaching

Document coordination of services or consultation with other members
of the interdisciplinary group (IDG)

For this and other noncancer diagnoses, document clearly the
symptoms and clinical and assessment findings that support the end
stage of the chronic illness process

Document patient changes, symptoms, and clinical information
identified from visits and team conferences that support hospice care
and limited life expectancy

9. **Queries for quality**
   - *Is patient's pain managed adequately?*
   - *Is patient's anxiety managed adequately?*
   - *What infection control measures are implemented?*
   - *What symptoms is the patient experiencing?*
   - *Have you documented to the interdisciplinary POC?*

10. **Resources for hospice care and practice**
    - The CDC National AIDS Clearinghouse has a free resource catalog
      and a 35-page booklet entitled. Caring for Someone with AIDS at
      Home, which has sections about symptoms in the final stages,
      hospice care, final arrangements, and dying at home. This can be
      ordered free by calling 1-800-458-5231.
    - Another helpful resource is the NHPCO's latest edition of Medical
      Guidelines for Determining Prognoses in Selected Non-Cancer
      Diseases. Call the NHPCO at 1-800-646-6460 for more information.
    - Positively Aware is a publication that provides information and
      support to anyone concerned with AIDS and HIV issues. For infor-
      mation, call (773) 989-9400.
    - *A Clinical Guide to Supportive and Palliative Safe Care for
      HIV/AIDS* (2003) is available free of charge from the Health
      Resources and Services Administration (HRSA) online at
      http://hab.hrsa.gov or may be ordered from the HRSA Information
      Center at 1-888-ASK-HRSA (1-888-275-4772).

ALZHEIMER'S DISEASE AND OTHER DEMENTIAS CARE

1. General considerations

As increasing numbers of elderly patients are cared for by their families or other caregivers in the home, the presence of Alzheimer's disease, organic brain syndrome, and other problems characterized by confusion has risen dramatically. According to the National Institute on Aging, Alzheimer's disease alone currently affects an estimated 4 million Americans. The skills of the hospice team are important to the safety and care of these patients and their families. Patients with Alzheimer's disease and other dementias may be appropriate candidates for hospice care when patients and their families face the final stages. Compassion and care are then directed toward comfort and support of the patient and family or caregivers.

2. Needs for visit

Physician order for hospice care, specific to the hospice program's admission criteria and policies

Standard precautions supplies

Vital signs equipment for baseline assessment

Other supplies or equipment, based on physician orders

3. Safety considerations

Infection control/standard precautions

Night-light

Removal of scatter rugs

Tub rail, grab bars for bathroom safety

Supportive and nonskid shoes

Wandering precautions

Smoking with supervision only

Handrail on stairs

Fall precautions

Protective skin measures

Stairway precautions

Smoke detector and fire evacuation plan

Assistance with ambulation

Supervised care and medication regimen

Others, based on the patient's unique condition and environment

4. Potential diagnoses and codes

AIDS dementia	042 and 294.10
Alzheimer's disease	331.0
Amyotrophic lateral sclerosis	335.20
Anxiety state	300.00
Aphasia	784.3

4

Atherosclerosis	440.9
Bladder incontinence	788.30
Constipation	564.00
Creutzfeldt-Jakob disease and dementia	046.1 and 294.10
CVA	436
Dehydration	276.5
Dementia	331.0 and 294.10
Depressive disorder	311
Depressive psychosis	296.20
Failure to thrive, adult	783.7
Huntington's chorea	333.4
Korsakoff's dementia	294.0
Multiple sclerosis	340
Nonpsychotic brain syndrome	310.9
Organic brain sydrome	310.9
Parkinson's disease	332.0
Pernicious anemia	281.0
Pneumonia	486
Presenile dementia	290.10
Pressure (decubitus) ulcer	707.0
Psychosis	298.9
Senile dementia	290.0
Subdural hematoma (nontraumatic)	432.1
Subdural hematoma (traumatic)	852.20
Transient ischemic attack (TIA)	435.9
Unipolar affective disorder	296.99
Urinary incontinence	788.30
Urinary tract infections	599.0

4

5. Skills and services identified

- *Hospice nursing*

a. *Comfort and symptom control*

   Complete initial assessment of all systems of patient with Alzheimer's
   admitted to hospice for _____ (specify problem necessitating
   care)

   Presentation of hospice philosophy and services

   Explain patient rights and responsibilities

   Assess patient, family, and caregiver wishes and expectations regarding
   care

   Assess patient, family, and caregiver resources available for care

   Provision of volunteer support to patient and family

   Teach family or caregiver physical care of patient

   Assess pain and other symptoms, including site, duration, characteristics,
   and relief measures

   Skilled assessment of the patient with dementia and support/coping
   skills of family and caregiver

   Skilled observation and assessment of all systems

Teach family and caregivers about disease and management
Comfort measures of backrub and hand or other therapeutic massage
Assess pain or other problems/complaints
Assess pain, and evaluate the pain management's effectiveness
Measure vital signs, including pain, q visit
Assess cardiovascular, pulmonary, and respiratory status
Teach new pain and symptom control medication regimen
Teach caregivers symptom control and relief measures
RN to assess patient's pain or other symptoms q visit to identify need
   for change, addition, or other plan or dose adjustment
RN to provide and teach effective oral care and comfort measures
Identify and monitor pain, symptoms, and relief measures
Teach caregiver or family care of weak, terminally ill patient
RN to instruct in pain control measures and medications
Teach patient and family about realistic expectations of disease process
Teach care of dying and identification of signs/symptoms of impending
   death
Presence and support
Other interventions, based on patient/family needs

b. *Safety and mobility considerations*
   Provide caregiver with home safety information and instruction related
      to _____ and documented in the clinical record
   Teach family regarding importance of observation of patient's safety
   Teach family regarding safety of patient in home
   Teach family regarding energy conservation techniques
   Other interventions, based on patient/family needs

c. *Emotional/Spiritual considerations*
   Psychosocial assessment of patient and family regarding disease and
      prognosis
   Provide emotional support to patient and family
   Spiritual counseling/support offered to patient and caregivers, who are
      verbalizing the reason for or meaning of suffering
   Assess mental status and sleep disturbance changes
   Other interventions, based on patient/family needs

d. *Skin care*
   Observation of skin and patient's physical status
   Teach caregiver regarding skin care needs, including the need for
      frequent position changes, appropriate pressure pads and mattresses,
      and the prevention of breakdown
   Pressure ulcer care as indicated
   Assess skin integrity
   Observation and evaluation of wound and surrounding skin
   Evaluate patient's need for equipment, supplies to decrease pressure,
      alternating pressure mattress, gel foam seat cushion, and heel and
      elbow protectors
   Teach family to perform dressing changes between RN visits, specifically

4

Teach patient, family, or caregiver about proper body alignment and positioning in bed to prevent skin tears from shearing skin

Observe and apply skilled assessment of areas for possible breakdown, including heels, hips, elbows, ankles, and other pressure-prone areas

Other interventions, based on patient/family needs

e. *Elimination considerations*

Assess bowel regimen, and implement program as needed

Implement and monitor bowel regimen, and teach program to family

Observation and evaluation of bladder elimination habits and management of incontinence, and assess need for indwelling catheter

Check for and remove impaction as needed

Condom catheter or indwelling catheter as indicated

Teach catheter care to caregiver

RN to teach caregiver daily catheter care

RN to evaluate the patient's bowel patterns and need for stool softeners, laxatives, and dietary adjustments and develop bowel management plan

Assess amount and frequency of urinary output

Other interventions, based on patient/family needs

f. *Hydration/Nutrition*

Encourage hand-held foods to encourage self-feeding (e.g., sandwiches, cookies)

Monitor hydration and nutrition intake

Assess nutrition and hydration status

Diet counseling for patient with anorexia

Nutrition/hydration supported by offering patient's choice of favorite or desired foods or liquids

Nutrition/hydration to be maintained by offering patient high-protein diet and foods of choice as tolerated

Teach feeding tube care to family

Teach patient and family to expect decreased nutritional and fluid intake as disease progresses

Other interventions, based on patient/family needs

g. *Therapeutic/Medication regimens*

Medication management to monitor antipsychotic behavior and other effects of therapy and/or interactions

RN monitor effects of tranquilizers given for severe agitation/anxiety

Evaluate for weight loss, weigh patient q visit, and record weight

Monitor patient's BP and compliance with medication regimen

RN to assess the patient's unique response to treatments or interventions, and report changes or unfavorable responses or reactions to the physician

Medication assessment and management

Obtain venipuncture and lab results as ordered q _____ (ordered frequency)

Teach patient and family about new medications and effects

Assess for electrolyte imbalance

Nonpharmacological interventions such as progressive muscle relaxation, imagery, positive visualization, music, massage and touch, and humor therapy of patient's choice implemented
Other interventions, based on patient/family needs

h. *Other considerations*
Assist family in setting up patient-centered routine and stress the importance of adhering to the routine once established
Assess progression of disease process
RN to assess the patient's response to treatments and interventions and to report changes, unfavorable responses, and reactions to physician
Other interventions, based on patient/family needs

- *Home health aide or certified nursing assistant*
Effective and safe personal care
Safe ADL assistance and support, ambulation and transfers
Respite care
Observation and reporting
Meal preparation
Homemaker services
Comfort care
Other duties

- *Social worker*
Caregiver role strain necessitating respite/relief measures/support
Psychosocial assessment of patient and family/caregiver, including adjustment to illness and its implications and the need for care
Identification of optimal coping strategies
Financial assessment and counseling regarding food acquisition, ability to prepare, and costs of needed medications
Intervention/support related to terminal illness and loss
Emotional/spiritual support
Facilitate communication among patient, family, and hospice team
Identification of optimal coping strategies
Referral/linkage to community services and resources as indicated
Grief counseling and intervention/support related to illness/loss
Patient/caregiver counseling and support
Identification of illness-related psychiatric condition necessitating care
Funeral and burial planning assistance

4

- *Volunteer(s)*
Support, friendship, companionship, and presence
Errands and transportation
Other services, based on interdisciplinary team recommendations and patient/caregiver needs

- *Spiritual counselor*
Spiritual assessment and care
Counseling, intervention, and support dimension of life related to life's meaning (consistent with patient's beliefs)

Pray with or for the patient/family, using prayers familiar to patient's
religious background (per their wishes)

Support, listening, and presence

Participation in sacred or spiritual rituals or practices

Funeral planning assistance

Other supportive care, based on patient/family needs and belief systems

- *Dietitian/Nutritional counseling*
   Assessment of patient with decreased caloric intake, weight loss,
   anorexia, and nausea

   Assessment and recommendations for swallowing difficulties

   Teaching and support of family members and caregivers

   Support and care with food and nourishment as desired by patient

   Assessment of family's view of benefits/burdens of tube feeding to
   prolong life

- *Occupational therapist*
   Evaluation of ADL and functional mobility

   Assess for need for adaptive equipment and assistive devices

   Safety assessment of patient's environment and ADL

   Assessment for energy conservation training

   Assessment of upper extremity function, retraining motor skills and/or
   splinting for contracture(s)

- *Physical therapy*
   Evaluation

   Safety assessment of patient's environment

   Instruct and supervise caregivers and volunteers on home exercise
   program/ROM and safe transfers

- *Bereavement counselor*
   Assessment of the needs of the bereaved family and friends

   Support and intervention, based on assessment and ongoing findings

   Presence and counseling

   Supportive visits and follow-up, other interventions (e.g., mailings, calls)

   Services related to bereavement work and support

- *Music, massage, art, or other therapies or services*
   Evaluation and intervention based on patient's and caregiver's unique
   wishes and needs that support care, comfort, and death in the setting
   of the patient's choice

   Pet therapy (including patient's pet, if available) and therapeutic
   intervention

   Assessment plan to engage patient and support comfort, quality,
   enjoyment, and dignity

6. Outcomes for care

- *Hospice nursing*
   Patient/caregiver verbalizes satisfaction with care

   Educational tools/plans incorporated in daily care, and patient/caregiver
   verbalizes understanding of safe, needed care

Patient will decide on care, interventions, and evaluation

Caregiver effective in care management and knows whom to call for questions/concerns

Patient will express satisfaction with hospice support received and will experience increased comfort

Patient will be made comfortable at home through death in accordance with the patient's wishes

Effective pain control and symptom control verbalized by patient

Patient verbalizes understanding of and adheres to care and medication regimens

Patient and caregiver supported through patient's death

Comfort maintained through course of care

The patient and family receive hospice support and care, and family members and friends are able to spend quality time with the patient

Caregiver able and verbalizes comfort with role and lists when to call hospice team members

Patient supported through and receives the maximum benefit from palliative chemotherapy and radiation with minimal complications

Patient and caregiver list adverse reactions, potential complications, signs/symptoms of infection (e.g., sputum change, chest congestion)

Comfort maintained through death with dignity

Pain effectively managed, and patient verbalizes comfort

Patient has stable respiratory status with patent airway (e.g., no dyspnea, infection free)

Comfort and individualized intervention of patient with immobility/bedbound status (e.g., skin, urinary, musculature, vascular)

Spiritual and psychosocial needs met (specify) as defined by patient and caregiver throughout course of care

Teaching program related to the prevention of infection and injuries demonstrated by caregivers

Family and caregivers taught and supported regarding the need for a safe, consistent, and nurturing physical environment

Caregivers demonstrate information taught, including the role of reassurance and consistency in activities and schedules

Patient will be comfortable; caregiver reports no or decreased fear, anxiety, and frustration

Patient and caregiver will demonstrate _____ % compliance with instructions related to care

Patient and caregiver demonstrate and practice effective handwashing and other infection control measures (specify, e.g., disposal of waste, cleaning linens)

Adherence to POC by patient and caregivers, and able to demonstrate safe and supportive care

Nutritional needs maintained/addressed as evidenced by patient's weight maintained/increased by _____ lbs

Patient will be maintained in home with caregiver stating/demonstrating adherence to POC

Adherence to medication regimen

Caregiver and family taught to care for patient as demonstrated by observation/interviews

Patient's daily, consistent routine maintained as noted in caregiver log/notes

Family and caregiver integrate information and care regarding implications of disease and terminal nature

Death with dignity and symptoms controlled in setting of patient/family choice

Death with maximum comfort through effective symptom control with specialized hospice support

Symptoms controlled in setting of patient/family choice

Effective pain relief and control (e.g., a peaceful and comfortable death)

Maximizing the patient's quality of life (e.g., patient is alert and pain free)

Pharmacological and nonpharmacological interventions such as localized heat application, positioning, relaxation methods, music and others

Patient cared for and family supported through death with physical, psychosocial, spiritual, and other needs acknowledged/addressed

Patient and family-centered hospice care provided based on the patient/family unique situation and needs

Infection control and palliation through death

Patient states pain is at _____ on 0–10 scale by next visit

- *Home health aide or certified nursing assistant*
  Effective and safe hygiene, personal care, and comfort
  ADL assistance
  Safe environment maintained

- *Social worker*
  Psychosocial support and counseling provided
  Financial/access problems addressed, resources identified as demonstrated by food in the refrigerator and medication availability to patient per POC
  Linkage with community services, support groups, and other resources
  Referral of patient and caregiver to _____ (specify)
  Adjustment to long-term implications of disease as stated in plan for continued care by RN and social worker
  Caregiver able to demonstrate/verbalize effective coping skills
  Resources identified, community linkage as appropriate for patient/family
  Funeral and burial planning assistance

- *Volunteer(s)*
  Patient and caregiver support provided as defined by needs of patient and caregiver
  Support, friendship, companionship, presence
  Comfort and dignity maintained/provided to patient and family

- *Spiritual counselor*
  Intervention and support provided related to that dimension of life related to life's meaning (consistent with patient's beliefs)

Spiritual support offered and provided as defined by needs of patient/caregiver

Provision of spiritual support and care as based on the assessed and ongoing needs of the patient and family

Support, listening, and presence

Spiritual support offered, and patient and family needs met

Participation in sacred or spiritual rituals or practices

Patient/family express a relief of symptoms of spiritual suffering

Other outcomes, based on the patient's/family's unique beliefs and needs

Pray with or for the patient/family, using prayers familiar to the patient's religious background (per their wishes)

- ***Dietitian/Nutritional counseling***

    Family and caregiver integrate recommendations into nutrition teaching (where appropriate)

    Patient and caregiver know whom to call for nutrition- and hydration-related questions/concerns

    Patient and family verbalize comprehension of nutritional needs

- ***Occupational therapist***

    Maximize independence in ADLs for patient/caregiver

    Optimal function maintained/attained

    Patient and caregiver demonstrates ADL program for maximum safety

- ***Physical therapist***

    Safe ambulation, transfers

    Home exercise program supports optimal function/mobility

- ***Bereavement counselor***

    Grief support services provided to patient and family

    Well-being and resolution process of grief initiated and followed through bereavement services

- ***Music, massage, art, or other therapies or services***

    Therapeutic massage/touch effective for patient as self-reported or observed by caregivers/family

    Improved muscle tone, relaxation, and/or sleep

    Patient comfortable and relaxed (e.g., sleeping) after therapy

    Music therapy intervention based on assessment to decrease pain perception, provide emotional expression and support

    Maintenance of comfort, physical, psychosocial, and spiritual health

    Patient has pet's presence as desired—in all care sites, when possible

    Holistic health maintained and comfort achieved through
    _____ (specify modality)

4

7. Patient, family and caregiver educational needs

Educational needs are the care regimens that contribute to safe and effective care at home between the hospice team's visits. These include the following:

   The basic tenets of hospice and the availability of support 24 hours a day, 7 days a week

Home safety assessment and counseling

The patient's medication regimen

Safe and proper body mechanics to promote patient comfort and prevent caregiver safety problems

Other teaching specific to the patient's and family's unique needs

Support groups available to patient's family, such as the hospice program's "Caregiver Support Group" meetings for family members and friends of the patient

Home safety concerns, issues, and teaching

The prevention of infection/skin problems by regularly inspecting patient's skin

Multiple medications and their relationship to each other

The importance of maintaining the patient's daily, consistent routines, when possible

Anticipated disease progression

8. Specific tips for quality and reimbursement

For this and other noncancer diagnoses, document clearly the symptoms and clinical and assessment findings that support the end stage of the chronic illness process

Document patient changes, symptoms, and clinical information identified from visits and team conferences that supports hospice care and limited life expectancy

Clearly support in the documentation the rationale that supports/explains the progression of the illness from the chronic to terminal stages

Document mentation, behavioral, and cognitive changes

Document dysphagia, weight loss, increased shortness of breath, dyspnea, infection, sepsis, and new or changed medications, etc.

Document skin changes (e.g., inflamed, painful, weeping skin site[s])

Document coordination of services and consultation with other members of the IDG

Unless the patient is in a hospice insurance program, some insurers will not pay for a skilled nurse visit that is made at death if the patient is dead when the nurse arrives at the home. From a Medicare home care perspective, the visit at the time of death may be covered when the orders and clinical record document assessment of the patient's status and signs of death/life or state law allows, pronouncement of death by an RN.

Document any variances to expected outcomes. Many models of hospice programs exist.

The Medicare hospice benefit does not require that the patient be homebound or have identified skilled needs. For further information on this benefit, please refer to CMS Hospice Manual 21.

Should the patient's status deteriorate and increased personal care be needed, obtain a telephone order for the increased service, noting frequency and estimating the duration.

Obtain a telephone order for all medication and treatment changes of the medical regimen and document these in the clinical record.

Document patient deterioration

Document dehydration, dehydrating
Document patient change or instability
Document pain, other symptoms not controlled
Document status after acute episode of _____ (specify)
Document positive urine, sputum, etc. culture; patient started
on _____ (specify ordered antibiotic therapy)
Document patient impacted; impaction removed manually
Document RN in frequent communication with physician regarding
_____ (specify)
Document febrile at _____, pulse change at _____, irr., irr.
Document change noted in _____
Document bony prominences red, opening
Document RN contacted physician regarding _____ (specify)
Document marked SOB
Document alteration in mental status
Document medications being adjusted, "perform", or monitored
Document unable to perform ADLs, personal care
Document all interdisciplinary team meetings and communications in
the POC and in the progress notes of the clinical record
All team members should have input into the POC and document their
interventions and goals

9. **Queries for quality**

   Alzheimer's disease and care for other dementias
   • *Is the patient's pain managed adequately?*
   • *Is the patient's anxiety managed adequately?*
   • *Is the patient's functional ability/status clearly documented?*
   • *Have you documented to the interdisciplinary POC?*
   • *What are the patient's symptoms?*

   Dementia care
   • *Is the patient's pain managed adequately?*
   • *Is the patient's anxiety managed adequately?*
   • *Is the patient's functional ability/status clearly documented?*
   • *Have you documented to the interdisciplinary POC?*
   • *What are the patient's symptoms?*

   Organic brain syndrome care
   • *Is the patient's pain managed adequately?*
   • *Is the patient's anxiety managed adequately?*
   • *Is the patient's functional ability/status clearly documented?*
   • *Have you documented to the interdisciplinary POC?*
   • *What are the patient's symptoms?*

4

10. **Resources for hospice care and practice**
    The book *The 36 Hour Day,* by Nancy L. Mace and Peter V. Rabins,
    MD, addresses all aspects of the difficulties encountered by families
    and friends as they care for their loved ones with Alzheimer's disease or
    other dementias. Call 1-800-537-5487.

In addition, the National Institute of Health, National Institute on Aging, has an Alzheimer's Disease Education and Referral Center. This center has information such as home safety booklets available to both professionals and families caring for patients with dementias. Its number is 1-800-438-4380.

Another helpful resource is the NHPCO's latest edition of *Medical Guidelines for Determining Prognoses in Selected Non-Cancer Diseases.* Call the NHPCO at 800-646-6460 for more information.

The American Hospice Foundation offers a pamphlet entitled Alzheimer's Disease and Hospice that can be obtained by calling (202) 223-0204 or writing to American Hospice Foundation, 1130 Connecticut Avenue NW, Suite 700, Washington, DC 20036-4101.

The Alzheimer's Association has created fact sheets entitled "Ethical Considerations" to assist with ethical questions that may occur when caring for patients with Alzheimer's disease. "Issues in Death and Dying" and "Issues of Diagnostic Disclosure" are available free by calling 1-800-272-3900.

4

AMYOTROPHIC LATERAL SCLEROSIS (ALS) AND OTHER NEUROMUSCULAR CARE

1. General considerations

Amyotrophic lateral sclerosis (ALS) is usually known as *Lou Gehrig's disease*. This rare neurological disease occurs usually between 40 and 70 years of age and affects twice as many men as women. Unfortunately, the prognosis is poor with this disease, with patients progressively degenerating toward respiratory failure.

2. Needs for visit

Physician order for hospice care, specific to the hospice program's admission criteria and policies
Standard precautions supplies
Vital signs equipment for baseline assessment
Other supplies or equipment based on physician orders

3. Safety considerations

Infection control/standard precautions
Night-light
Removal of scatter rugs
Tub rail, grab bars for bathroom safety
Oxygen precautions (if ordered)
Supportive and nonskid shoes
Handrail on stairs
Fall precautions
Identification and reporting of any skin problems
Smoke detector and fire evacuation plan
Assistance with ambulation
Others, based on the patient's unique condition and environment

4. Potential diagnoses and codes

Amyotrophic lateral sclerosis	335.20
Dysarthria	784.5
Dysphagia	787.2
Failure to thrive, adult	783.7
Joint contracture	718.40
Muscular dystrophy	359.1
Multiple sclerosis	340
Parkinson's disease	332.0
Seizure disorder	780.39

5. Skills and services identified

- *Hospice nursing*

a. *Comfort and symptom control*
   Complete initial assessment of all systems of patient with ALS admitted hospice for _____ (specify problem necessitating care)

4

Presentation of hospice philosophy and services

Explain patient rights and responsibilities

Assess patient, family, and caregiver wishes and expectations regarding care

Assess patient, family, and caregiver resources available for care

Provision of volunteer support to patient and family

Teach family or caregiver physical care of patient

Assess pain and other symptoms, including site, duration, characteristics, and relief measures

RN to provide and teach effective oral care and comfort measures

RN to assess and observe all systems and symptoms q visit and report changes, new symptoms to physician

Care coordination, teaching related to mechanical/respiratory support devices, ventilator, suction, etc.

Observation with assessment of pain and other symptoms to be managed within parameters of disease process

Comfort measures provided to patient who is essentially bedbound and alert, including backrub, hand massage, and music of choice

Teach family and caregiver signs, changes to report to nurse and physician

Assess pain, and evaluate the pain management's effectiveness

Teach care of the bedridden patient

Measure vital signs, including pain, q visit

Assess cardiovascular, pulmonary, and respiratory status

Teach caregivers symptom control and relief measures

Teach caregiver or family care of weak, terminally ill patient

RN to assess patient's pain or other symptoms q visit to identify need for change, addition, or other plan or dose adjustment

Oxygen at _____ liters per _____ (specific physician orders)

RN to instruct in pain control measures and medications

Teach patient and family about realistic expectations of disease process

Teach care of dying, signs/symptoms of impending death

Presence and support

Other interventions, based on patient/family needs

b. *Safety and mobility considerations*

Provide patient with home safety information and instruction related to _____ and documented in the clinical record

Rehabilitation management related to safe bed mobility and transfers

Teach family regarding safety of patient in home

Teach patient and family regarding energy conservation techniques

Teach caregiver to observe for increased secretions, and teach safe suctioning when needed

Other interventions, based on patient/family needs

c. *Emotional/Spiritual considerations*

Psychosocial assessment of patient and family regarding disease and prognosis

Provide emotional support to patient and family

Spiritual counseling/support offered to patients and caregivers who are verbalizing the reason for or meaning of suffering

Patient and family assisted through grieving process

Other interventions, based on patient/family needs

d. *Skin care*

Teaching and training of family and caregivers about skin care, positioning, and feeding regimens

Observation and evaluation of wound and surrounding skin

Assess skin and pressure-prone areas

Evaluate patient's need for equipment, supplies to decrease pressure, alternating pressure mattress, gel foam seat cushion, and heel and elbow protectors

Teach family to perform dressing changes between RN visits, specifically _____

Teach patient and family or caregiver about proper body alignment and positioning in bed to prevent skin tears from shearing skin

Observe and apply skilled assessment of areas for possible breakdown, including heels, hips, elbows, ankles, and other pressure-prone areas

Teach caregiver about skin care needs, including the need for frequent position changes, pressure pads, appropriate mattresses, and the prevention of breakdown

Other interventions, based on patient/family needs

e. *Elimination considerations*

Assess bowel regimen, and implement program as needed

RN to change catheter every 4 weeks and 3 pm visits for catheter problems, including patient complaints, signs and symptoms of infection, and other factors necessitating evaluation and possible catheter change

Observation and complete systems assessment of the patient with an indwelling catheter

RN to monitor bowel and bladder function

Check for and remove impaction as needed

Condom catheter or indwelling catheter as indicated

RN to teach caregiver daily catheter care

RN to evaluate the patient's bowel patterns, need for stool softeners, laxatives, and dietary adjustments and develop bowel management plan

Other interventions, based on patient/family needs

f. *Hydration/Nutrition*

Monitor patient who has nutritional supplements and water via nasogastric/gastric (NG/G) tube daily

Assess nutrition and hydration status

Diet counseling for patient with anorexia

Nutrition/hydration provided by offering patient's choice of favorite or desired foods or liquids

Nutrition/hydration to be maintained by offering patient high-protein diet and foods of choice as tolerated

Teach feeding-tube care to family

Teach patient and family to expect decreased nutritional and fluid
  intake as disease progresses

Other interventions, based on patient/family needs

g. *Therapeutic/Medication regimens*

Medication management of patient receiving morphine, antibiotic,
  muscle relaxant, and prednisone via NG/G tube

RN to assess the patient's unique response to treatments or interventions, and report changes or unfavorable responses or reactions to
  the physician

Teach new pain- and symptom-control medication regimen

Nonpharmacological interventions such as progressive muscle relaxation, imagery, positive visualization, music, massage and touch, and
  humor therapy of patient's choice implemented

Medication assessment and management

Other interventions, based on patient/family needs

h. *Other considerations*

Assess disease progression process

Comfort/safety through ongoing assessment related to swallowing and
  other changes

RN to assess the patient's response to treatments and interventions and to
  report to physician any changes, unfavorable responses, or reactions

Other interventions, based on patient/family needs

• **Home health aide or certified nursing assistant**

Effective and safe personal care

Safe ADL assistance and support

Observation and reporting

Respite care

Meal preparation

Homemaker services

Comfort care

Other duties

• **Social worker**

Psychosocial assessment of patient and family/caregiver, including
  adjustment to illness and its implications and the need for care

Identification of optimal coping strategies

Financial assessment and counseling regarding food acquisition, ability
  to prepare, and costs of needed medications

Intervention/support related to terminal illness and loss

Emotional/spiritual support

Depression/fear assessed and addressed

Facilitate communication among patient, family, and hospice team

Identification of caregiver role strain necessitating respite/relief
  measures and support

Referral/linkage to community services and resources as indicated

Grief counseling and intervention/support related to illness/loss

Assessment/intervention related to depression and fear
Patient/caregiver counseling and support
For patients who live alone with no support system (e.g., able, available, willing caregiver[s]), obtain linkage with community resources to allow patient to remain in the home
Identification of illness-related psychiatric condition necessitating care
Funeral and burial planning assistance

- *Volunteer(s)*
  Support, friendship, companionship, and presence
  Comfort and dignity maintained/provided for patient and family
  Errands and transportation
  Other services, based on interdisciplinary team recommendations and patient/caregiver needs

- *Spiritual counselor*
  Spiritual assessment and care
  Counseling, intervention, and support related to that dimension of life related to life's meaning (consistent with patient's beliefs)
  Support, listening, and presence
  Participation in sacred or spiritual rituals or practices
  Funeral planning assistance
  Other supportive case, based on patient/family needs and belief systems
  Pray with or for the patient/family, using prayers familiar to the patient's religious background (per their wishes)

- *Dietitian/Nutritional counseling*
  Assessment of patient with decreased intake, weight loss, anorexia, and nausea
  Assessment and recommendations for swallowing difficulties
  Teaching and support of family members and caregivers
  Support and care with soft foods and nourishment as desired by patient
  Evaluation of patient on G-tube or NG tube feedings and teach feeding safety techniques
  Monitoring and management of patient
  Teach caregiver regarding aspects of nutritional support system
  Evaluation/management of nutritional and fluid deficits and needs
  Encourage nutritional supplements and snacks to increase protein and caloric intake, as appropriate
  Food, dietary recommendations incorporating patient choice and wishes
  Care coordination with care team to decrease tube feeding near time of death to avoid choking, increased fluids, etc.

- *Occupational therapist*
  Evaluation of ADL and functional mobility
  Assess for need for adaptive equipment and assistive devices
  Safety assessment of patient's environment and ADL
  Assessment for energy conservation training
  Assessment of upper extremity function, retraining motor skills

4

- *Physical therapist*
  Evaluation
  Assessment of motor strength, presence of flaccidity or spasticity, contractures
  Safety assessment of patient and patient's environment
  Safe transfer training
  Strengthening exercises/program
  Assessment of gait safety
  Instruct/supervise caregiver and volunteers with regard to home exercise program for conditioning and strength
  Assistive, adaptive devices of equipment and teaching
  Assessment of upper body strength for trapeze or other methods to maintain function/bed mobility

- *Speech-language pathologist*
  Evaluation for speech/swallowing problems
  Teach communication techniques

- *Bereavement counselor*
  Assessment of the needs of the bereaved family and friends
  Support and intervention, based on assessment and ongoing findings
  Presence and counseling
  Supportive visits and follow-up and other interventions (e.g., mailings, calls)
  Services related to bereavement work and support

- *Music, massage, art, or other therapies or services*
  Evaluation and intervention based on patient's/caregiver's unique wishes and needs that support care and death in the setting of the patient's choice
  Therapeutic massage/touch effective for patient as self-reported or observed by caregivers/family
  Improved muscle tone, relaxation, and/or sleep
  Patient comfortable and relaxed (e.g., sleeping) after therapy
  Music therapy intervention based on assessment to decrease pain perception, provide emotional expression and support
  Pet therapy (including patient's pet, if available) and therapeutic intervention
  Assessment plan to engage patient and support comfort, quality, enjoyment, and dignity
  Maintenance of comfort and physical, psychosocial, and spiritual health
  Holistic health maintained and comfort achieved through _____ (specify modality)

6. Outcomes for care

- *Hospice nursing*
  Patient will be comfortable and pain free through illness and death, and interdisciplinary team members will work together to improve/maintain patient's quality of life

Patient/caregiver verbalizes satisfaction with care

Educational tools/plans incorporated in daily care, and patient/caregiver verbalizes understanding of safe, needed care

Patient will decide on care, interventions, and evaluation

Caregiver effective in care management and knows whom to call for questions/concerns

Patient will express satisfaction with hospice support received and will experience increased comfort

Patient will be made comfortable at home through death in accordance with the patient's wishes

Effective pain control and symptom control indicated by patient

Patient indicates understanding of and adheres to care and medication regimens

Patient and caregiver supported through patient's death

Comfort maintained through course of care

The patient and family receive hospice support and care, and family members and friends are able to spend quality time with the patient

Caregiver able and verbalizes comfort with role and lists when to call hospice team members

Patient or caregiver lists adverse reactions, potential complications, signs/symptoms of infection (e.g., sputum change, chest congestion)

Comfort maintained through death with dignity

Pain effectively managed, and patient verbalizes comfort

Patient has stable respiratory status with patent airway

Patient protected from injury, stable respiratory status, and compliant with medication, safety, and care regimens

Comfort and individualized intervention of patient with immobility/bedbound status (e.g., skin, urinary, musculature, vascular)

Spiritual and psychosocial needs met (specify) as defined by patient and caregiver throughout course of care

Patient states pain is at _____ on 0–10 scale by next visit

Death with dignity, and symptoms controlled in setting of patient/family choice

Death with maximum comfort through effective symptom control with specialized hospice support

Symptoms controlled in setting of patient/family choice

Effective pain relief and control (e.g., a peaceful and comfortable death)

Maximizing the patient's quality of life (e.g., patient is alert and pain free)

Pharmacological and nonpharmacological interventions such as localized heat application, positioning, relaxation methods, music, and others

Patient cared for, and family supported through death with physical, psychosocial, spiritual, and other needs acknowledged/addressed

Patient- and family-centered hospice care provided based on the patient's/family's unique situation and needs

Infection control and palliation through death

4

- *Home health aide or certified nursing assistant*
  Effective hygiene, personal care, and comfort
  ADL assistance
  Safe environment maintained

- *Social worker*
  Psychosocial assessment and counseling of patient and family,
    including adjustment to illness and its implications
  Emotional support
  Facilitate communication among patient, family, and staff
  Referrals to resources as indicated
  Grief counseling
  Patient/caregiver able to cope adaptively with illness and death
  Identification and addressing/resolution of problems impeding the
    successful implementation of the POC
  Adaptive adjustment to changed body and body image
  Psychosocial support and counseling offered/initiated to patient and
    caregivers experiencing grieving process
  Resources identified, community linkage as appropriate for patient/family
  Funeral and burial planning assistance

- *Volunteer(s)*
  Comfort, companionship, and friendship extended to patient/family
  Support provided as defined by the needs of the patient/caregiver
  Respite support

- *Spiritual counselor*
  Spiritual support offered and provided as defined by needs of
    patient/caregiver
  Provision of spiritual support and care as based on the assessed and
    ongoing needs of the patient and family
  Spiritual support offered and patient and family needs met
  Patient/caregiver express a relief of symptoms of spiritual suffering
  Intervention and support provided related to that dimension of life
    related to life's meaning (consistent with patient's beliefs)
  Participation in sacred or spiritual rituals or practices
  Support, listening, and presence
  Other outcomes, based on the patient's/family's unique beliefs and needs
  Pray with or for the patient/family, using prayers familiar to the
    patient's religious background (per their wishes)

- *Dietitian/Nutritional counseling*
  Family and caregiver integrating recommendations into nutrition
    teaching (where appropriate)
  Patient and caregiver know whom to call for nutrition- and
    hydration-related questions/concerns
  G-tube or NG tube is patent, and patient is receiving safe and
    maximum nutrition as ordered; no side effects reported by patient,
    caregiver, or clinician
  Patient and family verbalize comprehension of changing nutritional needs

- *Occupational therapist*
    Patient and caregiver demonstrate maximum functioning with ADLs
        adaptive techniques, and assistive devices
    Patient and caregiver demonstrate maximum safety in ADLs and
        functional mobility
    Patient and caregiver demonstrate effective use of energy conservation
        techniques
    Verbalization/demonstration of improved functional activity level and
        enhanced quality of life
    Patient and caregiver demonstrate effective use of diaphragmatic
        breathing to reduce shortness of breath and relaxation techniques to
        help in pain/symptom management
    Maximize independence in ADLs for patient and caregiver
    Optimal function maintained or attained
    Patient and caregiver demonstrate ADL program for maximum safety

- *Physical therapist*
    Maintenance of balance, mobility, and endurance as verbalized and
        demonstrated by patient
    Prevention of complications
    Safety in mobility and transfers

- *Speech-language pathologist*
    Safe swallowing and functional communication

- *Bereavement counselor*
    Grief support services provided to patient and family
    Well-being and resolution process of grief initiated and followed
        through bereavement services

- *Music, massage, art, or other therapies or services*
    Therapeutic massage/touch effective for patient as self-reported or
        observed by caregivers/family
    Improved muscle tone, relaxation, and/or sleep
    Patient comfortable and relaxed (e.g., sleeping) after massage
    Music therapy intervention based on assessment to decrease pain
        perception, provide emotional expression and support
    Maintenance of comfort and physical, psychosocial, and spiritual health
    Holistic health maintained, and comfort achieved through
        _____ (specify modality)
    Patient has pet's presence as desired—in all care sites, when possible

7. **Patient, family, and caregiver educational needs**
    Educational needs are the care regimens that contribute to safe and effec-
    tive care at home between the hospice team's visits. These include the
    following:
        The basic tenets of hospice and the availability of support 24 hours a
            day, 7 days a week
        Home safety assessment and counseling
        The patient's medication regimen

Safe and proper body mechanics to promote patient comfort and
prevent caregiver safety problems

Other teaching specific to the patient's and family's unique needs

Support groups available to patient's family, such as the hospice
program's "Caregiver Support Group" meetings for family members and friends of the patient

Anticipated disease progression

8. Specific tips for quality and reimbursement

Document any variances to expected outcomes. There are many models
of hospice programs.

The Medicare hospice benefit does not require that the patient be
homebound or have identified skilled needs. For further information on
this benefit, please refer to CMS Hospice Manual 21.

Should the patient's status deteriorate and increased personal care
be needed, obtain a telephone order for the increased service, noting
frequency and estimating the duration.

Obtain a telephone order for all medication and treatment changes of
the medical regimen, and document these in the clinical record.

Unless the patient is in a hospice insurance program, some insurers
will not pay for a skilled clinician visit that is made at death if the patient
is dead when the nurse arrives at the home. From a Medicare home
hospice care perspective, the visit at the time of death may be covered
when the orders and clinical record document assessment of the patient's
status or signs of death/life or state law allows pronouncement of death
by an RN.

Document patient deterioration

Document dehydration, dehydrating

Document patient change or instability

Document pain, other symptoms not controlled

Document status after acute episode of _____ (specify)

Document positive urine, sputum, etc. culture; patient started
on _____ (specify ordered antibiotic therapy)

Document patient impacted; impaction removed manually

Document RN in frequent communication with physician regarding
_____ (specify)

Document febrile at _____, pulse change at _____, irr., irr.

Document change noted in _____

Document bony prominences red, opening

Document RN contacted physician regarding _____ (specify)

Document marked SOB

Document alteration in mental status

Document medications being adjusted, regulated, or monitored

Document unable to perform own ADLs, personal care

Document all interdisciplinary team meetings and communications in
the POC and in the progress notes of the clinical record

All disciplines involved should have input into the POC and document
their interventions and goals

Document need for G-tube feeding, inability to swallow without choking, or history of aspiration

Document coordination of services and consultation with other members of the IDG

Remember that the clinical documentation is key to measuring compliance for quality and reimbursement purposes. Care coordination, timely verbal and initial physician orders, and assessment and addressing of spiritual and psychosocial needs should be ongoing and documented in the patient's clinical record

The documentation should support that all hospice care supports comfort and dignity while meeting patient/family needs

The documentation should include ongoing assessment and management of pain and other symptoms and the anticipation and prevention of secondary symptoms such as constipation

It is important to note that all team members, including clinicians and social workers, should assess, identify, and "hear" spiritual needs that the patient and family want to be addressed. These spiritual issues are key to the provision of quality hospice care and cannot be addressed effectively and promptly by the spiritual counselor only

Document clearly symptoms, clinical changes, and assessment findings related to pain and patient care

Document weight loss, increased shortness of breath, dyspnea, infection, sepsis, new or changed medications, etc.

Document any skin changes (e.g., inflamed, painful, weeping skin site[s])

Remember that the "litmus test" of care coordination rests on the quality of the clinical documentation by all team members. Review one of your patient's clinical records and ask yourself the following: "If I was unable to give a verbal report/update on this patient's/family's course of care, would a peer be able to pick up and provide the same level of care and know (from the documentation) the current orders, medications, and other details that contribute to effective hospice care?"

This patient population usually has many clinical changes that should be documented. These include weight loss, frequent upper respiratory infections (URIs), and multiple and changed medication regimens with varying routes. Side effects to the drug regimen should be observed, noted, documented, and reported

Your assessments, observations, and clinical findings assist in painting a picture to support coverage, accreditation, and documentation requirements for hospice care

Document any hospitalizations and changed clinical findings

Document patient changes, symptoms, and psychosocial issues impacting the patient and family and plan of care

Document coordination of care with other care providers, such as skilled healthcare facility, nursing home, and hired caregiver

4

9. Queries for quality

- *Is patient's pain managed adequately?*
- *Is patient's anxiety managed adequately?*
- *Is the patient's functional ability/status clearly documented?*
- *Have you documented to the interdisciplinary POC?*
- *What are the patient's symptoms?*

10. Resources for hospice care and practice

The Amyotrophic Lateral Sclerosis (ALS) Association offers resources for patients, families, and health care professionals. They have local chapters throughout the United States and offer support groups. All the services provided to patients and family are provided at no cost. The phone number for the ALS association is 1-800-782-4747.

The Muscular Dystrophy Association has a comprehensive guide available for caregivers of people affected by ALS, *When a Loved One Has ALS: A Caregiver's Guide* is a 94-page, illustrated manual filled with practical advice for meeting the medical, emotional, financial, and everyday challenges faced by those who are primary caregivers for family members or others with ALS. *When a Loved One Has ALS* can be ordered through your local MDA office, listed in the phone directory. If you have difficulty locating the office nearest you, call MDA national headquarters at 1-800-572-1717, or visit MDA's Web site, www.mdausa.org.

4

BEDBOUND CARE

1. **General considerations**

   Many hospice patients spend their last days in bed, depending on their diagnosis and health history. Though bedbound status is not a diagnosis, it is an important factor that affects all body systems and results in many teaching and guidance implications for family members and other caregivers.

   With more patients choosing to be cared for at home, the number of patients who are essentially bedridden continues to increase. While being bedridden is not a diagnosis, it is an important factor with implications for all body systems. Caregivers and family members are the key to these patients being cared for safely and effectively in their own home setting.

   Please refer to "Acquired Immuned Deficiency Syndrome (AIDS) Care," "Cancer Care," and "Cardiac Care (End Stage)," or another specific patient problem for a more in-depth discussion of these possible patient care needs.

2. **Needs for visit**

   Physician order for hospice care, specific to the hospice program's admission criteria and policies
   Standard precautions supplies
   Vital signs equipment for baseline assessment
   Other supplies or equipment, based on physician orders

3. **Safety considerations**

   Infection control/standard precautions
   Side rail use and position
   Supervised medication administration
   Wheelchair/fall precautions
   Prevention of injury related to proper positioning
   The need for meticulous skin care and observation
   Disposal of soiled dressings
   Multiple medications (e.g., side effects, interactions, safe storage)
   Night-light
   Safety for home medical equipment (e.g., bed, lift)
   Symptoms that necessitate immediate reporting/assistance
   Smoke detector and fire evacuation plan
   Extra caution on slippery surfaces
   Removal of scatter rugs
   Tub rail, grab bars for bathroom safety
   Supportive and nonskid shoes
   Handrail on stairs
   Fall precautions
   Protective skin measures
   Identify and report any skin problems

4

Assistance with ambulation
Others, based on the patient's unique condition and environment

4. Potential diagnoses and codes

Acute myocardial infarction	410.90
Adenocarcinoma, metastatic	199.1
Adrenal cancer	194.0
AIDS	042
ALS	335.20
Alzheimer's	331.0
Anorexia	783.0
Aphasia	784.3
Ascites, malignant	197.6
Bladder atony	596.4
Bladder cancer	188.9
Bone metastates	198.5
Brain, cancer of	198.3
Brain tumor	239.6
Breast cancer	174.9
Cancer of the head or neck	195.0
Cardiomyopathy	425.4
Cerebral vascular accident	436
Cervix, cancer of the	180.9
Cirrhosis of the liver	571.5
CHF	428.0
Colon, cancer	153.9
Colon lymphoma	202.83
Colostomy, attention to	V55.3
Constipation	564.00
COPD	496
Cor pulmonale	416.9
Coronary artery disease (CAD)	414.00
CVA	436
Decubitus (pressure) ulcer	707.0
Dehydration	276.5
Depression	311
Diabetes mellitus (NIDDM)	250.00
Diabetes mellitus (IDDM)	250.01
Dysphagia due to CVA	438.82
Esophagus, cancer of the	150.9
Failure to Thrive, adult	783.7
Fracture, pathological	733.10
Gastric cancer, metastatic	197.8
Gastric leiomyosarcoma with metastasis	151.9 and 199.1
Gastrostomy, attention to	V55.1
Heart disease, end stage	429.9
Heart failure	428.9
Hemiplegia	342.90

Huntington's disease	333.4
Hyperalimentation (procedure)	99.15
Hypertension	401.9
Ileostomy, attention to	V55.2
Ileus	560.1
Impaction, fecal	560.39
Incontinence of feces	787.6
Incontinence of urine	788.30
Kaposi's sarcoma	176.9
Kaposi's sarcoma with AIDS	042 and 176.9
Kidney, cancer of the (renal)	189.0
Laryngectomy (procedure)	30.4
Larynx, cancer of the	161.9
Leukemia, acute	208.00
Leukopenia	288.0
Liver, end-stage disease	571.8
Lou Gehrig's disease (ALS)	335.20
Lung cancer squamous cell	162.9
Lupus, systemic	710.0
Lymphoma with bone metastases	202.80 and 198.5
Mastectomy, radical	85.45
Mastectomy, simple	85.41
Metastases, general	199.1
Multiple myeloma	203.00
Multiple sclerosis	340
Myocardial infarction	410.90
Nasopharyngeal cancer	147.9
Oropharyngeal cancer	146.9
Osteoporosis	733.00
Ovarian cancer	183.0
Pain, low back	724.2
Pancreas, cancer of the	157.9
Paralysis	344.9
Paraplegia	344.1
Parkinson's disease	332.0
Pathological fracture	733.10
Peripheral vascular disease	443.9
Pharynx, cancer of the	149.0
Pleural effusion	511.9
Pneumocystis carinii	136.3
Pneumonia	486
Pneumonia, aspiration	507.0
Pressure (decubitus) ulcer	707.0
Prostate, cancer of	185
Protein-caloric malnutrition	263.9
Pulmonary edema	514
Pulmonary edema with cardiac disease	428.1
Pulmonary fibrosis	515

4

Quadriplegia	344.00
Radiation enteritis	558.1
Radiation myelitis	323.8 and E879.2
Rectosigmoid, cancer of	154.0
Rectum, cancer of the	154.1
Renal cell cancer, metastatic	198.0
Renal failure, chronic	585
Respirator, dependence on	V46.1
Respiratory failure, acute	518.81
Respiratory insufficiency (acute)	518.82
Seizure disorder	780.39
Septicemia	038.9
Skin cancer	173.9
Spinal cord tumor	239.7
Squamous cell carcinoma	199.1
Stomach, cancer of the	151.9
TIAs	435.9
Tongue, cancer of the	141.9
TPN (procedure)	99.15
Trachea, cancer of	162.0
Tracheostomy, attention to	V55.0
Urinary incontinence	788.30
Urinary retention	788.20
Urinary tract infection	599.0
Uterine sarcoma, metastatic	198.82
Uterus, cancer of the	179.

5. Skills and services identified

- ***Hospice nursing***

a. *Comfort and symptom control*

Complete initial assessment of all systems of patient who is bedbound admitted to hospice for _____ (specify problem)

Presentation of hospice philosophy and services

Explain patient rights and responsibilities

Assess patient, family, and caregiver wishes and expectations regarding care

Assess patient, family, and caregiver resources available for care

Provision of volunteer support to patient and family

Teach family or caregiver physical care of patient

Assess pain and other symptoms, including site, duration, characteristics, and relief measures

Teach caregiver aspects of care and management

Comprehensive assessment and observation of cardiovascular and other systems in bedridden patient with _____

RN to instruct on all aspects of care of the immobilized patient

Observation and assessment of blood pressure and other vital signs

Comfort measures provided to patient for pain and other symptom relief, including backrub, hand massage, and soothing music of patient's choice, when possible

Assess pain, and evaluate the pain management's effectiveness

Measure vital signs, including pain, q visit

Assess cardiovascular, pulmonary, and respiratory status

Teach caregivers symptom control and relief measures

Oxygen on at _____ liter per _____ (specify according to physicianorders)

RN to provide and teach effective oral care and comfort measures

Identify and monitor pain, symptoms, and relief measures

Teach caregiver or family care of weak, terminally ill patient

RN to instruct in pain control measures and medications

RN to assess patient's pain or other symptoms q visit to identify need for change, addition, or other plan or dose adjustment

RN to observe and assess patient for signs, symptoms of infection

Antiembolus hose applied and application method taught to caregiver

Teach patient and family about realistic expectations of disease process

Teach care of dying, signs/symptoms of impending death

Presence and support

Other interventions, based on patient/family needs

b. *Safety and mobility considerations*

Teach safe PO intake (especially liquids)

Monitor for choking/aspiration if PO intake possible

Provide caregiver with home safety information and instruction related to _____ and documented in the clinical record

Teach caregiver effective and safe suctioning of patient

Teach family regarding safety of patient in home

Teach family regarding energy conservation techniques

Safety related to safe bed mobility and transfers

Other interventions, based on patient/family needs

c. *Emotional/Spiritual considerations*

Psychosocial assessment of patient and family regarding disease and prognosis

RN to provide emotional support to patient and family with _____, an illness of a terminal nature

Assess mental status and sleep disturbance changes

Spiritual counseling/support offered to patients and caregiver who are verbalizing to clinician and aide team members the reason or meaning of suffering

Provide support to patient and family-member caregivers

Other interventions, based on patient/family needs

d. *Skin care*

Teach proper positioning and techniques for turning

Teach caregiver effective use of turn/pull sheet to avoid friction, skin tears, and burns

4

RN to change dressing at wound site using aseptic technique of
_____ (define ordered care)

Observation of the wound site and healing

Teach family and caregiver proper, safe wound care and signs and
symptoms of infection to watch for and report to RN or physician

Teach caregiver importance of and all aspects of effective skin care
regimens to prevent (further) breakdown. Include the need for
position changes every 1 to 2 hours, pressure pads or mattresses,
and other measures for prevention

RN to culture wound and urine for C and S and send to lab

RN enterostomal therapist to visit patient and evaluate wound for
specific care needs

Pressure ulcer care as indicated

Assess skin integrity

Evaluate patient's need for equipment and supplies to decrease
pressure, including alternating pressure mattress, gel foam seat
cushion, and heel and elbow protectors

Observation and evaluation of wound and surrounding skin

Teach family to perform dressing changes between RN visits, specifically

Teach family or caregiver about proper body alignment and positioning
in bed to prevent skin tears from shearing skin

Instruct patient and family regarding safety and standard precautions

Teach patient/caregiver all aspects of wound care, including safe
disposal of soiled supplies

Observe and apply skilled assessment of areas for possible breakdown,
including heels, hips, elbows, ankles, and other pressure-prone areas

Teaching and training of family caregivers about skin care, positioning,
and feeding regimens

Teach caregiver regarding skin care needs, including the need for
frequent position changes, appropriate pressure pads and mattresses,
and the prevention of breakdown

Other interventions, based on patient/family needs

e. *Elimination considerations*

Assess bowel regimen, and implement program as needed

Monitor bowel patterns, including frequency of bowel movements, and
evaluate bowel regimen (e.g., stool softeners, laxatives, and dietary
changes)

Check for and remove impaction per physician orders

RN to implement bladder training program

Teach caregiver daily catheter care and equipment care and signs and
symptoms that necessitate calling the RN/physician

RN to change catheter (specify type, size, and frequency)

Condom catheter or indwelling catheter as indicated

Assess amount and frequency of urinary output

RN to evaluate the patient's bowel patterns, need for stool softeners,
laxatives, and dietary adjustments and develop bowel management plan

Other interventions, based on patient/family needs

f. *Hydration/Nutrition*
Monitor hydration/nutrition status
Assess nutrition/hydration statuses
Diet counseling for patient with anorexia
Teach feeding-tube care to family
Nutrition/hydration supported by offering patient's choice of favorite or desired foods or liquids
Nutrition/hydration to be maintained by offering patient high-protein diet and foods of choice as tolerated
Teach patient and family to expect decreased nutritional and fluid intake as disease progresses
Other interventions, based on patient/family needs

g. *Therapeutic/Medication regimens*
RN to instruct on all medications, including schedule, functions of specific drugs and their side effects
RN to monitor and assess for complications of new medication regimen
Medication management related to drug/drug, drug/food side effects
RN to monitor patient's response to medications for pain and other symptom control
RN to assess the patient's unique response to treatments or interventions, and report changes or unfavorable responses or reactions to the physician
Medication assessment and management
Teach new pain and symptom control medication regimen
Teach new medication and effects
Obtain venipuncture as ordered q _____ (ordered frequency)
Teach patient and caregiver use of PCA pump
Assess for electrolyte imbalance
Nonpharmacological interventions such as progressive muscle relaxation, imagery, positive visualization, music, massage and touch, and humor therapy of patient's choice implemented
Other interventions, based on patient/family needs

4

h. *Other considerations*
Teach proper positioning and techniques for turning
Teach caregiver effective use of turn/pull sheet to prevent friction, skin tears, or burns
Assess disease progression process
RN to assess the patient's response to treatments and interventions and to report to the physician any changes, unfavorable responses, or reactions.
Other interventions, based on patient/family needs

• ***Home health aide or certified nursing assistant***
Effective and safe personal care
Safe ADL assistance and support, ambulation and transfers
Respite care
Observation and reporting

Meal preparation
Homemaker services
Comfort care
Other duties

- **Social worker**
  Psychosocial assessment of patient and family/caregiver, including
      adjustment to illness and its implications
  Financial assessment and counseling regarding food acquisition, ability
      to prepare, and costs of needed medications
  Intervention/support related to terminal illness and loss
  Emotional/spiritual support
  Depression/fear assessed and addressed
  Facilitate communication among patient, family, and hospice team
  Identification of optimal coping strategies
  Referral/linkage to community services and resources as indicated
  Grief counseling and intervention/support related to illness/loss
  Patient/caregiver counseling and support
  For patients who live alone with no support system (e.g., able,
      available, willing caregiver[s]): obtain linkage to necessary
      community resources to allow patient to remain in the home
  Illness-related psychiatric condition necessitating care, support, and
      intervention
  Identification of caregiver role strain necessitating respite/relief/support
  Funeral and burial planning assistance

- **Volunteer(s)**
  Support, friendship, companionship, and presence
  Comfort and dignity maintained/provided for patient and family
  Errands and transportation
  Other services, based on interdisciplinary team recommendations and
      patient/caregiver needs

- **Spiritual counselor**
  Spiritual assessment and care
  Pray with or for the patient/family, using prayers familiar to patient's
      religious background (per their wishes)
  Counseling, intervention, and support related to that dimension of life
      related to life's meaning (consistent with patient's beliefs)
  Support, listening, and presence
  Participation in sacred or spiritual rituals or practices
  Funeral and burial planning assistance
  Other supportive care, based on patient/family needs and belief
      systems

- **Dietitian/Nutritional counseling**
  Assessment of patient with decreased intake, weight loss, anorexia, and
      nausea
  Assessment and recommendations for swallowing difficulties
  Teaching and support of family members and caregivers

Support and care with food and nourishment as desired by patient

Teach safe PO and tube feeding techniques to prevent choking, aspiration, or overhydration (if on TPN)

Evaluation/management of nutritional deficits and needs

Encourage nutritional supplements and snacks to increase protein and caloric intake

Food, dietary recommendations incorporated into patient choice and wishes

Evaluation of patient on enteral/nutritional feedings

- *Occupational therapist*
  Evaluation of ADL's, functional mobility
  Assess for need for adaptive equipment and assistive devices
  Safety assessment of patient's environment and ADL's
  Assessment for energy conservation training
  Assessment of upper extremity function, retraining motor skills, and/or splinting for contractures

- *Physical therapist*
  Evaluation
  Safety assessment of patient's environment
  Safe transfer training
  Strengthening exercises/program
  Teach transfer safety/lift use
  Bed mobility exercises, as tolerated
  Instruct and supervise caregiver and volunteers on home exercise regimen

- *Speech-language pathologist*
  Evaluation for speech/swallowing problems
  Food texture recommendations
  Speech dysphagia program
  Alternate communication program

- *Bereavement counselor*
  Assessment of the needs of the bereaved family and friends
  Support and intervention, based on assessment and ongoing findings
  Presence and counseling
  Supportive visits and follow-up, other interventions (e.g., mailings, calls)
  Other services related to bereavement work and support

- *Music, massage, art, or other therapies or services*
  Evaluation and intervention based on patient's and caregiver's unique wishes and needs that support care, comfort, and death in the setting of the patient's choice
  Pet therapy (including patient's pet, if available) and therapeutic intervention
  Assessment plan to engage patient and support comfort, quality, enjoyment, and dignity

4

6. Outcomes for care

- *Hospice nursing*
    Patient and caregiver verbalize satisfaction with care
    Adherence to POC as demonstrated by caregiver demonstrations and
        verbalizations and patient findings by _____ (specify date)
    Caregiver effective in care management and knows whom to call for
        questions/concerns
    Skin integrity maintained as evidenced by problem-free skin
    Patient uses catheter without complaints or signs/symptoms of infection
    Patient will exhibit a reduction in problems such as pain, SOB, clot
        formation, urinary infection, and decreased function caused by
        immobility/disease processes
    Regulated bowel program, as evidenced by regular bowel movements
    Patient will express satisfaction with hospice support received and will
        experience increased comfort
    Patient will be made comfortable at home through death in accordance
        with the patient's wishes
    Effective pain control and symptom control verbalized by patient
    Patient verbalizes understanding of and adheres to care and medication
        regimens
    Patient and caregiver supported through patient's death
    Comfort maintained through course of care
    The patient and family receive hospice support and care, and family
        members and friends are able to spend quality time with the
        patient
    Caregiver able and verbalizes comfort with role and lists when to call
        hospice team members
    Patient supported through and receives the maximum benefit from
        palliative chemotherapy and radiation with minimal complications
    Patient or caregiver lists adverse reactions, potential complications,
        signs/symptoms of infection (e.g., sputum change, chest congestion)
    Comfort maintained through death with dignity
    Pain effectively managed, and patient verbalizes comfort
    Comfort and individualized intervention of patient with immobility/
        bedbound status (e.g., skin, urinary, musculature, vascular)
    Spiritual and psychosocial needs met (specify) as defined by patient
        and caregiver throughout course of care
    Caregiver, by _____ (date), will verbalize care of patient
    Symptom relief and supportive intervention and care
    Compliance to care program as evidenced by observation and
        demonstration during nurse's and other team members' visits
    Patient can describe medication regimen and side effects and knows
        when and for what symptoms to call the clinician
    Catheter patent and infection free
    Comfort through death with dignity at home with loved ones
    Patient or caregiver will express increased patient comfort
    Patient able to spend quality time with family and friends through
        illness and death

4

Death with dignity, and symptoms controlled in setting of patient/
family choice

Death with maximum comfort through effective symptom control with
specialized hospice support

Symptoms controlled in setting of patient/family choice

Effective pain relief and control (e.g., a peaceful and comfortable death)

Maximizing the patient's quality of life (e.g., patient is alert and pain free)

Pharmacological and nonpharmacological interventions, such as localized
heat application, positioning, relaxation methods, music, and others

Patient cared for, and family supported through death with physical,
psychosocial, spiritual, and other needs acknowledged/addressed

Patient- and family-centered hospice care provided based on the
patient's/family's unique situation and needs

Infection control and palliation through death

- *Home health aide or certified nursing assistant*
  Effective hygiene, personal care, and comfort
  ADL assistance
  Safe environment maintained
  Safe ambulation and transfers

- *Social worker*
  Resources identified, community linkage as appropriate for patient/family
  Problems are identified and addressed, and patient and caregiver are
  linked with appropriate support services. Plan of care successfully
  implemented
  Patient and caregiver cope adaptively with illness and death
  Adaptive adjustment to changed body and body image
  Psychosocial support and counseling offered to patient and caregivers
  experiencing loss and grief
  Optimal care for patient in home environment
  Funeral and burial planning assistance

- *Volunteer(s)*
  Comfort, companionship, and friendship extended to patient/family
  Support and respite provided as defined by the needs of the
  patient/caregiver

- *Spiritual counselor*
  Spiritual support offered and provided as defined by needs of
  patient/caregiver
  Provision of spiritual support and care as based on the assessed and
  ongoing needs of the patient and family
  Spiritual support offered, and patient and family needs met
  Intervention and support provided related to that dimension of life
  related to life's meaning (consistent with patient's beliefs)
  Support, listening, and presence
  Participation in sacred rituals or practices
  Other outcomes, based on the patient's/family's unique beliefs and needs
  Pray with or for the patient/family, using prayers familiar to the
  patient's religious background (per their wishes)

4

- *Dietitian/Nutritional counseling*
  Family and caregiver integrate dietary recommendations into nutrition-related care and intervention
  Patient and caregiver know whom to call for nutrition- and hydration-related questions/concerns
  Patient and family verbalize comprehension of changing nutritional needs

- *Occupational therapist*
  Patient and caregiver demonstrate effective use of energy conservation
  Verbalization/demonstration of improved functional activity level and enhanced quality of life
  Patient demonstrates effective use of diaphragmatic breathing to reduce shortness of breath and relaxation techniques to help in pain/symptom management
  Patient and caregiver demonstrate correct use of exercise and splints for maximum upper extremity function and joint position

- *Physical therapist*
  Prevention of complications
  Home exercise and upper extremity program taught to caregiver
  Optimal strength and mobility maintained/achieved
  Compliance with home exercise program by _____ (date)
  Safety in bed mobility

- *Speech-language pathologist*
  Communication method implemented, and patient able to be understood as self-reported or reported by family/caregivers
  Swallowing safety evaluated and maintained

- *Bereavement counselor*
  Support services related to grief provided to patient and family
  Well-being and resolution process of grief initiated and followed through bereavement services

4

- *Music, massage, art, or other therapies or services*
  Therapeutic massage/touch effective for patient as self-reported or observed by caregivers/family
  Improved muscle tone, relaxation, and/or sleep
  Patient comfortable and relaxed (e.g., sleeping) after massage
  Music therapy intervention based on assessment to decrease pain perception and provide emotional expression and support
  Maintenance of comfort, physical, psychosocial, and spiritual health
  Patient has pets present as desired—in all care sites, when possible
  Holistic health maintained and comfort achieved through _____ (specify modality)

7. **Patient, family, and caregiver educational needs**
   Educational needs are the care regimens that contribute to safe and effective care at home between the hospice team's visits. These include the following:
   The basic tenets of hospice and the availability of support 24 hours a day, 7 days a week

Home safety assessment and counseling
Safe and proper body mechanics to promote patient comfort and
    prevent caregiver safety problems
Other teaching specific to the patient's and family's unique needs
Support groups available to patient's family, such as the hospice
    program's "Caregiver Support Group" meetings for family
    members and friends of the patient
Skin care regimens
Catheter and wound care programs
Effective personal hygiene habits
Home exercise program, including ROM
Safety measures in the home when the patient is immobilized
Prevention of infections
Medication program and the medications' relationships to each other
Importance of medical follow-up
When to call the hospice or the physician
Anticipated disease progression
Other information based on the patient's/family's unique needs

8. Specific tips for quality and reimbursement

Document any variances to expected outcomes. There are many models
of hospice programs.

The Medicare hospice benefit does not require that the patient be
homebound or have identified skilled needs. For further information on
this benefit, please refer to CMS Hospice Manual 21.

Should the patient's status deteriorate and increased personal care be
needed, obtain a telephone order for the increased service, noting
frequency and estimating the duration.

Obtain a telephone order for all medication and treatment changes of
the medical regimen and document these in the clinical record.

Remember that nutritional solutions/supplements are usually covered
by Medicare or other third-party payors when they are the *sole* source of
nutrition. (They usually cannot be supplementary.) Also, they are generally covered when taken by routes other than PO—for example, enteral
tube feedings.

Unless the patient is in a hospice insurance program, some insurers will
not pay for a skilled clinician visit that is made at death if the patient is
dead when the clinician arrives at the home. From a Medicare home care
perspective, the visit at the time of death may be covered when the orders
and clinical record document assessment of the patient's status or signs
of death/life or state law allows pronouncement of death by an RN.

Document patient deterioration
Document dehydration, dehydrating
Document patient change or instability
Document pain, other symptoms not controlled
Document status after acute episode of _____ (specify)
Document positive urine, sputum, etc. culture; patient started on
    _____ (specify ordered antibiotic therapy)

Document patient impacted; impaction removed manually

Document RN in frequent communication with physician regarding
_____ (specify)

Document febrile at _____, pulse change at _____, irr., irr.

Document change noted in _____

Document bony prominences red, opening

Document RN contacted physician regarding _____ (specify)

Document marked SOB

Document alteration in mental status

Document medications being adjusted, regulated, or monitored

Remember that the clinical documentation is key to measuring
compliance for quality and reimbursement purposes. Care
coordination, timely verbal and initial physician orders, and
assessment and addressing of spiritual and psychosocial needs
should be ongoing and documented in the patient's clinical record

The documentation should support that all hospice care supports
comfort and dignity while meeting patient/family needs

The documentation should include ongoing assessment and
management of pain and other symptoms and the anticipation and
prevention of secondary symptoms such as constipation

It is important to note that all team members, including nurses and
social workers, should assess, identify, and "hear" spiritual needs
that the patient and family want to be addressed. These spiritual
issues are key to the provision of quality hospice care and cannot be
addressed effectively and promptly by the spiritual counselor only

Document clearly symptoms, clinical changes, and assessment findings
related to pain and patient care

Document weight loss, increased shortness of breath, dyspnea,
infection, sepsis, new or changed medications and the patient's
response, etc.

Document any skin changes (e.g., inflamed, painful, weeping skin
site[s])

Remember that the "litmus test" of care coordination rests on the
quality of the clinical documentation by all team members. Review
one of your patient's clinical records and ask yourself the following:
"If I was unable to give a verbal report/update on this patient'/family's
course of care, would a peer be able to pick up and provide the same
level of care and know (from the documentation) the current orders,
including specific medications, and other details that contribute to
effective hospice care?"

This patient population usually has many clinical changes that should
be documented. These include weight loss and multiple and changed
medication regimens with varying routes. Side effects to the drug
regimen should be observed, noted, documented, and reported

Your assessments, observations, and clinical findings assist in painting
a picture to support coverage and documentation requirements for
hospice care

Document any hospitalizations and changed clinical findings

Document patient changes, symptoms, and psychosocial issues
impacting the patient and family and plan of care
Document coordination of services or consultation with other members
of the IDG

9. Queries for quality

Bedbound care
- *Is patient's pain managed adequately?*
- *Is patient's anxiety managed adequately?*
- *Is the patient's functional ability/status clearly documented?*
- *What is the condition of the patient's skin?*
- *Have you documented to the interdisciplinary POC?*

Immobility care
- *Is patient's pain managed adequately?*
- *Is patient's anxiety managed adequately?*
- *Is the patient's functional ability/status clearly documented?*
- *What is the condition of the patient's skin?*
- *Have you documented to the interdisciplinary POC?*

10. Resources for hospice care and practice

Available free from the Agency for Healthcare and Research Quality
(AHRQ) are *Clinical Practice Guideline Number 3: Preventing
Pressure Ulcers: Patient Guide, Pressure Ulcers in Adults: Prediction
and Prevention, and Pressure Ulcers in Adults: Prediction and
Prevention. Treating Pressure Sores: Consumer Guide Number 15* and
*Pressure Ulcer Treatment: Quick Reference Guide for Clinicians
Number 15* are also available. The patient guides are available in
English and Spanish, and all can be ordered by calling 1-800-358-9295
or visit online at www.AHRQ.gov.

The pamphlet *Get Relief From Cancer Pain* is available from the
National Cancer Institute's Cancer Information Service. Call 1-800-4-
CANCER.

The 76-page booklet *Questions and Answers About Pain Control* is
available free from the National Cancer Institute's Cancer Information
Service. Call 1-800-4-CANCER.

4

BRAIN TUMOR CARE

1. General considerations

Hospice clinicians use all their skills in the care of patients with brain tumors and their family members. The many symptoms and problems may be overwhelming to the family and caregivers. The patient's care needs vary depending on the tumor site and specific type. The support and assurance provided to these patients and families may be as important as control of seizures or other symptoms that can be difficult to manage at home.

Please refer also to "Cancer Care," "Bedbound Care," or "Pain Care" should these sections also pertain to your patient.

2. Needs for visit

Physician order for hospice care, specific to the hospice program's
     admission criteria and policies
Standard precautions supplies
Vital signs equipment for baseline assessment
Other supplies or equipment, based on physician orders

3. Safety considerations

Infection control/standard precautions
Side rail use and position
Supervised medication administration
Wheelchair/fall/seizure precautions and postseizure actions
     to take
Prevention of injury related to proper position
Need for meticulous skin care and observation
Multiple medications (e.g., side effects, interactions,
     safe storage)
Night-light
Safety for home medical equipment (e.g., bed, lift)
Symptoms that necessitate immediate reporting/assistance
Smoke detector and fire evacuation plan
Extra caution on slippery surfaces
Removal of scatter rugs
Tub rail, grab bars for bathroom safety
Supportive and nonskid shoes
Handrail on stairs
Fall precautions
Protective skin measures
Identification and report of any skin problems
Phone number of whom to call with a care problem
Smoke detector and fire evacuation plan
Assistance with ambulation
Others, based on the patient's unique condition
     and environment

4. Potential diagnoses and codes

Acoustic neuroma	225.1
Astrocytoma	191.9
Bone marrow transplant (surgical)	41.00
Bone metastases	198.5
Brain tumor, recurrent	239.6
Cancer of the brain	198.3
Cerebrovascular accident	436
Depression, reactive	300.4
Failure to thrive, adult	783.7
Glioblastoma	191.9
Meningitis	322.9
Metastases (general)	199.1
Metastatic brain tumor	198.3
Pathological fracture	733.10
Pneumonia	486
Seizures	780.39
Radiation enteritis	558.1
Radiation myelitis	323.8 and E879.2
Transient ischemic attacks	435.9
Urinary tract infection	599.0

5. Skills and services identified

- *Hospice nursing*

a. *Comfort and symptom control*

Complete initial assessment of all systems of patient with seizures admitted to hospice for _____ (specify problem)

Skilled observation, and complete systems assessment of the patient with seizures and a brain tumor

Presentation of hospice philosophy and services

Explain patient rights and responsibilities

Assess patient, family, and caregiver wishes and expectations regarding care

Assess patient, family, and caregiver resources available for care

Provision of volunteer support to patient and family

Teach family or caregiver physical care of patient

Assess pain and other symptoms, including site, duration, characteristics, and relief measures

Monitor for signs and symptoms of infection

Observation and assessment of patient's pain and other symptoms

RN to conduct neurological checks q visit, including levels of consciousness, pupil checks, and others as ordered

Comfort measures of backrub and hand massages

Observe for alopecia, and implement management regimen

RN to monitor blood pressure and other vital signs

RN to monitor patient for seizure activity and teach seizure and associated safety precautions

Monitor for fluid retention

Pain assessment and management

Observe oral mucosa for breakdown and other problems

Assess effectiveness of pain relief program

Comfort measures of backrub and hand or other therapeutic massage

RN to provide and teach effective oral care and comfort measure

Assess pain and evaluate effectiveness of pain management

Teach care of bedridden patient

Measure vital signs, including pain, q visit

Assess cardiovascular, pulmonary, and respiratory status

Teach caregivers symptom control and relief measures

Oxygen on at _____ liter per _____ (specify physician orders)

Identify and monitor pain, symptoms, and relief measures

Assess neurological status

Teach patient and family seizure precautions

RN to assess patient's pain with other symptoms q visit to identify need for dose addition or other plan or dose adjustment

Teach signs and symptoms of TIA or stroke

Seizure precautions interventions

RN to assess patient's pain or other symptoms q visit to identify need for change, addition, or other plan or dose adjustment

Teach caregiver or family care of weak, terminally ill patient

Teach patient/family about realistic expectations of disease process

Teach care of dying, signs/symptoms of impending death

Presence and support

Other interventions, based on patient/family needs

b. *Safety and mobility considerations*

Assess need for a personal emergency response system

Provide caregiver with home safety information and instruction related to _____ and documented in the clinical record

Teach family regarding safety patient in home

Teach family regarding energy-conservation techniques

Patient and caregiver provided with home safety information and instruction related to seizures and documented in clinical record

Other interventions, based on patient/family needs

c. *Emotional/Spiritual considerations*

Psychosocial assessment of patient and family regarding disease and prognosis

RN to provide emotional support to patient and family with _____, a terminal illness

Assess mental status and sleep disturbance changes

Provide emotional support to patient and spouse

Provide support to patient and family-member caregivers

Other interventions, based on patient/family needs

d. *Skin care*

Teach caregiver regarding skin care needs, including the need for frequent position changes, appropriate pressure pads and mattresses, and the prevention of breakdown

Pressure ulcer care as indicated

RN to teach patient regarding care of irradiated skin sites

Assess skin integrity

Observation and evaluation of wound and surrounding skin

Evaluate patient's need for equipment and supplies to decrease pressure, including alternating pressure mattress, gel foam seat cushion, and heel and elbow protectors

Observation and evaluation of wound and surrounding skin

Teach family to perform dressing changes between RN visits, specifically _____

Teach patient and family or caregiver about proper body alignment and positioning in bed to prevent skin tears from shearing skin

Observe and apply skilled assessment of areas for possible breakdown, including heels, hips, elbows, ankles, and other pressure-prone areas

Other interventions, based on patient/family needs

e. *Elimination considerations*

Assess bowel regimen, and implement program as needed

Monitor bowel patterns, including frequency of bowel movements, and evaluate bowel regimen (e.g., stool softeners, laxatives, and dietary changes)

RN to teach caregiver daily care of catheter

Observation and complete systems assessment of the patient with an indwelling catheter

Check for and remove impaction as needed

Condom catheter or indwelling catheter as indicated

Assess amount and frequency of urinary output

Teach catheter care to caregiver

RN to evaluate the patient's bowel patterns, need for stool softeners, laxatives, and dietary adjustments and develop bowel management plan

Other interventions, based on patient/family needs

f. *Hydration/Nutrition*

Assess nutrition and hydration statuses

Diet counseling to patient with anorexia

Teach feeding-tube care to family

Nutrition/hydration supported by offering patient's choice of favorite or desired foods or liquids

Teach patient and family to expect decreased nutritional and fluid intake as disease progresses

Other interventions, based on patient/family needs

g. *Therapeutic/Medication regimens*

Teach about and observe side effects of palliative chemotherapy, including constipation, anemia, and fatigue

Monitor weight gain caused by steroids (potential for diabetes and edema)

4

RN to instruct caregiver on all aspects of medication management, including schedule, functions, and side effects

RN to assess the patient's unique response to treatments or interventions, and report changes or unfavorable responses or reactions to the physician

Medication assessment and management

Teach new pain and symptom control medication regimen

Teach about new medication and effects

Teach new medication regimen

Obtain venipuncture as ordered q _____ (ordered frequency)

Teach patient and caregiver use of PCA pump

Assess for electrolyte imbalance

Nonpharmacological interventions such as progressive muscle relaxation, imagery, positive visualization, music, massage and touch, and humor therapy of patient's choice implemented

Assess effectiveness and side effects of new medication regimen, including food/drug and possible drag/drug interactions

Other interventions, based on patient/family needs

h. *Other considerations*

Teach patient radiation therapy regimen and schedule

Support patient/caregiver through radiation, chemotherapy, and other modalities for tumor reduction

Teach patient and caregiver about steroid therapy and side effects to watch for

Assess disease progression process

RN to assess the patient's response to treatments and interventions and to report to the physician any changes, unfavorable responses, or reactions

Other interventions, based on patient/family needs

- **Home health aide or certified nursing assistant**

Effective and safe personal care

Safe ADL assistance, support, ambulation, and transfer assist

Respite care and active listening skills

Observation and reporting

Meal preparation

Homemaker services

Comfort care

Other duties

- **Social worker**

Psychosocial assessment of patient and family/caregiver, including adjustment to illness and its implications and the need for care

Identification of optimal coping strategies

Financial assessment and counseling regarding food acquisition, ability to prepare, and costs of needed medications

Identification of caregiver role strain necessitating respite/relief measures or support

Intervention/support related to terminal illness and loss

Emotional/spiritual support

Depression/fear assessed and addressed

Facilitate communication among patient, family, and hospice team

Referral/linkage to community services and resources as indicated

Grief counseling and intervention/support related to illness/loss

Patient/caregiver counseling and support

For patients who live alone with no support system (e.g., able, available, willing caregiver[s]), linkage to necessary community resources to allow patient to remain in home.

Illness-related psychiatric condition necessitating care/support/intervention

Counseling support to patient/family regarding patient's behavioral changes

Assessment of depression, fears, or anxiety

Funeral and burial planning assistance

- *Volunteer(s)*

  Support, friendship, companionship, and presence

  Comfort and dignity maintained/provided for patient and family

  Errands and transportation

  Other services, based on interdisciplinary team recommendations and patient/caregiver needs

- *Spiritual counselor*

  Spiritual assessment and care

  Counseling, intervention, and support related to that dimension of life related to life's meaning (consistent with patient's beliefs)

  Pray with or for the patient/family, using prayers familiar to patient's religious background (per their wishes)

  Support, listening, and presence

  Participation in sacred or spiritual rituals or practices

  Funeral planning assistance

  Other supportive care, based on patient/family needs and belief systems

- *Dietitian/Nutritional counseling*

  Assessment of patient with decreased intake, weight loss, anorexia, weight gain or loss caused by steroids, and nausea

  Assessment and recommendations for swallowing difficulties

  Teaching and support of family members and caregivers

  Support and care with food and nourishment as desired by patient

- *Occupational therapist*

  Evaluation of ADL and functional mobility

  Assess for need for adaptive equipment and assistive devices

  Safety assessment of patient's environment and ADLs

  Assessment for energy conservation training

  Assessment of upper extremity function, retraining motor skills, and/or splinting for contracture(s)

4

- *Physical therapist*
  Evaluation
  Assessment of patient's environment for safety
  Safe transfer training
  Strengthening exercises/program
  Assessment of gait safety
  Instruct and supervise caregiver and volunteers on home exercise
      program for conditioning and strength
  Assistive, adaptive devices or equipment and teaching

- *Speech-language pathologist*
  Evaluation for speech/swallowing problems

- *Bereavement counselor*
  Assessment of the needs of the bereaved family and friends
  Support and intervention, based on assessment and ongoing findings
  Presence and counseling
  Supportive visits and follow-up, other interventions (e.g., mailings, calls)
  Other services related to bereavement work and support

- *Pharmacist*
  Evaluation of hospice patient on multiple medications for possible
      food/drug, drug/drug interactions
  Medication monitoring regarding therapeutic levels and dosages
  Pain consult and input into interdisciplinary plan of care related to pain
      control, palliation, and symptom management
  Assessment of medication regimen and plan for safety and compliance

- *Music, massage, art, or other therapies or services*
  Evaluation and intervention based on patient's and caregiver's unique
      wishes and needs that support care, comfort, and death in the setting
      of the patient's choice
  Pet therapy (including patient's pet, if available) and therapeutic
      intervention
  Assessment plan to engage patient and support comfort, quality,
      enjoyment, and dignity

6. Outcomes for care

- *Hospice nursing*
  Seizures controlled throughout illness and death
  Death with dignity, and symptoms controlled in setting of patient/
      family choice
  Death with maximum comfort through effective symptom control with
      specialized hospice support
  Symptoms controlled in setting of patient/family choice
  Effective pain relief and control (e.g., a peaceful and comfortable
      death)
  Maximizing the patient's quality of life (e.g., patient is alert and
      pain free)

Pharmacological and nonpharmacological interventions, such as localized heat application, positioning, relaxation methods, and music

Patient cared for, and family supported through death with physical, psychosocial, spiritual, and other needs acknowledged/addressed

Patient- and family-centered hospice care provided based on the patient's/family's unique situation and needs

Infection control and palliation

Patient states pain is at _____ on 0–10 scale by next visit

Patient and caregiver verbalize satisfaction with care

Educational tools/plans incorporated in daily care, and patient and caregiver verbalize understanding of safe, needed care

Patient will decide on care, interventions, and evaluation

Caregiver effective in care management and knows whom to call for questions/concerns

Patient will express satisfaction with hospice support received and will experience increased comfort

Patient will be made comfortable at home through death in accordance with the patient's wishes

Effective pain control and symptom control verbalized by patient

Patient verbalizes understanding of and adheres to care and medication regimens

Patient and caregiver supported through patient's death

Comfort maintained through course of care

The patient and family receive hospice support and care, and family members and friends are able to spend quality time with the patient

Caregiver able and verbalizes comfort with role and knows when to call hospice team members

Patient supported through and receives the maximum benefit from palliative chemotherapy and radiation with minimal complications

Patient and caregiver list adverse reactions, potential complications, signs/symptoms of infection (e.g., sputum change, chest congestion)

Comfort maintained through death with dignity

Pain effectively managed and patient verbalizes comfort

Patient protected from injury, has stable respiratory status, and compliant with medication, safety, and care regimens

Comfort and individualized intervention of patient with immobility/bed-bound status (e.g., skin, urinary, musculature, vascular)

Spiritual and psychosocial needs met (specify) as defined by patient and caregiver throughout course of care

Injury protection related to patient with seizures

Seizures controlled, patient is protected from injury, patient has stable neurological status, and patient complies with medication and care regimens (e.g., steroids)

Patient and caregiver knowledgeable about side effects (e.g., constipation) and interventions needed

Patient and caregiver knowledgeable about and compliant with seizure care regimen and care for optimal control, when possible

4

Early detection and intervention of problems related to patients with
immobility/bedbound status (e.g., skin, urinary, musculature, vascular)
Patient will be comfortable and pain free through illness and death, and
IDT will work together to improve/maintain the patient's quality of life
Caregiver and patient, when able, express satisfaction with care
Caregiver, by _____ (date), will verbalize specific care of patient
Compliance to care program as evidenced by observation and
demonstration during visits by clinician and other team members

- *Home health aide or certified nursing assistant*
Effective hygiene, personal care, and comfort
Safe ADL assistance and ambulation
Safe environment maintained

- *Social worker*
Problems are identified and addressed with patient and caregiver, and
they are linked with appropriate support services. Plan of care
successfully implemented
Patient and caregiver cope adaptively with illness and death
Adaptive adjustment to changed body and body image
Psychosocial support and counseling offered to patients and caregivers
experiencing loss and grief
Resources identified, and community linkage is provided as appropriate
for patient and family
Funeral and burial planning assistance

- *Volunteer(s)*
Comfort, companionship, and friendship extended to patient/family
Support provided as defined by the needs of the patient/caregiver

- *Spiritual counselor*
Spiritual assessment and care
Counseling, intervention, and support related to that dimension of life
related to life's meaning (consistent with patient's beliefs)
Support, listening, and presence
Intervention and support provided related to that dimension of life
related to life's meaning (consistent with patient's beliefs)
Participation in sacred or spiritual rituals or practices
Other supportive care, based on patient/family needs and belief systems
Spiritual support offered and provided as defined by needs of
patient/caregiver
Provision of spiritual support and care as based on the assessed and
ongoing needs of the patient and family
Spiritual support offered and patient and family needs met
Pray with or for the patient/family, using prayers familiar to the
patient's religious background (per their wishes)

- *Dietitian/Nutritional counseling*
Family and caregiver integrating dietary recommendations into nutrition
teaching (where appropriate)

Patient and caregiver know whom to call for nutrition- and
hydration-related questions/concerns

Nutrition and hydration per patient's choices

Caregiver integrating dietary recommendations into daily meal planning

Patient and family verbalize comprehension of changing nutritional needs

- *Occupational therapist*
  Optimal functional and safe mobility maintained or enhanced

  Patient demonstrates maximum independence with ADLs, adaptive
  techniques, and assistive devices

  Patient and caregiver demonstrate maximum safety in ADLs and
  functional mobility

  Patient demonstrates effective use of energy conservation

  Verbalization/demonstration of improved functional activity level and
  enhanced quality of life

  Patient demonstrates effective use of diaphragmatic breathing to reduce
  shortness of breath and relaxation techniques to help in pain/
  symptom management

  Patient and caregiver demonstrate correct use of exercise and splints for
  maximum upper-extremity function and joint position

- *Physical therapist*
  Prevention of complications

  Home exercise and upper-extremity program taught to caregiver

  Optimal strength and mobility maintained or achieved

  Compliance with home exercise program by _____ (date)

  Safety in mobility and transfers

- *Speech-language pathologist*
  Communication method implemented, and patient able to be
  understood as self-reported or reported by family/caregivers

  Safe swallowing and functional communication

  Recommended lists of foods/textures for safety and patient choice

- *Bereavement counselor*
  Support services related to grief provided to patient and family

  Well-being and resolution process of grief initiated and followed
  through bereavement services

- *Pharmacist*
  Multiple-drug regimen reviewed for food/drug and drug/drug
  interactions in patient on steroids and other medications

  Stability and safety in complex medication regimen

  Effective pain control and symptom management as reported by
  patient/caregiver

- *Music, massage, art, or other therapies or other services*
  Therapeutic massage/touch effective for patient as self-reported or
  observed by caregivers/family

  Improved muscle tone, relaxation, and/or sleep

  Patient comfortable and relaxed (e.g., sleeping) after massage

4

Music therapy intervention based on assessment to decrease pain
   perception, provide emotional expression and support
Maintenance of comfort and physical, psychosocial, and spiritual health
Patient has pet's presence as desired—in all care sites, when possible
Holistic health maintained and comfort achieved through
   _____ (specify modality)

7. Patient, family, and caregiver educational needs

Educational needs are the care regimens that contribute to safe and effective
care at home between the hospice team's visits. These include the following:

   The basic tenets of hospice and the availability of support 24 hours a
      day, 7 days a week
   Home safety assessment and counseling
   The patient's medication regimen
   Safe and proper body mechanics to promote patient comfort and
      prevent caregiver safety problems
   Other teaching specific to the patient's and family's unique needs
   Support groups available to the patient's family, such as the hospice
      program's "Caregiver Support Group" meetings for family mem-
      bers and friends of the patient
   Effective personal hygiene habits
   Avoidance of infections
   Pain and other symptom control measures and management
   Patient's medications and their relationship to each other
   Information about the disease process and seizure activity care
   Importance of taking the prescribed seizure medications
   Need to report new symptoms to the physician immediately
   Home safety related to mental status, stairs in home, ambulation
   Importance of steroids and other medications
   Catheter care
   Anticipated disease progression
   Other information based on the patient's pathology from the tumor
      and the patient's unique needs

8. Specific tips for quality and reimbursement

For this and other diagnoses, clearly document the symptoms and
   clinical and assessment findings that support the end stage of the
   chronic illness process
Document patient changes, symptoms, and clinical information
   identified from visits and team conferences that support hospice care
   and limited life expectancy
Clearly support in the documentation the rationale that supports/explains
   the progression of the illness from the chronic to terminal stages
Document mentation, behavioral, and cognitive changes
Document dysphagia, weight loss, increased shortness of breath,
   dyspnea, infection, sepsis, new or changed medications, etc.
Document skin changes (e.g., inflamed, painful, weeping skin site[s])
Unless the patient is in a hospice insurance program, some insurers will
   not pay for a skilled clinician visit that is made at death if the patient

4

is dead when the clinician arrives at the home. From a Medicare home care perspective, the visit at the time of death may be covered when the orders and clinical record document assessment of the patient's status or signs of death/life or state law allows pronouncement of death by an RN.

Document any variances with expected outcomes. There are many models of hospice programs.

The Medicare hospice benefit does not require that the patient be homebound or have identified skilled needs. For further information on this benefit, please refer to CMS Hospice Manual 21.

Should the patient's status deteriorate and increased personal care be needed, obtain a telephone order for the increased service, noting frequency and estimating the duration.

Obtain a telephone order for all medication and treatment changes of the medical regimen and document these in the clinical record.

Document patient deterioration

Document dehydration, dehydrating

Document patient change or instability

Document pain, other symptoms not controlled

Document status after acute episode of _____ (specify)

Document positive urine, sputum, etc. culture; patient started on _____ (specify ordered antibiotic therapy)

Document patient impacted; impaction removed manually

Document RN in frequent communication with physician regarding _____ (specify)

Document fertile at _____, pulse change at _____, irr., irr.

Document change noted in _____

Document bony prominences red, opening

Document that RN contacted physician regarding _____ (specify)

Document marked SOB

Document alteration in mental status

Document medications being adjusted, regulated, or monitored

Document unable to perform own ADLs, personal care

Document all interdisciplinary team meetings and communications in the POC and in the progress notes of the clinical record

Document coordination of services and consultation with other members of the IDG

4

9. Queries for quality
- *Is patient's pain managed adequately?*
- *Is patient's anxiety managed adequately?*
- *Is the patient's functional ability/status clearly documented?*
- *What are the patient's symptoms?*
- *Have you documented to the interdisciplinary POC?*

10. Resources for hospice care and practice
The Epilepsy Foundation offers *Seizure Recognition and First Aid*, which can be ordered by calling 1-800-332-1000.

The American Cancer Society has support groups such as "I Can Cope" and other programs. To locate the chapter nearest your patient, call 1-800-ACS-2345.

The American Cancer Society also has a "Look Good ... Feel Better Program" for women undergoing chemotherapy or radiation. They can be reached at 1-800-395-LOOK.

The Brain Tumor Association can be reached at 1-800-886-2282. The National Brain Tumor Foundation can be reached at 1-800-934-CURE (2873).

4

BREAST CANCER CARE

1. General considerations

The high incidence of breast cancer is appropriately alarming to all women. In addition, breast cancer is diagnosed in approximately 1300 men each year, with nearly 400 deaths annually.

Patients with breast cancer need physical care and psychosocial support from the hospice team.

Please refer to "Cancer Care" or "Pain Care" should these sections also pertain to your patient.

2. Needs for visit

Physician order for hospice care, specific to the hospice program's admission criteria and policies
Standard precautions supplies
Vital signs equipment for baseline assessment
Other supplies or equipment, based on physician orders

3. Safety considerations

Infection control/standard precautions
Supervised medication administration
Multiple medications (e.g., side effects, interactions, safe storage)
Night-light
Safety for home medical equipment (e.g., bed, lift)
Symptoms that necessitate immediate reporting/assistance
Smoke detector and fire evacuation plan
Extra caution on slippery surfaces
Removal of scatter rugs
Tub rail, grab bars for bathroom safety
Supportive and nonskid shoes
Handrail on stairs
Fall precautions
Protective skin measures
Identification and report of any skin problems
Others, based on the patient's unique condition and environment

4

4. Potential diagnoses and codes

Bone marrow transplant (surgical)	41.00
Bone metastases	198.5
Breast cancer	174.9
Cancer of the breast	174.9
Failure to thrive, adult	783.7
Fibrocystic disease	610.1
Fracture (pathological)	733.10
Lumpectomy (partial mastectomy)	85.21
Lymphedema (postmastectomy)	457.0

Malignant neoplasms of the breast	174.9
Mastectomy (radical)	85.45
Mastectomy (simple)	85.41
Metastatic lung cancer	197.0
Paget's disease	731.0
Pneumonia	486
Radiation enteritis	558.1
Radiation myelitis	323.8 and E879.2
Secondary malignant neoplasm breast	198.81
Wound dehiscence	998.32
Wound infection	998.59

5. Skills and services identified

- *Hospice nursing*

a. *Comfort and symptom control*

Complete initial assessment of all systems of patient with breast cancer admitted to hospice for _____ (specify problem necessitating care)

Skilled observation and complete systems assessment of the patient with breast cancer, including nutrition, hydration, pain and other symptoms, as well as patient and family coping skills

Comprehensive assessment of the patient after mastectomy with diagnosis of cancer

Presentation of hospice philosophy and services

Explain patient rights and responsibilities

Assess patient, family, and caregiver wishes and expectations regarding care

Assess patient, family, and caregiver resources available for care

Provision of volunteer support to patient and family

Teach family or caregiver physical care of patient

Assess pain and other symptoms, including site, duration, characteristics, and relief measures

RN to provide and teach effective oral care and comfort measures

Pain assessment and management q visit

RN to teach about and observe for signs, symptoms of infection

RN to evaluate amount and type of drainage

Teach about pain regimen, including care for phantom sensations such as itching, tingling, and pain, and relief of these sensations

Patient to elevate affected arm

Check affected arm for edema or circulatory problems

Teach use/care of drain/mechanism

RN to assess and monitor pain after reconstructive surgery and patient's response to interventions and effective pain and other symptom relief measures

RN to assess blood pressure, other vital signs, including pain, q visit

Comfort measures of backrub and hand or other therapeutic massage

Teach about and observe side effects of palliative chemotherapy, including constipation, anemia, and fatigue

Assess weight as ordered
Assess pain and evaluate effectiveness of pain management
Teach care of bedridden patient
RN to instruct in pain control measures and medication
Measure vital signs, including pain, q visit
Assess cardiovascular, pulmonary, and respiratory status
Teach caregivers symptom control and relief measures
Oxygen on at _____ liter per _____ (specify physician orders)
Identify and monitor pain, symptoms, and relief measures
RN to assess patient's pain or other symptoms q visit to identify need
  for change, addition, or other plan or dose adjustment
RN to teach about compression garments or pneumatic pumping
Effective management of pain and prevention of secondary symptoms
Interventions of symptoms directed toward comfort and palliation
Teach caregiver or family care of weak, terminally ill patient
Teach patient and family about realistic expectations of disease
  process
Teach care of dying, signs/symptoms of impending death
Presence and support
Other interventions, based on patient/family needs

b. *Safety and mobility considerations*
  Provide caregiver with home safety information and instruction related
    to _____ and documented in the clinical record
  Teach family about safety of patient in home
  Teach family about energy conservation techniques
  Instruct patient and caregiver to protect arm from infection and injury
  RN to teach patient to avoid venipunctures, blood pressure readings,
    etc., in affected arm
  Other interventions based on patient/family needs

c. *Emotional/Spiritual considerations*
  Psychosocial assessment of patient and family regarding disease and
    prognosis
  RN to provide emotional support to patient with significant body image
    change
  Assess mental status and sleep disturbance changes
  RN to provide emotional support to patient and family
  Ongoing acknowledgment of spirituality and related concerns of
    patient/family
  Other interventions, based on patient/family needs

d. *Skin care*
  RN to evaluate for deterrents to wound healing (e.g., radiation, poor
    nutrition)
  Teach patient and caregiver wound care, including infection control
    measures
  RN to provide skilled observation and assessment of surgical site
  RN to teach patient about care of irradiated skin sites
  RN to assess healing in reconstruction of breast site

4

Pressure ulcer care as indicated

Assess skin integrity

Observation and evaluation of wound and surrounding skin

Evaluate patient's need for equipment and supplies to decrease pressure, including alternating pressure mattress, gel foam seat cushion, and heel and elbow protectors

Teach family to perform dressing changes between RN visits, specifically _____

Teach patient and family or caregiver about proper body alignment and positioning in bed to prevent skin tears from shearing skin

Observe and apply skilled assessment of areas for possible breakdown, including heels, hips, elbows, ankles, and other pressure-prone areas

Teach caregiver about skin care needs, including the need for frequent position changes, appropriate pressure pads and mattresses, and the prevention of breakdown

Other interventions, based on patient/family needs

e. *Elimination considerations*

Assess bowel regimen, and implement program as needed

Monitor bowel patterns, including frequency of bowel movements, and evaluate bowel regimen (e.g., stool softeners, laxatives, dietary changes)

RN to teach caregiver daily care of catheter

Observation and complete systems assessment of the patient with an indwelling catheter

Check for and remove impaction as needed

Condom catheter or indwelling catheter as indicated

Assess amount and frequency of urinary output

Teach catheter care to caregiver

RN to evaluate the patient's bowel patterns, need for stool softeners, laxatives, and dietary adjustments, and develop bowel management plan

Other interventions, based on patient/family needs

f. *Hydration/Nutrition*

RN to instruct patient and spouse in importance of adequate hydration and nutrition needed for effective postoperative healing

Assess nutrition/hydration status

Diet counseling for patient with anorexia

Teach feeding-tube care to family

Nutrition/hydration supported by offering patient's choice of favorite or desired foods or liquids

Nutrition/hydration to be maintained by offering patient high-protein diet and foods of choice as tolerated

Teach patient and family to expect decreased nutritional and fluid intake as disease progresses

Other interventions, based on patient/family needs

g. *Therapeutic/Medication regimens*

Teach about chemotherapy regimen, if appropriate

RN to instruct caregiver on all aspects of medications, including schedule, functions, possible side effects, and drug/drug and drug/food interactions

RN to assess the patient's unique response to treatments or interventions and report changes or unfavorable responses or reactions to the physician

Medication assessment and management

Measure abdominal girth for ascites and edema, and document sites and amount

Obtain venipuncture as ordered q _____ (ordered frequency)

Teach new medication regimen and side effects

Teach new pain and symptom control medication regimen

Assess for electrolyte imbalance

Teach patient and caregiver use of PCA pump

Nonpharmacological interventions such as progressive muscle relaxation, imagery, positive visualization, music, massage and touch, and humor therapy of patient's choice implemented

Other interventions, based on patient/family needs

h. *Other considerations*

Instruct patient in increased risk of infection and lymphedema in affected arm, including signs and symptoms of cellulitis

Teach importance of Medic Alert bracelet and the need to avoid venipunctures, blood tests, and other procedures on affected arm

RN to assess the patient's response to treatments and interventions and to report to physician any changes, unfavorable responses, or reactions

Assess disease process progression

Other interventions, based on patient/family needs

- *Home health aide or certified nursing assistant*

4

Effective and safe personal care

Safe ADL assistance and support

Observation and reporting

Respite care and active listening skills

Meal preparation

Homemaker services

Comfort care

Other duties

- *Social worker*

Psychosocial assessment of patient and family/caregiver, including adjustment to illness and its implications

Identification of optimal coping strategies

Financial assessment and counseling regarding food acquisition, ability to prepare, and costs of needed medications

Identification of caregiver role strain necessitating respite/relief measures or support

Intervention/support related to terminal illness and loss

Emotional/spiritual support

Depression/fear assessed and addressed

Facilitate communication among patient, family, and hospice team

Referral/linkage to community services and resources as indicated

Grief counseling and intervention/support related to illness/loss

Patient/caregiver counseling and support

For patients who live alone with no support system (e.g., able, available, willing caregiver[s]), obtain linkage to community resources to enable patient to remain in the home

Identification of illness-related psychiatric condition necessitating care, support, and intervention

Counseling regarding body image changes

Funeral and burial planning assistance

- *Volunteer(s)*

Support, friendship, companionship, and presence

Comfort and dignity maintained for patient and family

Errands and transportation

Other services, based on interdisciplinary team recommendations and patient/caregiver needs

- *Spiritual counselor*

Spiritual assessment and care

Counseling, intervention, support related to that dimension of life related to life's meaning (consistent with patient's beliefs)

Pray with or for the patient/family, using prayers familiar to patient's religious background (per their wishes)

Support, listening, and presence

Participation in sacred or spiritual rituals or practices

Funeral and burial planning assistance

Other supportive care, based on patient's/family's needs and beliefs

- *Dietitian/Nutritional counseling*

Assessment of patient with decreased intake, weight loss, anorexia, and nausea

Teaching and support of family members and caregivers

Support and care with food and nourishment as desired by patient

Evaluation/management of nutritional deficits and needs

Encouragement of nutritional supplements and snacks to increase protein and caloric intake

Food, dietary recommendations incorporating patient choice and wishes (if patient on tube feeding, teach safe tube feeding techniques)

Assessment of and instruction in use of alternative nutritional therapies, such as herbs, vitamin/mineral supplements, and macrobiotic diets

- *Occupational therapist*

Evaluation of ADL and functional mobility

Assess for need for adaptive equipment and assistive devices

Safety assessment of patient's environment and ADLs

Assessment for energy conservation training

Assessment of upper extremity function, retraining motor skills

Measures to improve function and problems with body image, such as the breast prosthesis and altered upper-extremity function

- *Physical therapist*

  Evaluation

  Assessment of patient's environment for safety

  Safe transfer training

  Strengthening exercises/program

  Assessment of gait safety

  Instruct/supervise caregiver and volunteers on home exercise program for conditioning and strength

  Assistive, adaptive devices of equipment and teaching

- *Bereavement counselor*

  Assessment of the needs of the bereaved family and friends

  Support and intervention, based on an assessment and ongoing findings

  Presence and counseling

  Supportive visits, follow-up, and other interventions (e.g., mailings, calls)

  Other services related to bereavement work and support

- *Music, massage, art, or other therapies or services*

  Evaluation and intervention based on patient's and caregiver's unique wishes and needs that support care, comfort, and death in the setting of the patient's choice

  Pet therapy (including patient's pet, if available) and therapeutic intervention

  Assessment plan to engage patient and support comfort, quality, enjoyment, and dignity

6. Outcomes for care

- *Hospice nursing*

  Death with dignity and symptoms controlled in setting of patient/family choice

  Death with maximum comfort through effective symptom control with specialized hospice support

  Symptoms controlled in setting of patient/family choice

  Effective pain relief and control (e.g., a peaceful and comfortable death)

  Maximizing the patient's quality of life (e.g., patient is alert and pain free per patient wishes)

  Pharmacological and nonpharmacological interventions, such as localized heat application, positioning, relaxation methods, and music

  Patient cared for and family supported through death with physical, psychosocial, spiritual, and other needs acknowledged/addressed

  Patient- and family-centered hospice care provided based on the patient's/family's unique situation and needs

  Infection control and palliation

  Patient states pain is at _____ on a scale of 0–10 by next visit

4

Patient/caregiver verbalizes satisfaction with care

Adherence to POC as demonstrated by caregiver demonstrations and verbalizations and patient findings by _____ (specify date)

Caregiver effective in care management and knows whom to call for questions/concerns

Skin integrity maintained as evidenced by problem-free skin

Pain controlled and comfort needs met throughout POC

IV access site remains patent, and flushing/dressing care is provided per protocol without signs/symptoms of infection

Patient's weight will be maintained/increased/decreased by _____

Regulated bowel program, as evidenced by regular bowel movements

Wound site healing tracked through measurements of site and amount and type of drainage. Date projected for healing is _____ (specify date)

Patient will report being comfortable _____ % of the day (comfortable defined as pain free)

Complications/side effects of chemotherapy/radiation, including infection, bleeding, dehydration, nausea, and vomiting, controlled by _____ as reported by patient/caregiver

Compliance with and adherence to interdisciplinary care plan as demonstrated by observation and reporting by caregiver/patient

Caregiver demonstrates ability to manage pain, where applicable

Patient maintains comfort and dignity throughout illness

Patient protected from injury, stable respiratory status, and compliant with medication, safety, and care regimens

Comfort and individualized intervention of patient with immobility/bedbound status (e.g., skin, urinary, musculature, vascular)

Spiritual and psychosocial needs met (specify) as defined by patient and caregiver throughout course of care

Educational tools/plans incorporated in daily care and patient/caregiver verbalizes understanding of safe, needed care

Patient will decide on care, interventions, and evaluation

Caregiver effective in care management and knows whom to call for questions/concerns

Patient will express satisfaction with hospice support received and will experience increased comfort

Patient will be made comfortable at home through death in accordance with the patient's wishes

Effective pain control and symptom relief verbalized by patient

Patient verbalizes understanding of and adheres to care and medication regimens

Patient and caregiver supported through patient's death

Comfort maintained through course of care

The patient and family receive hospice support and care, and family members and friends are able to spend quality time with the patient

Caregiver able and verbalizes comfort with role and lists when to call hospice team members

Patient supported through and receives the maximum benefit from palliative chemotherapy and radiation with minimal complications

Patient/caregiver lists adverse reactions, potential complications, signs/symptoms of infection (e.g., sputum change, chest congestion)

Comfort maintained through death with dignity

Pain effectively managed, and patient verbalizes comfort

Patient has stable respiratory status with patent airway (e.g., no dyspnea, infection free)

Complications from chemotherapy and radiation therapy are reduced

Patient and caregiver demonstrate compliance with care instructions

Patient is able to maintain comfort and dignity throughout illness

Patient verbalizes self-care regimen and comfort level

Patient verbalizes and demonstrates care identified on plan, including medication regimen, exercise program, and diet instructions

Other goals/outcomes based on the patient's unique needs and problems

- ***Home health aide or certified nursing assistant***
  Effective hygiene, personal care, and comfort
  ADL assistance
  Safe environment maintained

- ***Social worker***
  Problem identified and addressed with patient/caregiver and linked with appropriate support services and plan of care successfully implemented

  Patient and caregiver cope adaptively with illness and death

  Adaptive adjustment to changed body and body image

  Psychosocial support and counseling offered to patient/caregivers experiencing loss and grief

  Needs of minor children assessed and incorporated into plan

  Resources identified, community linkage obtained as appropriate for patient/family

  Funeral and burial planning assistance

- ***Volunteer(s)***
  Comfort, companionship, and friendship extended to patient/family
  Support provided as defined by the needs of the patient/caregiver
  Support and respite provided as defined by patient/caregiver

- ***Spiritual counselor***
  Spiritual support offered and provided as defined by needs of patient/ caregiver

  Provision of spiritual support and care as based on the assessed and ongoing needs of the patient and family

  Intervention and support provided related to that dimension of life related to life's meaning (consistent with patient's beliefs)

  Spiritual support offered, and patient and family needs met

  Patient/family express a relief of symptoms of spiritual suffering

  Support, listening, and presence

  Participation in sacred or spiritual rituals or practices

  Other outcomes, based on the patient's/family's unique beliefs and needs

4

- *Dietitian/Nutritional counseling*
  Family and caregiver integrating recommendations into nutrition
    teaching (where appropriate)
  Patient and caregiver know whom to call for nutrition- and
    hydration-related questions/concerns
  Nutrition and hydration per patient's choices
  Caregiver integrating dietary recommendations into daily meal planning
  Patient and family verbalize comprehension of decreasing nutritional
    needs as disease progresses

- *Occupational therapist*
  Patient and caregiver demonstrate maximum independence with ADLs,
    adaptive techniques, and assistive devices
  Patient and caregiver demonstrate maximum safety in ADLs and
    enhanced functional mobility
  Patient and caregiver demonstrate effective use of energy conservation
  Verbalization/demonstration of improved functional activity level and
    enhanced quality of life
  Patient and caregiver demonstrate effective use of diaphragmatic
    breathing to reduce shortness of breath and relaxation techniques to
    help in pain/symptom management
  Patient and caregiver demonstrate correct use of exercise
  Patient and caregiver will be independent in prosthesis and
    upper-extremity exercise programs, and patient will verbalize
    improved body image

- *Physical therapist*
  Prevention of complications
  Home exercise and upper-extremity program taught to caregiver
  Optimal strength and mobility maintained/achieved
  Compliance with home exercise program by _____ (date)

- *Bereavement counselor*
  Support services related to grief provided to patient and family
  Well-being and resolution process of grief initiated and followed
    through bereavement services
  Support services offered/provided to children

- *Music, massage, art, or other therapies or services*
  Therapeutic massage/touch effective for patient as self-reported or
    observed by caregivers/family
  Improved muscle tone, relaxation, and/or sleep
  Patient comfortable and relaxed (e.g., sleeping) after massage
  Music therapy intervention based on assessment to decrease pain
    perception and provide emotional expression and support
  Maintenance of comfort and physical, psychosocial and spiritual
    health
  Patient has pet's presence as desired—in all care sites, when possible
  Holistic health maintained and comfort achieved through
    _____ (specify modality)

7. **Patient, family and caregiver educational needs**
   Educational needs are the regimens that the caregiver will be managing with the patient. These include the following:
   - The basic tenets of hospice and the availability of support 24 hours a day, 7 days a week
   - Home safety assessment and counseling
   - The patient's medication regimen
   - Safe and proper body mechanics to promote patient comfort and prevent caregiver safety problems
   - Other teaching specific to the patient's and family's unique needs
   - Support groups available to patient's family, such as the hospice program's "Caregiver Support Group" meetings for family members and friends of the patient
   - Home safety assessment and teaching
   - Effective personal hygiene habits
   - The avoidance of infections
   - Multiple medications and their relationship to one other
   - The importance of medical follow-up
   - Self-care observational aspects of care, particularly the postoperative wound site
   - Support groups in the community that are available to your patients and their caregivers
   - The importance of wearing a Medic Alert bracelet
   - Anticipated disease progression
   - Other information based on patient's unique needs

8. **Specific tips for quality and reimbursement**
   - Document in the clinical notes the symptoms and interventions that demonstrate the clear progression of care of a patient with terminal cancer.
   - Document when/if the patient has respiratory changes, shortness of breath, exacerbation of conditions, dysphagia, pain, and other symptoms and that they are identified and resolved
   - Remember that the clinical documentation is key to measuring ongoing compliance for quality and reimbursement purposes. Care coordination, timely verbal and initial physician orders, and assessment and addressing of spiritual and psychosocial needs should be clearly documented in the patient's clinical record
   - The documentation should support that all hospice care supports comfort and dignity while meeting patient/family needs
   - The documentation should include the ongoing assessment and management of pain and other symptoms and the anticipation and prevention of secondary symptoms such as constipation
   - It is important to note that all team members, including nurses and social workers, should assess, identify, and "hear" spiritual needs that the patient/family want to be addressed. These spiritual issues are key to the provision of high-quality hospice care and cannot be addressed effectively and promptly by the spiritual counselor only

4

Document clearly symptoms, clinical changes, and assessment findings that support the end stage of the disease process

Document patient changes, symptoms, and clinical information identified from visits and team conferences that supports hospice care and a limited life expectancy

Clearly support in the documentation the rationale that supports or explains the progression of the illness from the chronic to terminal stages

Document mentation, behavioral, and cognitive changes

Document dysphagia, weight loss, increased shortness of breath, dyspnea, infection, sepsis, new or changed medications, etc.

Document any skin changes (e.g., inflamed, painful, weeping skin site[s])

Document when the patient is actively dying, deteriorating, or progressing toward death

Remember that the "litmus test" of care coordination rests on the quality of the clinical documentation completed by all team members. Review one of your patient's clinical records, and ask yourself the following: "If I was unable to give a verbal report/update on this patient, would a peer be able to pick up and provide the same level of care and know (from the documentation) the current orders, including specific medications and other details that contribute to effective hospice care?"

Document any variances to expected outcomes. Although these patients have appropriate psychosocial needs, make sure that your documentation reflects what the particular third-party payor or insurer perceives as "skilled," hands-on nursing care. Be sure that in addition to the needed professional support you provide, the wound care, observation and assessment, or pain management is reflected in your notes.

There are many models of hospice programs.

The Medicare hospice benefit does not require that the patient be homebound or have identified skilled needs. For further information on this benefit, please refer to CMS Hospice Manual 21.

Should the patient's status deteriorate and increased personal care be needed, obtain a telephone order for the increased service, noting frequency and estimating the duration.

Obtain a telephone order for all medication and treatment changes of the medical regimen, and document these in the clinical record.

Document coordination of services and consultation with other members of the IDG

Obtain orders for any change in the POC and concurrence of other team members

9. Queries for quality

Breast cancer care
- *Is patient's pain managed adequately?*
- *Is patient's anxiety managed adequately?*

- *What are the patient's symptoms?*
- *Is the patient's functional ability/status clearly documented?*
- *Have you documented to the interdisciplinary POC?*

Mastectomy care
- *Is patient's pain managed adequately?*
- *Is patient's anxiety managed adequately?*
- *What are the patient's symptoms?*
- *Is the patient's functional ability/status clearly documented?*
- *Have you documented to the interdisciplinary POC?*

10. **Resources for hospice care and practice**
    The American Cancer Society (ACS) has a "Look Good... Feel Better Program" that offers support and make-over services by cosmetologists for women undergoing chemotherapy or radiation therapy. Call 1-800-395-LOOK for more information.

    "tlc" is a magazine/catalog available through the ACS. Items include bathing suits, wigs, hair pieces, mesh hair caps to catch hair lost at night from chemotherapy, and other specifically designed products to help women feel and look dignified and attractive after loss and change. Call the ACS at 1-800-850-9445 to obtain a free catalog.

    The Y-ME National Breast Cancer Organization provides information, support, and referrals. Whenever possible, trained breast cancer survivors are matched to callers by background and experience, 1-800-221-2141. Spanish language services are available, 1-800-986-9505.

    Contact the American Cancer Society (ACS) to learn about *Reach to Recovery,* a visitation program offered by trained breast cancer survivors for women and their families, 1-800-ACS-2345. Spanish language services are also available.

    Contact Y-ME's Wig and Prosthesis Bank for women with financial need, 1-800-221-2141. Spanish language services are available at 1-800-986-9505.

4

CANCER CARE

1. General considerations

Cancer care and the generalized care of patients with cancer are characterized by frequent contact with health care providers over a long period of time.

Please refer to "Breast Cancer and Mastectomy Care," "Brain Tumor Care," "Constipation Care," "Infusion Care," and "Head and Neck Cancer Care" should these sections also pertain to your patient.

2. Needs for visit

Physician order for hospice care, specific to the hospice program's admission criteria and policies

Standard precautions supplies

Vital signs equipment for baseline assessment

Other supplies or equipment, based on physician orders

3. Safety considerations

Infection control/standard precautions

Night-light

Extra caution on slippery surfaces

Removal of scatter rugs

Tub rail, grab bars for bathroom safety

Supportive and nonskid shoes

Handrail an stairs

Fall precautions

Protective skin measures

Identification and report of any skin problems

Smoke detector and fire evacuation plan

Assistance with ambulation

Disposal of soiled dressing/sharps, intravenous (IV)/infusion administration supplies

Symptoms that necessitate immediate reporting/assistance

Safety for home medical equipment (e.g., bed, lift)

Supervised medication administration

Multiple medications (e.g., side effects, interactions, safe storage)

Others, based on the patient's unique condition and environment

4. Potential diagnoses and codes

Attention to ileostomy	V55.2
Bladder cancer	188.9
Bone marrow transplantation (surgical)	41.00
Bone metastases	198.5
Bowel obstruction	560.9
Brain cancer	191.9
Breast cancer	174.9

Cervix, cancer of	180.9
Colon cancer	153.9
Colon lymphoma	202.83
Colostomy, attention to	V55.3
Colostomy (surgical)	46.10
Debility	799.3
Endometrial cancer	182.0
Esophagus, cancer of the	150.9
Ewing's sarcoma	170.9
Failure to thrive, adult	783.7
Fitting and adjustment of urinary devices	V53.6
Fracture, pathological	733.10
Gastric cancer, metastatic	197.8
Gastrostomy, attention to	V55.1
Gastrostomy, temporary (surgical)	43.19
Glioma	191.9
Head or neck, cancer of the	195.0
Hickman catheter insertion (surgical)	38.93
Hodgkin's disease	201.90
Ileostomy, attention to	V55.2
Intestinal obstruction	560.9
Kaposi's sarcoma	176.9
Kidney cancer	189.0
Laryngectomy, complete (surgical)	30.3
Leukemia, acute	208.00
Leukopenia	288.0
Liver cancer	155.2
Liver, metastatic cancer of	197.7
Lung, adenocarcinoma	162.9
Lung cancer, squamous cell	162.9
Lung resection, segmental (surgical)	32.3
Lymphoma (non-Hodgkin's)	202.80
Malaise and fatigue	780.79
Mastectomy, radical (surgical)	85.46
Mastectomy, simple (surgical)	85.42
Melanoma, malignant	172.9
Metastases, general	199.1
Multiple myeloma	203.00
Nasopharyngeal	147.9
Nausea with vomiting	787.01
Neuroblastoma, unspecified site	194.0
Obstruction, intestinal	560.9
Oropharyngeal	146.9
Osteosarcoma	170.9
Ovarian cancer	183.0
Pancreatectomy (surgical)	52.6
Pancreatic cancer	157.9
Pharynx cancer	149.0

4

Pleural effusion, right or left	511.9
Pneumonia	486
Pressure wound	707.0
Prostate, cancer of	185
Protein-caloric malnutrition	263.9
Radiation enteritis	558.1
Radiation myelitis	323.8 and E879.2
Rectosigmoid	154.0
Rectum, cancer of the	154.1
Renal (cancer of the kidney)	189.0
Renal cell cancer, metastatic	198.0
Sarcoma	171.9
Secondary malignant neoplasm breast	198.81
Septicemia	038.9
Skin carcinoma	173.9
Spinal cord compression	336.9
Spinal cord tumor	239.7
Stomach, cancer of the	151.9
Testis, cancer of	186.9
Tongue, cancer of the	141.9
Tracheostomy, attention to	V55.0
Urinary tract infection	599.0
Uterine sarcoma, metastatic	198.82
Uterus, cancer of the	179
Vulvar cancer	184.4
Wound dehiscence	998.32

5. Skills and services identified

• *Hospice nursing*

a. *Comfort and symptom control*

Complete initial assessment of all systems of patient with cancer admitted to hospice for _____ (specify problem necessitating care)

Observation and complete assessment of the patient with cancer of _____ (specify site/type)

Presentation of hospice philosophy and services

Explain patient rights and responsibilities

Assess patient, family, and caregiver wishes and expectations regarding care

Assess patient, family, and caregiver resources available for care

Assess pain and other symptoms including site, duration, characteristics, and relief measures (see Part Six)

Provision of volunteer support to patient and family

Teach family or caregiver physical care of patient

Assess pain and other symptoms

RN to provide and teach effective oral care and comfort measures

Teach care of bedridden patient

Measure vital signs, including pain, q visit

Assess cardiovascular, pulmonary, and respiratory status

Teach new pain- or symptom-control medication regimen

Teach caregivers symptom control and relief measures

Assess weight as ordered

Oxygen on at _____ liter per _____ (specify physician orders)

Teach caregiver or family care of weak, terminally ill patient

RN to instruct in pain control measures and medications

RN to assess patient's pain or other symptoms q visit to identify need for change, addition, or other plan or dose adjustment

RN to teach patient and caregiver about disease process and management

Comfort measures of backrub and hand or other therapeutic massage

Assess pain, and evaluate the pain management's effectiveness q visit

Effective management of pain and prevention of secondary symptoms

Interventions of symptoms directed toward comfort and palliation

Teach caregiver/patient use of pain assessment tool/scale and reporting mechanism(s)

Observation and assessment of patient with nausea and vomiting who is receiving palliative radiation and chemotherapy

Teach patient and family about realistic expectations of disease process

Teach care of dying and signs/symptoms of impending death

Presence and support

Other interventions, based on patient/family needs

b. *Safety and mobility considerations*

Provide caregiver with home safety information and instruction related to _____ and documented in the clinical record

Notify Fire Department (with permission from patient) of ventilator-dependent/tracheostomy patient

Teach family about safety

Teach family about energy conservation techniques

Teach patient and caregiver care needed for safe, effective management at home

Other interventions, based on patient/family needs

c. *Emotional/Spiritual considerations*

Psychosocial assessment of patient and family regarding disease and prognosis

Assess patient's and family's coping skills

Assess mental status, sleep disturbance changes

Inform patient/family/caregiver of available volunteer support

RN to provide emotional support to patient and family

Psychosocial aspects of pain control (e.g., depression) with team support/intervention

Ongoing acknowledgment of spirituality and related concerns of patient/family

Other interventions, based on patient/family needs

d. *Skin care*

Pressure ulcer care as indicated

RN to teach patient regarding care of irradiated skin sites

RN to assess skin site after radiation therapy and teach skin care regimen

Observation and evaluation of wound and surrounding skin

Evaluate patient's need for equipment and supplies to decrease
pressure, including alternating pressure mattress, gel foam seat
cushion, and heel and elbow protectors

Teach family to perform dressing changes between RN visits,
specifically _____

Teach patient and family or caregiver about proper body alignment and
positioning in bed to prevent skin tears from shearing skin

Observe and apply skilled assessment of areas for possible breakdown,
including heels, hips, elbows, ankles, and other pressure-prone areas

Teach caregiver about skin care needs, including the need for frequent
position changes, appropriate pressure pads and mattresses, and the
prevention of breakdown

Other interventions, based on patient/family needs

e. *Elimination considerations*

Assess bowel regimen, and implement program as needed

Rectal tube for increased flatulence/gas pain

Check for and remove impaction as needed

Condom catheter or indwelling catheter as indicated

Assess amount and frequency of urinary output

Teach catheter care to caregiver

RN to teach caregiver daily care of catheter

RN to evaluate bowel patterns and need for stool softeners, laxatives,
and dietary adjustments and develop bowel management plan

Other interventions, based on patient/family needs

f. *Hydration/Nutrition*

Instruct patient about specific diet _____ (specify physician orders)

Assess nutrition/hydration status

Diet counseling for patient with anorexia

Teach feeding-tube care to family

Nutrition/hydration supported by offering patient's choice of favorite or
desired foods or liquids

Nutrition/hydration to be maintained by offering patient high-protein
diet and foods of choice as tolerated

Clinician to teach family regarding patient's need for small, high-calorie,
and frequent meals of patient's choice

Teach patient and family to expect decreased nutritional and fluid
intake as disease progresses

Other interventions, based on patient/family needs

g. *Therapeutic/Medication regimens*

Medication review and management (e.g., drug/drug, drug/food
interactions)

Measure abdominal girth for ascites and edema, and document sites and amount

Obtain venipuncture as ordered q _____ (ordered frequency)

Teach new medication regimen and side effects

Teach new pain and symptom control medication regimen

Assess for fluid and electrolyte imbalance

Administer IM or SC injection for pain control

Nonpharmacological interventions such as progressive muscle relaxation, imagery, positive visualization, music, massage and touch, and humor therapy of patient's choice implemented

Assess the patient's unique response to treatments or interventions, and report changes or unfavorable responses or reactions to the physician

Teach about and observe side effects of chemotherapy, including constipation, anemia, and fatigue

Teach patient and caregiver use of PCA pump

Other interventions, based on patient/family needs

h. *Other considerations*

RN to assess the patient's response to treatments and interventions and to report to the physician changes, unfavorable responses, or reactions

Teach family or caregiver signs of bleeding, including hematuria and bruising

Observation and assessment, communication with physician related to signs and symptoms of oncologic emergencies (e.g., spinal cord compression, superior vena cava syndrome, hypercalcemia) and symptom treatment

Assess disease process progression

Other interventions, based on patient/family needs

• *Home health aide or certified nursing assistant*

Effective and safe personal care

Safe ADL assistance and support and ambulation and transfer assist

Observation and reporting

Respite care

Active listening skills

Meal preparation

Homemaker services

Comfort care

Other duties

• *Social worker*

Psychosocial assessment of patient and family/caregiver, including adjustment to illness and its implications

Identification of optimal coping strategies

Financial assessment and counseling regarding food acquisition, ability to prepare, and costs of needed medications

Intervention/support related to terminal illness and loss

Emotional/spiritual support
Depression/fear assessed and addressed
Facilitation of communication among patient, family, and hospice team
Identification of optimal coping strategies
Referral/linkage to community services and resources as indicated
Grief counseling and intervention/support related to illness/loss
Patient/caregiver counseling and support
For patients who live alone with no support system (e.g., able, available, willing caregiver[s]), obtain linkage with necessary community resources to allow patient to stay in the home
Identification of illness-related psychiatric condition necessitating care
Facilitation of completion of will and arrangements for funeral
Funeral and burial planning assistance

- *Volunteer(s)*
Support, friendship, companionship, and presence
Comfort and dignity maintained for patient and family
Errands and transportation
Other services, based on interdisciplinary team recommendations and patient/caregiver needs

- *Spiritual counselor*
Spiritual assessment and care
Counseling, intervention, and support related to that dimension of life related to life's meaning (consistent with patient's beliefs)
Support, listening, and presence
Pray with or for the patient/family, using prayers familiar to patient's religious background (per their wishes)
Participation in sacred or spiritual rituals or practices
Funeral planning assistance
Other supportive care, based on patient's/family's needs and belief systems

- *Dietitian/Nutritional counseling*
Assessment of patient with decreased intake, weight loss, anorexia, and nausea
Assessment and recommendations for swallowing difficulties
Teaching and support of family members and caregivers
Support and care with food and nourishment as desired by patient
Evaluation/management of nutritional deficits and needs
Encourage nutritional supplements and snacks to increase protein and caloric intake
Food and dietary recommendations incorporating patient choice and wishes
Counseling and instruction of family regarding patient's decreased appetite and possible eventual inability to eat
Assessment of and instruction in use of alternative nutritional therapies such as herbs, vitamin/mineral supplements, and macrobiotic diets

- *Occupational therapist*
  Evaluation of ADL and functional mobility
  Energy conservation techniques
  Adaptive, assistive, safety supports/devices and training
  ADL training
  Measures to improve function and body image (e.g., breast prosthesis),
  as patient requests
  Assess need for adaptive/equipment devices
  Teach compensatory techniques
  Safety assessment of patient's environment and ADL measures to
  improve function and body image, such as breast or other prosthesis
  and extremity function

- *Physical therapist*
  Evaluation
  Safety assessment of patient's environment
  Safe transfer training or bed mobility exercises
  Pain assessment/reduction factors
  Strengthening exercises/program
  Assessment of gait safety and home safety measures
  Instruct/supervise caregiver and volunteers on home exercise program
  for conditioning and strength
  Evaluation of equipment (e.g., assistive, adaptive devices) and
  teaching

- *Speech-language pathologist*
  Evaluation for speech/swallowing problems
  Food texture recommendations
  Alternate functional communication

- *Bereavement counselor*
  Assessment of the needs of the bereaved family and friends
  Support and intervention, based on assessment and ongoing findings
  Presence and counseling
  Supportive visits and follow-up, other interventions (e.g., mailings,
  calls)
  Other services related to bereavement work and support

4

- *Pharmacist*
  Evaluation of hospice patient on multiple medications for possible
  food/drug, drug/drug interactions
  Medication monitoring regarding therapeutic levels and dosages
  Pain consult and input into interdisciplinary POC related to pain
  control, palliation, and symptom management
  Assessment of medication regimen and plan for safety and compliance

- *Music, massage, art, or other therapies or services*
  Evaluation and intervention based on patient's and caregiver's unique
  wishes and needs that support care, comfort, and death in the setting
  of the patient's choice

Assessment plan to engage patient and support comfort, quality, enjoyment, and dignity

Pet therapy (including patient's pet, if available) and therapeutic intervention

6. Outcomes for care

- *Hospice nursing*

Death with dignity, and symptoms controlled in setting of patient/family choice

Optimal comfort, support, and dignity provided throughout illness

Death with maximum comfort through effective symptom control with specialized hospice support

Patient and caregiver able to list adverse drug/chemotherapy/radiation reactions and know whom to call for follow-up and resolution

Pain and symptoms managed/controlled in setting of patient/family choice (e.g., patient and family report ability to eat, sleep, perform other activities)

Patient's and family's privacy, independence, and choices supported with respect and maintained through death

Enhancement and support of quality of life

Effective pain relief and symptom control (e.g., a peaceful and comfortable death at home, some enjoyment of life) (see Box 4-1)

Maximizing the patient's quality of life (e.g., alert and pain free or as patient wishes)

Pharmacological and nonpharmacological interventions, such as localized heat application, positioning, relaxation methods, and music

Patient cared for and family supported through death with physical, psychosocial, spiritual, and other concerns/needs acknowledged/addressed

Patient- and family-centered hospice care provided based on the patient's/family's unique situation and needs

Infection control and palliation

Grief/bereavement expression and support provided

Caregiver demonstrates ability to manage pain, where applicable

Patient maintains comfort and dignity throughout illness

Patient will report being comfortable _____ % of the day (comfortable as defined by patient)

Complications/side effects of chemotherapy/radiation, including infection, bleeding, dehydration, nausea, and vomiting, controlled by _____, as reported by patient/caregiver

Planned and effective bowel program, as evidenced by regular bowel movement and patient/family report of comfort

Compliance with and adherence to interdisciplinary care plan as demonstrated by observation and reporting by caregiver/patient

Patient states pain is at _____ on a scale of 1–10 by next visit

Other goals/outcomes based on the patient's unique needs and problems

---

BOX 4-1

BARRIERS TO CANCER PAIN MANAGEMENT

Problems Related to Health Care Professionals
Inadequate knowledge of pain management
Poor assessment of pain
Concern about regulation of controlled substances
Fear of patient addiction
Concern about side effects of analgesics
Concern about patients becoming tolerant to analgesics

Problems Related to Patients
Reluctance to report pain
    Concern about distracting physicians from treatment of underlying
      disease
    Fear that pain means disease is worse
    Concern about not being a "good" patient
Reluctance to take pain medications
    Fear of addiction or of being thought of as an addict
    Worries about unmanageable side effects
    Concern about becoming tolerant to pain medications

Problems Related to the Health Care System
Low priority given to cancer pain treatment
Inadequate reimbursement
    The most appropriate treatment may not be reimbursed or may be
      too costly for patients and families
Restrictive regulation of controlled substances
Problems of availability of treatment or access to it

Modified from Cancer Pain Management Guideline Panel: *Management of cancer pain. Clinical practice guideline*, AHCPR Publication No. 94-0592, Rockville, Md, 1994, Agency for Health Care Policy and Research, Public Health Service, U.S. Department of Health and Human Services.

- *Home health aide or certified nursing assistant*
  Effective hygiene, personal care, and comfort
  Safe ADL assistance and ambulation
  Safe environment maintained

- *Social worker*
  Problem identified and addressed, with patient/caregiver linked with
      appropriate support services and POC successfully implemented
  Patient and caregiver cope adaptively with illness and death
  Adaptive adjustment to changed body and body image
  Psychosocial support and counseling offered to patient/caregivers
      experiencing loss and grief
  Facilitation of will and funeral arrangements

- *Volunteer(s)*
  Comfort, companionship, and friendship extended to patient/family
  Support provided as defined by the needs of the patient/caregiver
  Patient and family supported by team with care, comfort, and
      companionship

- *Spiritual counselor*
  Spiritual support offered and provided as defined by needs of
      patient/caregiver
  Provision of spiritual support and care as based on the assessed and
      ongoing needs of the patient and family
  Spiritual support offered and patient and family needs met
  Patient and family express relief of symptoms of spiritual suffering
  Support, listening, and presence
  Participation in sacred or spiritual rituals or practices
  Intervention and support provided related to that dimension of life
      related to life's meaning (consistent with patient's beliefs)
  Pray with or for the patient/family, using prayers familiar to the
      patient's religious background (per their wishes)

- *Dietitian/Nutritional counseling*
  Family/caregiver integrating recommendations into nutrition teaching
      (where appropriate)
  Patient and family verbalize understanding of changing nutritional needs
  Patient/caregiver know whom to call for nutrition- and
      hydration-related questions/concerns
  Nutrition/hydration per patient's choices
  Caregiver integrating recommendations into daily meal planning

- *Occupational therapist*
  Patient and caregiver demonstrate maximum independence with ADLs,
      adaptive techniques, and assistive devices
  Patient and caregiver demonstrate maximum safety in ADL and
      functional mobility
  Patient and caregiver demonstrate effective use of energy conservation
  Verbalization/demonstration of improved functional activity level and
      enhanced quality of life
  Patient and caregiver demonstrate effective use of diaphragmatic
      breathing to reduce shortness of breath and relaxation techniques to
      help in pain/symptom management
  Patient and caregiver will be independent in prosthesis and upper-
      extremity exercise programs, and will verbalize improved body
      image

- *Physical therapist*
  Prevention of complications
  Home exercise and upper-extremity program taught to caregiver
  Optimal strength and mobility maintained/achieved
  Compliance with home exercise program by _____ (date)

- *Speech-language pathologist*
  Communication method implemented, and patient able to be
  understood as self-reported or reported by family/caregivers
  Safe swallowing and functional communication
  Recommended list of food textures for safety and patient choice

- *Bereavement counselor*
  Grief support services provided to patient and family
  Well-being and resolution process of grief initiated and followed
  through bereavement services

- *Pharmacist*
  Multiple drug regimen reviewed for food/drug and drug/drug
  interactions in patient on steroids and other medications
  Stability and safety in complex medication regimen
  Effective pain and symptom control and symptom management as
  reported by patient/caregiver

- *Music, massage, art, or other therapies or services*
  Therapeutic massage/touch effective for patient as self-reported or
  observed by caregivers/family
  Improved muscle tone, relaxation, and/or sleep
  Patient comfortable and relaxed (e.g., sleeping) after massage
  Music therapy intervention based on assessment to decrease pain
  perception and provide emotional expression and support
  Maintenance of comfort and physical, psychosocial, and spiritual health
  Holistic health maintained and comfort achieved through
  _____ (specify modality)
  Patient has pet's presence as desired—in all care sites, when possible

7. **Patient, family, and caregiver educational needs**
   Educational needs are the care regimens that contribute to safe and
   effective care at home between the hospice team's visits. These include
   the following:
   The basic tenets of hospice and the availability of support 24 hours a
   day, 7 days a week
   Home safety assessment and counseling
   The patient's medication regimen
   Safe and proper body mechanics to promote patient comfort and
   prevent caregiver safety problems
   Anticipated disease progression
   Support groups available to patient's family, such as the hospice
   program's "Caregiver Support Group" meetings for family mem-
   bers and friends of the patient

8. **Specific tips for quality and reimbursement**
   Administer other teaching specific to the patient's and family's unique
   needs. Document any variances to expected outcomes. There are many
   models of hospice programs.

The Medicare hospice benefit does not require that the patient be homebound or have identified skilled needs. For further information on this benefit, please refer to CMS Hospice Manual 21.

Should the patient's status deteriorate and increased personal care be needed, obtain a telephone order for the increased service, noting frequency and estimating the duration.

Obtain a telephone order for all medication and treatment changes of the medical regimen and document these in the clinical record.

Document the clear progression of symptoms of the disease process and interventions that demonstrate caring for a patient with terminal cancer in the clinical notes

Document when/if the patient has respiratory changes, shortness of breath, exacerbation of conditions, dysphagia, pain, and other symptoms and that they are identified and resolved

Remember that the clinical documentation is key to measuring compliance for quality and reimbursement purposes. Care coordination, timely verbal and initial physician orders, and assessment and addressing of spiritual and psychosocial needs should be clearly documented in the patient's clinical record

Documentation should support that all hospice care supports comfort and dignity while meeting patient/family needs

Documentation should include the ongoing assessment and management of pain and other symptoms and the anticipation and prevention of secondary symptoms such as constipation

It is important to note that all team members, including clinicians and social workers, should assess, identify, and "hear" spiritual needs that the patient/family want to be addressed. These spiritual issues are key to the provision of high-quality hospice care and cannot be addressed effectively and promptly by the spiritual counselor only

Document clearly symptoms, clinical changes, and assessment findings that consitute evidence of the end stage of the cancer process

Document patient changes, symptoms, and clinical information identified from visits and team conferences that support the need for hospice care and that constitute evidence of a limited life expectancy

Clearly support in the documentation the rationale that supports/explains the progression of the illness from the chronic to terminal stages

Document mentation, behavioral, and/or cognitive changes

Document dysphagia, weight loss, increased shortness of breath, dyspnea, infection, sepsis, new or changed medications, etc.

Document any skin changes (e.g., inflamed, painful, weeping skin sites)

Document when the patient is actively dying, deteriorating, and progressing toward death

Remember that the "litmus test" of care coordination rests on the quality of the clinical documentation by all team members. Review one of your patient's clinical records, and ask yourself, "If I was unable to give a verbal report/update on this patient, would a peer be able to pick up and provide the same level of care and know (from the documentation) the current orders, medications, and other details that contribute to effective hospice care?"

Documentation of coordination of services and consultation with the other members of the IDG

Unless the patient is in a hospice insurance program, some insurers will not pay for a skilled nurse visit that is made at death if the patient is dead when the clinician arrives at the home. From a Medicare home care perspective, the visit at the time of death may be covered when the orders and clinical record allows pronouncement of death by a clinician.

Document patient deterioration

Document dehydration, dehydrating

Document patient change or instability

Document pain or uncontrolled symptoms not controlled

Document status after acute episode of _____ (specify)

Document positive urine, sputum, etc. culture; patient started on _____ (specify ordered antibiotic therapy)

Document any impaction; impaction removed manually

Document RN in frequent communication with physician regarding _____ (specify)

Document febrile at _____, pulse change at _____, irr., irr.

Document change noted in _____

Document bony prominences red, opening

Document RN contacted physician regarding _____ (specify)

Document marked SOB

Document alteration in mental status

Document medications being adjusted, regulated, or monitored

Document unable to perform ADLs, personal care

Document all IDT meetings and communications in the POC and in the progress notes of the clinical record

All disciplines involved should have input into the POC and document their interventions and goals

9. Queries for quality

Cancer care
- *Is patient's pain managed adequately?*
- *Is patient's anxiety managed adequately?*
- *What are the patient's symptoms?*
- *Does patient/family have access to appropriate community resources, and are they documented in the record?*
- *Have you documented to the interdisciplinary POC?*

Tumor care
- *Is patient's pain managed adequately?*
- *Is patient's anxiety managed adequately?*
- *What are the patient's symptoms?*

- *Does patient/family have access to appropriate community resources, and are they documented in the record?*
- *Have you documented to the interdisciplinary POC?*

10. Resources for hospice care and practice

The National Cancer Institute (NCI) offers a 37-page free publication entitled *Advanced Cancer: Living Each Day*, which can be ordered by calling 1-800-4-CANCER. The NCI and the American Cancer Society (ACS) offer a publication called *Caring for the Patient with Cancer at Home: A Guide for Patients and Families*. This 90-page publication covers many symptoms and problems associated with cancer and cancer therapy. This booklet can be ordered by calling the ACS at 1-800-ACS-2345 or the NCI at 1-800-4-CANCER.

The American Cancer Society has support groups such as "I Can Cope" and other programs. To locate the chapter nearest your patient, call 1-800-ACS-2345.

The American Cancer Society also has a "Look Good... Feel Better Program" for women undergoing chemotherapy or radiation. It can be reached at 1-800-395-LOOK.

A pamphlet entitled *Get Relief from Cancer Pain* is available from the National Cancer Institute's Cancer Information Service by calling 1-800-4-CANCER (1-800-422-6237).

Questions and Answers about Pain Control, a 76-page booklet, is available free from the Cancer Information Service by calling the toll-free number.

4

CARDIAC CARE (END STAGE)

1. General considerations

Patients and families may be referred to hospice for progressive and cardiac myopathies, severe congestive heart failure, angina, post myocardial infarctions, and many other cardiac problems. These patients and their families have usually had a long history of curative and aggressive treatment directed toward the cardiac disease. Supportive and skillful care is directed toward comfort and symptomatic relief of chest pain, shortness of breath, and other problems.

2. Needs for visit

Physician order for hospice care, specific to the hospice program's admission criteria and policies

Standard precautions supplies

Vital signs equipment for baseline assessment

Other supplies or equipment, based on physician orders

3. Safety considerations

Infection control/standard precautions

Disposal of soiled dressings, sharps, intravenous (IV) infusion administration supplies

Supervised medication administration

Tub rail, grab bars, shower seat for bathroom safety

Supportive and nonskid shoes

Fall precautions

Oxygen precautions

Identification and report of any skin problems/changes

Multiple medications (e.g., side effects, heparin precautions, interactions, safe storage)

Night-light

Safety for home medical equipment (e.g., bed, lift)

Cardiac or other symptoms that necessitate reporting/assistance

Smoke detector and fire evacuation plan

Pace activities

Change positions slowly

Protective skin measures

Others, based on the patient's unique condition and environment

4. Potential diagnoses and codes

Abdominal aortic aneurysm	441.4
Acute myocardial infarction	410.90
Anemia	285.9
Aneurysm repair (surgical)	39.52
Angina	413.9
Angina, unstable	411.1

Angioplasty (percutaneous) (surgical)	39.59
Aortic stenosis	424.1
Aortic valve disorder	424.1
Aortocoronary bypass (one vessel) (surgical)	36.11
Aortocoronary bypass (four vessls) (surgical)	36.14
Atherosclerosis (coronary)	414.00
Atrial fibrillation	427.31
Atrial flutter	427.32
Bacterial endocarditis	421.0
Cardiac dysrhythmia	427.9
Cardiac murmurs	785.2
Cardiomegaly	429.3
Cardiomyopathy	425.4
Chronic ischemic heart disease	414.9
Congestive heart failure	428.0
Chronic obstructive pulmonary disease (COPD)	496
Cor pulmonale	416.9
Coronary artherosclerosis (coronary artery disease)	414.00
Coronary artery bypass graft surgery	
two coronary arteries (surgical)	36.12
three coronary arteries (surgical)	36.13
four coronary arteries (surgical)	36.14
Coronary bypass syndrome	411.1
Cerebrovascular accident (CVA)	436
Depressive disorder	311
Diabetes (type I) juvenile, with complications	250.91
Diabetes (type II) adult, with complications	250.90
Digoxin toxicity	995.2 and E942.1
Electrolyte and fluid imbalance	276.9
Endocarditis	424.90
Failure to thrive, adult	783.7
HCVD with congestive heart failure (CHF)	402.91
Heart block	426.9
Heart disease, end stage	429.9
Heart transplant (surgical)	37.5
Hypertension with heart involvement	402.90
Ischemic heart disease	414.9
Left heart failure	428.1
Mediastinitis	519.2
Mitral valve disease	394.9
Mitral valve disorder	424.0
Myocardial infarction	410.92
Obesity	278.00
Other aftercare following surgery	V58.4
Pacemaker (S/P)	V45.00
Pericardial disease	423.9
Peripheral vascular disease	443.9
Pleural effusion	511.9

4

Pneumonia	486
Postsurgical status, aortocoronary bypass status	V45.81
Postsurgical status, presence of neuropacemaker or other electronic device (implanted automatic cardiac defibrillator)	V45.89
Pulmonary edema with cardiac disease	428.1
Respiratory arrest (S/P)	799.1
Respiratory failure, acute	518.81
Substernal wound infection	998.5
Transplant, heart (surgical)	37.51
Venous thrombosis	453.9
Wound dehiscence	998.32
Wound infection	998.59

5. Skills and services identified

• *Hospice nursing*

a. *Comfort and symptom control*

Observation and assessment of patient with long-standing congestive heart failure on multiple medications, admitted to hospice with severe edema, with poor activity tolerance, and on oxygen therapy 24 hours a day

Observation and complete system assessment of patient with cardiac disease _____ (specify physician's orders)

Presentation of hospice philosophy and services

Explain patient rights and responsibilities

Assess patient, family, and caregiver wishes and expectations regarding care

Assess patient, family, and caregiver resources available for care

Provision of volunteer support to patient and family

Teach family or caregiver physical care of patient

Assess pain and other symptoms, including site, duration, characteristics, and relief measures

RN to monitor for presence and amount of lower leg edema

Teach patient or caregiver record keeping for daily weights and other aspects of self-observational care skills

Assess site, amount, and frequency of chest pain episodes

Teach care of bedridden patient

Measure vital signs and pain q visit

Assess pain, and evaluate the pain management's effectiveness

RN to observe for signs and symptoms of digoxin toxicity, including GI symptoms such as vomiting or nausea and neurological changes such as visual disturbances, headache, and cardiovascular manifestations

RN to observe for signs and symptoms of infection

Teach patient signs and symptoms of pacemaker problems or failure, including increased SOB, cough, pulse change, and increased edema

RN to assess and monitor patient's pain, implement ordered pain control/relief measures, and assess patient's response to interventions—surgical or cardiac pain

Assess for orthostatic hypotension

Comprehensive patient/family education regarding signs, symptoms of CHF, daily records of weight, I & O, infusion pump care, etc.

Assess cardiovascular, pulmonary, and respiratory status

Assess for SOB and dyspnea, and promote rest and pacing of activities

Comfort measures of backrub and hand or other therapeutic massage

Oxygen on at _____ liters per _____ (specify physician orders)

Teach caregivers symptom control and relief measures

Pain assessment and management q visit

Identify and monitor pain, symptoms, and relief measures

Teach caregiver or family care of weak, terminally ill patient

RN to assess patient's pain or other symptoms q visit to identify need for change, addition, or other plan or dose adjustment

Observation and assessment, communication with physician related to signs and symptoms of continuing decompensation and increased symptoms, pain, discomfort, shortness of breath, and measures to alleviate and control

Teach caregiver/patient use of pain assessment tool/scale and reporting mechanism(s)

Effective management of pain and prevention of secondary symptoms

RN to provide and teach effective oral care and comfort measures

Intervention of symptoms directed toward comfort and palliation

Teach patient/family about realistic expectations of disease process

Teach care of dying and signs/symptoms of impending death

Presence and support

Other interventions, based on patient/family needs

b. *Safety and mobility considerations*

Patient provided with home safety information and instruction related to _____ and documented in the clinical record

Teach patient and family regarding energy conservation techniques

RN to teach care and safety regarding oxygen safety at home

Teach patient and family about planning and pacing activities

Teach family regarding safety of patient in home

Other interventions, based on patient/family needs

c. *Emotional/Spiritual considerations*

Psychosocial assessment of patient and family regarding disease and prognosis

Assess mental status and sleep disturbance changes

Psychosocial aspects of pain control (e.g., depression) assessed and acknowledged with team support/intervention

RN to provide emotional support to patient and family

Inform patient/family/caregiver of available volunteer support

Ongoing acknowledgment of spirituality and related concerns of patient/family

Other interventions, based on patient/family needs

d. *Skin care*

RN to provide skilled observation and assessment of surgical sites, post–cardiac surgery care

Observation and assessment of skin

RN to assess wound site, change dressing (specify dressing orders and frequency per physician orders, and teach caregiver about wound and infection control care)

RN to culture wound site and send to lab for C & S

Pressure ulcer care as indicated

Assess skin integrity

Evaluate patient's need for equipment and supplies to decrease pressure, including alternating pressure mattress, gel foam seat cushion, and heel and elbow protectors

Observation and evaluation of wound and surrounding skin

Teach family to perform dressing changes between RN visits, specifically _____

Teach patient, family, or caregiver about proper body alignment and positioning in bed to prevent skin tears from shearing skin

Observation and skilled assessment of areas for possible breakdown, including heels, hips, elbows, ankles, and other pressure-prone areas

Teach caregiver regarding skin care needs, including the need for frequent position changes, appropriate pressure pads and mattresses, and the prevention of breakdown

Other interventions, based on patient/family needs

e. *Elimination considerations*

Assess bowel regimen, and implement program as needed

Check for and remove impaction as needed (per physician orders)

Condom catheter or indwelling catheter as indicated

Assess amount and frequency of urinary output

RN to teach catheter care to caregiver

RN to teach caregiver daily care of catheter

RN to evaluate the patient's bowel patterns and need for stool softeners, laxatives, and dietary adjustments, and to develop bowel management plan

Other interventions, based on patient/family needs

f. *Hydration/Nutrition*

Instruct patient about specified diet _____ (specify physician orders)

Teaching and training regarding diet and exercise

Assess nutrition and hydration statuses, and provide nutritional information/education

Diet counseling for patient with anorexia

Teach feeding-tube care to family

Obtain weights as ordered to assist in comfort and medication regulation

Nutrition/hydration supported by offering patient's choice of favorite or desired foods or liquids

Nutrition/hydration maintained by offering patient high-protein diet and foods of choice as tolerated

Teach patient and family to expect decreased nutritional and fluid intake as disease progresses

Other interventions, based on patient/family needs

g. *Therapeutic/Medication regimens*

RN to instruct patient and caregiver regarding multiple medication, including schedule, functions, routes, knowledge, compliance, and possible side effects

RN to assess the patient's unique response to treatments or interventions, and to report changes, unfavorable responses, or reactions to the physician

Assess for nitroglycerin use, frequency, amount, and relief patterns

Patient education related to side effects and actions of multiple medications

Medication management related to complex regimen including beta blockers, anticoagulants, antihypertensives, etc. Consider drug/drug, drug/food interactions

Teach new pain and symptom control medication regimen

Medication assessment and management

Teach new medication regimen and side effects

Teach patient and caregiver use of PCA pump

RN to instruct in pain control measures and medications

Implement nonpharmacological interventions such as progressive muscle relaxation, imagery, positive visualization, music, massage and touch, and humor therapy of patient's choice

Other interventions, based on patient/family needs

h. *Other considerations*

Assess disease progression of process

RN to assess the patient's response to treatments and interventions and to report to the physician changes, unfavorable responses, or reactions

Other interventions, based on patient/family needs

- **Home health aide or certified nursing assistant**

Effective and safe personal care

Safe ADL assistance and support

Respite care and active listening skills

Observation and reporting

Meal preparation

Homemaker services

Comfort care

Other duties

- **Social worker**

Psychosocial assessment of patient and family/caregiver, including adjustment to illness and its implications

Identification of optimal coping strategies

Financial assessment and counseling regarding food acquisition, ability to prepare, and costs of needed medications

Intervention/support related to terminal illness and loss
Emotional/spiritual support
Depression/fear assessed and addressed
Facilitate communication among patient, family, and hospice team
Referral/linkage to community services and resources as
indicated
Grief counseling and intervention/support related to illness/loss
Patient/caregiver counseling and support
Identification of caregiver role strain necessitating respite/relief
measures/support
For patients who live alone with no support system (e.g., able,
available, willing caregiver[s]), obtain linkage with necessary
community resources to enable patient to remain in the home
Identification of illness related psychiatric condition
Funeral and burial planning assistance

- *Volunteer(s)*
  Support, friendship, companionship, and presence
  Comfort and dignity maintained/provided for patient and family
  Errands and transportation
  Other services, based on interdisciplinary team recommendations and
  patient/caregiver needs

- *Spiritual counselor*
  Spiritual assessment and care
  Counseling, intervention, and support related to that dimension of life
  related to life's meaning (consistent with patient's beliefs)
  Support, listening, and presence
  Pray with or for the patient/family, using prayers familiar to patient's
  religious background (per their wishes)
  Participation in sacred or spiritual rituals or practices
  Funeral planning assitance
  Other supportive care, based on patient/family needs and
  belief systems

- *Dietitian/Nutritional counseling*
  Assessment of patient with decreased intake, weight gain/loss, anorexia,
  and nausea
  Supportive counseling with patient/family indicating that patient will
  have a decreased appetite and usually at some point may not
  eat/drink
  Assessment and recommendations for swallowing difficulties
  Teaching and support of family members and caregivers
  Support and care with food and nourishment as desired by patient
  Evaluation/management of nutritional deficits and needs
  Encourage nutritional supplements and snacks to increase protein and
  caloric intake
  Food and dietary recommendations incorporating patient choice and
  wishes

4

- *Occupational therapist*
  Evaluation of ADL and functional mobility
  Assessment of need for adaptive equipment and assistive devices
  Safety assessment of patient's environment and ADLs
  Assessment for energy conservation training
  Energy conservation techniques

- *Physical therapist*
  Evaluation
  Safety assessment of patient's environment
  Safe transfer training or bed mobility exercises
  Pain assessment/reduction factors
  Strengthening exercises/program
  Assessment of gait safety and home safety measures
  Instruct/supervise caregiver and volunteers on home exercise program
      for conditioning and strength
  Assistive, adaptive devices and evaluation of equipment and teaching

- *Bereavement counselor*
  Assessment of the needs of the bereaved family and friends
  Support and intervention, based on assessment and ongoing findings
  Presence and counseling
  Supportive visits and follow-up, other interventions (e.g., mailings,
      calls)
  Other services related to bereavement work and support

- *Pharmacist*
  Evaluation of hospice patient on multiple cardiac medications for
      possible food/drug, drug/drug interactions
  Medication monitoring regarding therapeutic levels and dosages
  Pain consult and input into interdisciplinary plan of care related to pain
      control, palliation, and symptom management
  Assessment of medication regimen and plan for safety and compliance
  Other interventions, based on the unique needs of the patient/family

- *Music, massage, art, or other therapies or services*
  Evaluation and intervention based on patient's and caregiver's unique
      wishes and needs that support care, comfort, and death in the setting
      of the patient's choice
  Assessment plan to engage patient and support comfort, quality,
      enjoyment, and dignity
  Pet therapy (including patient's pet, if available) and therapeutic
      intervention
  Other interventions, based on the unique needs of the patient/family

6. **Outcomes for care**

- *Hospice nursing*
  Death with dignity and symptoms controlled in setting of patient/family
      choice

Optimal comfort, support, and dignity provided throughout illness

Death with maximum comfort through effective symptom control with specialized hospice support

Patient/caregiver able to list adverse cardiac drug reactions/problems with infusion pump/site and whom to call for follow-up and resolution

Patient reports decrease in SOB, chest pain by _____ (specify date)

Caregiver effective in care management and knows whom to call for questions/concerns

Skin integrity maintained as evidenced by problem-free skin

Pain controlled and comfort needs met throughout POC

IV access site remains patent without signs/symptoms of infection, and flushing/dressing care is provided per protocol

Patient verbalizes understanding of and adheres to medication regimens

Patient/caregiver verbalizes side effects and actions of anticoagulant therapy

Regulated bowel program, as evidenced by regular bowel movements

Patient will report being comfortable _____ % of the day (*comfortable* as defined by patient)

Compliance with and adherence to interdisciplinary care plan as demonstrated by observation and reporting by caregiver/patient

Patient and caregiver verbalize satisfaction with care

Educational tools/plans incorporated in daily care, and patient and caregiver verbalize understanding of safe, needed care

Patient will decide on care, interventions, and evaluation

Caregiver effective in care management and knows whom to call for questions/concerns

Patient will express satisfaction with hospice support received and will experience increased comfort

Patient will be made comfortable at home through death in accordance with the patient's wishes

Effective pain control and symptom control verbalized by patient

Patient verbalizes understanding of and adheres to care and medication regimens

Patient and caregiver supported through patient's death

Comfort maintained through course of care

The patient and family receive hospice support and care, and family members and friends are able to spend quality time with the patient

Caregiver able and verbalizes comfort with role and understands when to call hospice team members

Patient supported through and receives the maximum benefit from palliative chemotherapy and radiation with minimal complications

Patient and caregiver list adverse reactions, potential complications, signs/symptoms of infection (e.g., sputum change, chest congestion)

Comfort maintained through death with dignity

Pain effectively managed, and patient verbalizes comfort

Patient has stable respiratory status with patent airway (e.g., no dyspnea, infection free)

Optimal gas exchange and comfort as measured through oximetry and laboratory tests

Patient is protected from injury, has stable respiratory status, and is compliant with medication, safety, and care regimens

Comfort and individualized intervention of patient with immobility/bedbound status (e.g, skin, urinary, musculature, vascular)

Spiritual and psychosocial needs met (specify) as defined by patient and caregiver throughout course of care

Patient states pain is _____ on 0–10 scale by next visit

Patient and caregiver demonstrate appropriate backup or "rescue" therapies for breakthrough pain or other symptoms (e.g., dyspnea)

Pain and symptoms managed/controlled in setting of patient/family choice (e.g., patient/family report ability to eat, sleep, speak clearly with pacing)

Patient's/family's privacy, independence, and choices supported with respect and maintained through death

Enhancement and support of quality of life

Effective symptom relief and control (e.g., a peaceful and comfortable death at home, some enjoyment of life)

Maximizing the patient's quality of life (e.g., alert and pain free or as patient wishes)

Pharmacological and nonpharmacological interventions such as localized heat application, positioning, relaxation methods, and music

Patient cared for and family supported through death with physical, psychosocial, spiritual, and other concerns/needs acknowledged/addressed

Patient- and family-centered hospice care provided based on the patient's/family's unique situation and needs

Infection control and palliation

Grief/bereavement expression and support provided

Patient is pain free by next visit

Caregiver demonstrates ability to manage pain, where applicable

Patient maintains comfort and dignity throughout illness

Planned and effective bowel program, as evidenced by bowel movements and patient/family report of comfort

- *Home health aide or certified nursing assistant*
  Effective hygiene, personal care, and comfort
  ADL assistance
  Comfort and presence
  Observation and reporting
  Safe environment maintained

- *Social worker*
  Problem identified and addressed, with patient/caregiver linked with appropriate support services and plan of care successfully implemented
  Patient and caregiver cope adaptively with illness and death
  Adaptive adjustment to changed body and body image

Psychosocial support and counseling offered to patient/caregivers
experiencing loss and grief
Caregiver system assessed and development of stable caregiver plan
facilitated
Resources identified, community linkage as appropriate for patient/family
Funeral and burial planning assistance

- *Volunteer(s)*
   Comfort, companionship, and friendship extended to patient/family
   Patient and caregiver support as defined by needs of patient/family
   Support and respite provided as defined by the patient/caregiver

- *Spiritual counselor*
   Spiritual support assessed, offered, and provided as defined by needs of
   patient/caregiver
   Participation in sacred or spiritual rituals or practices (consistent with
   patient's beliefs)
   Provision of spiritual support and care as based on the assessed and
   ongoing needs of the patient and family
   Support, listening, and presence
   Spiritual support offered and patient/family needs met
   Patient/family express a relief of symptoms of spiritual suffering
   Intervention and support provided related to that dimension of life
   related to life's meaning (consistent with patient's beliefs)
   Pray with or for the patient/family, using prayers familiar to the
   patient's religious background (per their wishes)

- *Dietitian/Nutritional counseling*
   Family and caregiver integrating recommendations into nutrition
   teaching (where appropriate)
   Patient and caregiver know whom and where to call for nutrition- and
   hydration-related questions/concerns
   Nutrition/hydration per patient/caregiver choices
   Caregiver demonstrates use of recommendations into daily meal planning
   Patient/family verbalize comprehension of changing nutritional needs

4

- *Occupational therapist*
   Patient and caregiver demonstrate maximum independence with ADLs,
   adaptive techniques, and assistive devices
   Patient and caregiver demonstrate maximum safety in ADL and
   functional mobility
   Patient and caregiver demonstrate effective use of energy conservation
   Verbalization/demonstration of improved functional activity level and
   enhanced quality of life
   Patient and caregiver demonstrate effective use of diaphragmatic
   breathing to reduce shortness of breath and relaxation techniques to
   help in pain/symptom management

- *Physical therapist*
   Prevention of complications
   Home exercise and upper-extremity program taught to caregiver

Optimal strength, mobility, function maintained/achieved
Compliance with home exercise program by _____ (specify date)

- ***Bereavement counselor***
  Support services related to grief provided to patient and family
  Well-being and resolution process of grief initiated and followed
  through bereavement services

- ***Pharmacist***
  Multiple drug regimen reviewed for food/drug and drug/drug
  interactions in patient on dobutamine infusions for end stage cardiac
  disease and other medications
  Stability and safety in complex medication regimen with maximum
  benefit to patient
  Effective pain and symptom control and symptom management as
  reported by patient/caregiver
  Laboratory reports reviewed for therapeutic dosages and effective
  patient response

- ***Music, massage, art, or other therapies or services***
  Therapeutic massage/touch effective for patient as self-reported or
  observed by caregivers/family
  Improved muscle tone, relaxation, and/or sleep
  Patient comfortable and relaxed (e.g., sleeping) after massage
  Music therapy intervention based on assessment to decrease pain
  perception and provide emotional expression and support
  Maintenance of comfort and physical, psychosocial, and spiritual
  health
  Holistic health maintained and comfort achieved through
  _____ (specify modality)
  Patient has pet's presence as desired—in all care sites, when possible

4

7. **Patient, family, and caregiver educational needs**
   Educational needs are the care regimens that contribute to safe and effec-
   tive care at home between the hospice team's visits. These include the
   following:
   The basic tenets of hospice and the availability of support 24 hours a
   day, 7 days a week
   Home safety assessment and counseling
   The patient's medication regimen
   Safe and proper body mechanics to promote patient comfort and
   prevent caregiver safety problems
   Other teaching specific to the patient's and family's unique needs
   Support groups available to patient's family, such as the hospice
   program's "Caregiver Support Group" meetings for family mem-
   bers and friends of the patient
   Anticipated disease progression
   Effective use of oxygen, including use, ordered liter flow, and safety
   Other teaching specific to the patient and family/caregiver needs

8. Specific tips for quality and reimbursement

Document any variances to expected outcomes. There are many models of hospice programs.

The Medicare hospice benefit does not require that the patient be homebound or have identified skilled needs. For further information on this benefit, please refer to CMS Hospice Manual 21.

Should the patient's status deteriorate and increased personal care be needed, obtain a telephone order for the increased service, noting frequency and estimating the duration.

Obtain a telephone order for all medication and treatment changes of the medical regimen and document these in the clinical record.

Unless the patient is in a hospice insurance program, some insurers will not pay for a skilled clinician visit that is made at death if the patient is dead when the clinician arrives at the home. From a Medicare home care perspective, the visit at the time of death may be covered when the orders and clinical record document assessment of the patient's status or signs of death/life or state law allows pronouncement of death by an RN.

Document patient deterioration
Document dehydration, dehydrating
Document patient change or instability
Document pain, other symptoms not controlled
Document status after acute episode of _____ (specify)
Document positive urine, sputum, etc. culture; patient started
    on _____ (specify ordered antibiotic therapy)
Document patient impacted; impaction removed manually
Document RN in frequent communication with physician
    regarding _____ (specify)
Document febrile at _____, pulse change at _____, irr., irr.
Document change noted in _____
Document bony prominences red, opening
Document RN contacted physician regarding _____ (specify)
Document marked SOB
Document alteration in mental status
Document medications being adjusted, regulated, or monitored
Document unable to perform own ADLs, personal care
Document all interdisciplinary team meetings and communications in
    the POC and in the progress notes of the clinical record
All hospice team members should have input into the POC and
    document their interventions and goals
Remember that the clinical documentation is key to measuring
    compliance for quality and reimbursement purposes. Care
    coordination, timely verbal and initial physician orders, and
    assessment and addressing of spiritual and psychosocial needs
    should be ongoing and documented in the patient's
    clinical record
The documentation should support that all hospice care supports
    comfort and dignity while meeting patient/family needs

4

The documentation should include ongoing assessment and management of pain and other symptoms and the anticipation and prevention of secondary symptoms such as constipation

It is important to note that all team members, including clinicians and social workers, should assess, identify, and "hear" spiritual needs that the patient and family want to be addressed. These spiritual issues are key to the provision of high-quality hospice care and cannot be addressed effectively and promptly by the spiritual counselor only

Document clearly symptoms, clinical changes, and assessment findings related to pain and patient care

Document weight loss, increased shortness of breath, dyspnea, infection, sepsis, new or changed medications, etc.

Document any skin changes (e.g., inflamed, painful, weeping skin site[s])

Remember that the "litmus test" of care coordination rests on the quality of the clinical documentation by all team members. Review one of your patient's clinical records and ask yourself the following: "If I was unable to give a verbal report/update on this patient's/family's course of care, would a peer be able to pick up and provide the same level of care and know (from the documentation) the current orders, medications, and other details that contribute to effective hospice care?"

This patient population usually has many clinical changes that should be documented. These include weight loss and multiple and changed medication regimens with varying routes. Side effects of the drug regimen should be observed, noted, documented, and reported

Your assessments, observations, and clinical findings assist in painting a picture to support coverage and documentation requirements for hospice care

Document any hospitalizations and changed clinical findings

Document patient changes, symptoms, and psychosocial issues impacting the patient and family and plan of care

Document changes to the plan of care such as medications, services, frequency, communications, and concurrence of other team members

Document coordination of services or consultation of the other members of the IDT

Document communications and care coordination with other care providers, such as skilled health care facility or nursing home staff, inpatient team members, and hired caregivers

Document any hospitalizations and changed clinical findings

In the clinical documentation, paint the picture of your end-stage cardiac patient. The patient may be on multiple cardiac medications, have bad multiple cardiac events or surgeries, have chronic edema, need oxygen at all times, be very short of breath, and have poor or no activity tolerance or energy. This is the kind of specificity in the clinical documentation that clearly shows why the hospice team was called in at this point along the patient's illness continuum and supports coverage and documentation requirements of an insurance provider, such as Medicare

For this and other noncancer diagnoses, document clearly the symptoms and clinical and assessment findings that support the end stage of the chronic illness process

Document patient changes, symptoms, psychosocial issues impacting the care, and information gathered at the patient/family visits and during team meetings

The documentation should reflect ongoing effects of the terminal condition, the patient's/family's difficulty with care or coping, and the continued desire for hospice care

Document angina episodes and relief interventions

Note easy fatigability or any episodes of palpitations

Document dyspnea, with or without activity

Document orthopnea, lower extremity or other edema

Document decreased tolerance to activity or other changes

9. Queries for quality

- *Is patient's pain managed adequately?*
- *Is patient's anxiety managed adequately?*
- *Is patient's functional ability/status clearly documented?*
- *What are the patient's symptoms?*
- *Have you documented to the interdisciplinary POC?*

10. Resources for hospice care and practice

A helpful resource is the National Hospice on Palliative Care Organization's latest edition of *Medical Guidelines for Determining Prognoses in Selected Non-Cancer Diseases.* Call NHPCO at 1-800-646-6460.

www.lungusa.org, The American Lung Association's web site, offers "Traveling with Oxygen," a fact sheet. For more information, call (212)315-8700.

CEREBRAL VASCULAR ACCIDENT (CVA) CARE

1. General considerations

Because of the high prevalence of hypertension, cerebral vascular accident (CVA), or **stroke**, continues to be a leading cause of illness and death.

Please refer to "Bedbound Care," "Cardiac Care," or "Pain Care" should these sections pertain to your patient.

2. Needs for visit

Physician order for hospice care, specific to the hospice program's admission criteria and policies

Standard precautions supplies

Vital signs equipment for baseline assessment

Other supplies or equipment, based on physician orders

3. Safety considerations

Infection control/standard precautions

Night-light

Extra caution on slippery surfaces

Removal of scatter rugs

Tub rail, grab bars for bathroom safety

Supportive and nonskid shoes

Handrail on stairs

Fall precautions/protocol

Protective skin measures

Identification and report of any skin problems

Protection of affected extremities from injury

Bathroom safety supports, including shower bench, tub rails

Wheelchair precautions/assisted ambulation and transfers

Safety for home medical equipment (e.g., bed, cane)

The phone number and name of person to call with a care problem

Smoke detector and fire evacuation plan

Others, based on the patient's unique condition and environment

4. Potential diagnoses and codes

AMI	410.92
Angina	413.9
Aphasia	784.3
Atrial fibrillation	427.31
Carotid artery occlusion	433.1
Catheter, indwelling	57.94
Cerebrovascular disease	437.9
CHF	428.0
COPD	496
Cor pulmonale	416.9
CVA	436

CVA with dysphasia	436 and 784.5
Diabetes mellitus, with complications, NIDDM	250.90
Diabetes mellitus, with complications, IDDM	250.91
Dysphagia	787.2
Dysphagia and CVA	782.2 and 436.0
Emphysema	492.8
Endarterectomy (surgical)	38.10
Esophageal stricture	530.3
Failure to thrive, adult	783.7
Fluid and electrolyte imbalance	276.9
Foley catheter	57.94
Gastrostomy	43.19
Gastrostomy, tube insertion	43.11
Heart disease, chronic ischemic	414.9
Hemiplegia or hemiparesis	342.9
Hypertension	401.9
Hypertension, accelerated	401.0
Hypertensive nephrosclerosis	403.90
Incontinence of feces	787.6
Incontinence of urine	788.30
Left-sided heart failure	428.1
Nasogastric tube feeding	96.6
Nasogastric tube insertion	96.07
Obesity	278.00
Paralysis agitans (Parkinson's disease)	332.0
Pneumonia	486
Pneumonia aspiration	507.0
Pressure (decubitus) ulcer	707.0
Protein-caloric malnutrition	263.9
Quadriplegia	436 and 344.00
Seizure disorder	780.3
TLA	435.9
Urinary retention	788.20
Urinary tract infection	599.0

4

5. Skills and services identified

- *Hospice nursing*

a. *Comfort and symptom control*

   Skilled assessment and observation of all systems of patient S/P CVA
      and terminal prognosis

   Observation and assessment of patient with _____ on
      multiple medications, admitted to hospice with increasing debility,
      right-sided weakness, and seizures in hospital

   Presentation of hospice philosophy and services

   Explain patient rights and responsibilities

   Assess patient, family, and caregiver wishes and expectations regarding
      care

Assess patient, family, and caregiver resources available for care

Provision of volunteer support to patient and family

Teach family or caregiver physical care of patient

RN to provide and teach effective oral care and comfort measures

Assess pain and other symptoms, including site, duration, characteristics, and relief measures

Assess pain, and evaluate pain management's effectiveness

Teach care of bedridden patient

Measure vital signs, including pain, q visit

Assess cardiovascular, pulmonary, and respiratory status

Teach new pain or symptom control medication regimen

Teach caregivers symptom control and relief measures

Oxygen on at _____ liter per _____ (specify physician orders)

Identify and monitor pain, symptoms, and relief measures

Teach caregiver or family care of weak, terminally ill patient

RN to instruct in pain control measures and medications

Teach family or caregiver care of the immobilized or bedridden patient

Assess neurological status

Assess respiratory, cardiovascular statuses and other systems

Observe and monitor for neurological deficits

Teach patient/family use of standardized form/tool to use between hospice team members' visits (and for care coordination among team members)

Teach patient/family principles of effective pain management

Observation and assessment, communication with physicians related to signs and symptoms of continuing decompensation and increased symptoms, pain, discomfort, shortness of breath, and measures to alleviate and control

Effective management of pain and prevention of secondary symptoms

Interventions of symptoms directed toward comfort and palliation

Pain assessment and management q visit, including source of pain (e.g., cancer pain, infection, pathological fracture, other medical problems such as cardiac or arthritis pain)

RN to teach patient and caregiver about disease process and management

Teach patient and family about realistic expectations of disease process

Teach care of dying and signs/symptoms of impending death

Presence and support

Other interventions, based on patient/family needs

b. *Safety and mobility considerations*

Provide caregiver with home safety information and instruction related to _____ and documented in the clinical record

Teach family or caregiver about oxygen therapy, utilization, and associated safety information

Teach family regarding safety of patient in home

Teach family regarding energy conservation techniques

Other interventions, based on patient/family needs

c. *Emotional/Spiritual considerations*

Psychosocial assessment of patient and family regarding disease and prognosis

RN to provide emotional support to patient and family

Assess mental status and sleep disturbance changes

RN to provide support and intervention for depression

Psychosocial aspects of pain control (e.g., depression, others) assessed and acknowledged with team support/intervention

Assess for and manage plans for psychosocial and/or spiritual pain (e.g., all pain, anxiety, interpersonal difficulties, other distress)

Teach patient/family about depression and signs/symptoms of exacerbation, needing more intervention

Ongoing acknowledgment of spirituality and related concerns of patient/family

Inform patient/family/caregiver of available volunteer support

Other interventions, based on patient/family needs

d. *Skin care*

Pressure ulcer care as indicated

Assess skin integrity

Observation and evaluation of wound and surrounding skin

Evaluate patient's need for equipment, including supplies to decrease pressure, alternating pressure mattress, gel foam seat cushion, and heel and elbow protectors

Teach family to perform dressing changes between RN visits, specifically ＿＿＿＿＿＿

Teach patient and family or caregiver about proper body alignment and positioning in bed to prevent skin tears from shearing skin

Observe and apply skilled assessment of areas for possible breakdown, including heels, hips, elbows, ankles, and other pressure-prone areas

Teach caregiver about patient's skin care needs, including the need for frequent position changes, appropriate pressure pads and mattresses, and the prevention of breakdown

Other interventions, based on patient/family needs

4

e. *Elimination considerations*

Assess bowel regimen, and implement program as needed

Check for and remove impaction as needed

Condom catheter or indwelling catheter as indicated

Assess amount and frequency of urinary output

Teach catheter care to caregiver

RN to teach caregiver daily care of catheter

RN to evaluate the patient's bowel patterns and need for stool softeners, laxatives, and dietary adjustments, and to develop bowel management plan

Check for and remove fecal impactions prn, per physician orders

Implement bowel and bladder training regimen

RN to change catheter (specify type, size) q ＿＿＿ (specify ordered frequency)

Observation and complete systems assessment of patient with an
indwelling catheter

RN to change catheter every 4 weeks and 3 prn visits for catheter
problems, including patient complaints, signs and symptoms of
infection, and other factors necessitating evaluation and possible
catheter change

Teaching and ongoing assessment related to early prevention and
identification of constipation and its correction/resolution

Initiate bowel management program per physician

Implement bowel assessment management program

Teach patient, family, and aide the importance of observing and noting
bowel movements between scheduled nursing visits

Obtain patient history related to norms for bowel movements to date
(e.g., "All my life I go only every other day")

Consider stool softeners and offer laxative of choice, Fleet's enemas
prn, and other methods per patient wishes and physician orders

Other interventions, based on patient/family needs

f. *Hydration/Nutrition*

Instruct patient about specified diet _____ (specify physician
orders)

Assess nutrition and hydration statuses

Diet counseling for patient with anorexia

Teach family or caregiver about feeding tubes or pumps

Nutrition/hydration supported by offering patient's choice of favorite or
desired foods or liquids

Nutrition/hydration maintained by offering patient high-protein diet and
foods of choice as tolerated

Assessment and plan related to anorexia/cachexia, tube feedings,
difficulty/painful swallowing, and/or transitional feedings
(e.g., TPN to oral)

Teach patient and family to expect decreased nutritional and fluid
intake as disease progresses

Other interventions, based on patient/family needs

g. *Therapeutic/Medication regimens*

Medication assessment and management q visit

Teach new medications and effects

Assess for electrolyte imbalance

Teach patient and caregiver use of PCA pump

Nonpharmacological interventions such as progressive muscle
relaxation, imagery, positive visualization, music, massage and
touch, and humor therapy of patient's choice implemented

Teach new medication regimen

Assessment of effectiveness of new therapeutic medical regimen

RN to assess the patient's response to therapeutic treatments and interventions and to report to the physician any changes or unfavorable
responses

Encourage family/caregivers to give the patient medications on the
schedule and around the clock

Medications changed using equianalgesic conversion tables/physician orders (e.g., from oral morphine to an equianalgesic dose of transdermal fentanyl)

Other interventions, based on patient/family needs

h. *Other considerations*

Observation and assessment of hospice patient with CVA and mental status changes, signs/complaints of depression

Observation of patient for neuropsychiatric complications of illness, including confusion, depression, and anxiety

Assess progression of disease process

RN to assess the patient's response to treatments and interventions and to report to the physician changes, unfavorable responses, or reactions

Other interventions, based on patient/family needs

- ***Home health aide or certified nursing assistant***
  Effective and safe personal care
  Safe ADL assistance and support
  Observation and reporting
  Respite care and active listening skills
  Meal preparation
  Homemaker services
  Comfort care
  Other duties

- ***Social worker***
  Psychosocial assessment of patient and family/caregiver, including adjustment to long-term illness and its implications
  Identification of optimal coping strategies/caregiver role strain
  Financial assessment and counseling regarding food acquisition, ability to prepare, and costs of needed medications
  Intervention/support related to terminal illness and loss
  Emotional/spiritual support
  Depression/fear assessed and addressed
  Facilitate communication among patient, family, and hospice team
  Referral/linkage to community services and resources as indicated
  Grief counseling and intervention/support related to illness/loss
  Patient/caregiver counseling and support
  Patient lives alone with no support system (e.g., able, available, willing caregiver[s]), obtain necessary resources to allow patient to remain in home
  Identification of illness-related psychiatric condition necessitating care
  Facilitation of will/funeral arrangements

- ***Volunteer(s)***
  Support, friendship, companionship, and presence
  Comfort and dignity maintained/provided for patient and family
  Errands and transportation
  Other services, based on IDT recommendations and patient/caregiver needs

4

- *Spiritual counselor*
  Spiritual assessment and care
  Counseling, intervention, and support related to that dimension of life related to life's meaning (consistent with patient's beliefs)
  Support, listening, and presence
  Pray with or for the patient/family, using prayers familiar to patient's religious background (per their wishes)
  Participation in sacred or spiritual rituals or practices
  Funeral planning assistance
  Other supportive care, based on patient/family needs and belief systems

- *Dietitian/Nutritional counseling*
  Assessment of patient with decreased intake, weight loss, anorexia, and pressure ulcer
  Supportive counseling with patient/family indicating that patient will have a decreased appetite and usually at some point may not eat/drink
  Assessment and recommendations for swallowing difficulties
  Teaching and support of family members and caregivers
  Support and care with soft food and nourishment as desired by patient
  Evaluation/management of nutritional deficits and needs
  Encourage nutritional supplements and snacks to increase protein and caloric intake
  Food and dietary recommendations incorporate patient choice and wishes
  Evaluation for tube feeding/TPN if condition warrants and per plan of care

- *Occupational therapist*
  Evaluation of ADL and functional mobility
  Assess for need for adaptive equipment and assistive devices
  Safety assessment of patient's environment and ADLs
  Assessment for energy conservation training
  Assessment of upper-extremity function, retraining motor skills, and/or splinting for contracture(s)

- *Physical therapist*
  Evaluation
  Safety assessment of patient's environment
  Safe transfer training or bed mobility exercises
  Pain assessment/reduction factors
  Strengthening exercises/program
  Assessment of gait safety and home safety measures
  Instruct/supervise caregiver and volunteers on home exercise program for conditioning and strength
  Assistive, adaptive devices and evaluation of equipment and teaching

- *Speech-language pathologist*
  Evaluation for speech/swallowing problems
  Food texture recommendations
  Alternative functional communication

- *Bereavement counselor*
  Assessment of the needs of the bereaved family and friends
  Support and intervention, based on assessment and ongoing findings
  Presence and counseling
  Supportive visits and follow-up, other interventions (e.g., mailings, calls)
  Other services related to bereavement work and support

- *Pharmacist*
  Evaluation of hospice patient with constipation on cathartics, stool softeners, and other medications for possible food/drug, drug/drug interactions
  Medication monitoring regarding therapeutic levels and dosages
  Pain consult and input into interdisciplinary POC related to pain control, palliation, and symptom management
  Assessment of medication regimen and plan for safety and compliance

- *Music, massage, art, or other therapies or services*
  Evaluation and intervention based on patient's and caregiver's unique wishes and needs that support care, comfort, and death in the setting of the patient's choice
  Pet therapy (including patient's pet, if available) and therapeutic intervention
  Assessment plan to engage patient and support comfort, quality, enjoyment, and dignity

6. Outcomes for care

- *Hospice nursing*
  Supportive care and scopolamine patches per physician order
  Mental distress, depression, and fear of dying addressed throughout care by hospice team
  Patient and family able to care for and support patient
  Patient and caregiver can verbalize symptoms, changes, or accelerations that necessitate call to physician
  Patient and family demonstrate compliance to medication and other therapeutic interventions
  Patient demonstrates stabilization and increased or enhanced coping skills related to functioning and depression
  Pain and symptoms managed/controlled in setting of patient/family choice (e.g., patient/family report ability to eat, sleep, speak with pacing)
  Planned and effective bowel program, as evidenced by regular bowel movements and patient/family report of comfort
  Death with dignity, and pain/symptoms controlled in setting of patient/family choice
  Optimal comfort, support, and dignity provided throughout illness
  Death with maximum comfort through effective symptom control with specialized hospice support

4

Patient and caregiver able to list adverse drug reactions/problems with medication regimen and whom to call for follow-up and resolution

Patient's/family's privacy, independence, and choices supported with respect and maintained through death

Enhancement and support of quality of life

Effective symptom relief and control (e.g., a peaceful and comfortable death at home, depression controlled, some enjoyment of life)

Maximizing the patient's quality of life (e.g., alert and pain free or as patient wishes)

Pharmacological and nonpharmacological interventions such as localized heat application, biofeedback, massage, positioning, relaxation methods, and music

Patient states pain is at _____ on 0–10 scale by next visit

Patient and caregiver verbalize satisfaction with care

Educational tools/plans incorporated in daily care, and patient/caregiver verbalizes understanding of safe, needed care

Patient will decide on care, interventions, and evaluation

Caregiver effective in care management and knows whom to call for questions/concerns

Patient will express satisfaction with hospice support received and will experience increased comfort

Patient will be made comfortable at home through death in accordance with the patient's wishes

Effective pain control and symptom control verbalized by patient

Patient verbalizes understanding of and adheres to care and medication regimens

Patient and caregiver supported through patient's death

Comfort maintained through course of care

Patient and family receive hospice support and care, and family members and friends are able to spend quality time with the patient

Caregiver is able and verbalizes comfort with role and lists when to call hospice team members

Patient supported through and receives the maximum benefit from palliative chemotherapy and radiation with minimal complications

Patient and caregiver list adverse reactions, potential complications, signs/symptoms of infection (e.g., sputum change, chest congestion)

Comfort maintained through death with dignity

Pain effectively managed, and patient verbalizes comfort

Patient is protected from injury, has stable respiratory status, and is compliant with medication, safety, and care regimens

Comfort and individualized intervention of patient with immobility/bedbound status (e.g., skin, urinary, musculature, vascular)

Spiritual and psychosocial needs met (specify) as defined by patient and caregiver throughout course of care

Adherence to POC as demonstrated and verbalized by caregiver and demonstrated by patient findings by _____ (specify date)

Wound healed by _____ with stabilization of site and no infection

Patient/caregiver demonstrates compliance with instructions related to medications, extremity elevation, and wound care

Lab values (e.g., CBC) will be within normal limits for patient by _____ (date)

Patient and family will report optimal function S/P CVA by _____

Weight lost/maintained/gained _____ lbs by _____ (date)

Patient reports decrease in SOB, chest pain by _____

Patient's catheter will remain infection free and patent

Caregiver is effective in care management and knows whom to call for questions/concerns

Pain controlled and comfort needs met throughout POC

IV access site remains patent without signs/symptoms of infection, and flushing/dressing care is provided per protocol

Patient verbalizes understanding of and adheres to medication regimens

Regulated bowel program, as evidenced by regular bowel movements

Patient will report being comfortable _____ % of the day (*comfortable* defined as pain free)

Patient cared for and family supported through death with physical, psychosocial, spiritual, and other concerns/needs acknowledged/addressed

Patient- and family-centered hospice care provided based on the patient's/family's unique situation and needs

Infection control and palliation

Grief/bereavement expression and support provided

Caregiver demonstrates ability to manage pain, where applicable

Patient maintains comfort and dignity throughout illness

- *Home health aide or certified nursing assistant*
  Effective hygiene, personal care, and comfort
  ADL assistance
  Safe environment maintained

- *Social worker*
  Problems identified and addressed, with patient and caregiver linked with appropriate support services and plan of care successfully implemented
  Patient and caregiver cope adaptively with illness and death
  Adaptive adjustment to changed body and body image
  Psychosocial support and counseling offered to patient/caregivers experiencing loss and grief
  Funeral and burial planning assitance

- *Volunteer(s)*
  Comfort, companionship, and friendship extended to patient/family
  Support and respite provided as defined by the needs of the patient/caregiver
  Patient and family supported by team with care, comfort, and companionship

4

- *Spiritual counselor*
  Support, listening, and presence
  Spiritual support offered and provided as defined by needs of
      patient/caregiver
  Participation in sacred or spiritual rituals or practices
  Provision of spiritual support and care based on the assessed and
      ongoing needs of the patient and family
  Spiritual support offered, and patient and family needs met
  Patient and family express relief of symptoms of spiritual suffering
  Pray with or for the patient/family using prayers familiar to the
      patient's religious background (per their wishes)

- *Dietitian/Nutritional counseling*
  Family and caregiver integrate recommendations into nutrition teaching
      (where appropriate)
  Patient and caregiver know whom to call for nutrition- and
      hydration-related questions/concerns
  Nutrition/hydration per patient's choices
  Caregiver integrates recommendations into daily meal planning

- *Occupational therapist*
  Patient and caregiver demonstrate maximum independence with ADLs,
      adaptive techniques, and assistive devices
  Patient and caregiver demonstrate maximum safety in ADL and
      functional mobility
  Patient and caregiver demonstrate effective use of energy conservation
  Verbalization/demonstration of improved functional activity level and
      enhanced quality of life
  Patient and caregiver demonstrate effective use of diaphragmatic
      breathing to reduce shortness of breath and relaxation techniques to
      help in pain/symptom management
  Patient and caregiver demonstrate correct use of exercise and splints for
      maximum upper extremity function and joint position

- *Physical therapist*
  Prevention of complications
  Home exercise and upper extremity program taught to caregiver
  Optimal strength, mobility, and function maintained/achieved
  Compliance with home exercise program by _____ (specify date)
  Safety in mobility and transfers

- *Speech-language pathologist*
  Communication method implemented, and patient able to be
      understood as self-reported or reported by family/caregivers
  Safe swallowing and functional communication
  Recommended lists of food/textures for safety and patient choice

- *Bereavement counselor*
  Grief support services provided to patient and family
  Well-being and resolution process of grief initiated and followed
      through bereavement services

4

- *Music, massage, art, or other therapies or services*
  Therapeutic massage/touch effective for patient as self-reported or
      observed by caregivers/family
  Improved muscle tone, relaxation, and/or sleep
  Patient comfortable and relaxed (e.g., sleeping) after massage
  Music therapy intervention based on assessment to decrease pain
      perception and provide emotional expression and support
  Patient has pet's presence as desired—in all care sites, when possible
  Maintenance of comfort and physical, psychosocial, and spiritual health
  Holistic health maintained and comfort achieved through
      _____ (specify modality)

7. **Patient, family, and caregiver educational needs**
   Educational needs are the care regimens that contribute to safe and effective care at home between the hospice team's visits. These include the
   following:
       The basic tenets of hospice and the availability of support 24 hours a
           day, 7 days a week
       Home safety assessment and counseling
       The patient's medication regimen
       Safe and proper body mechanics to promote patient comfort and
           prevent caregiver safety problems
       Other teaching specific to the patient's and family's unique needs
       Support groups available to patient's family, such as the hospice
           program's "Caregiver Support Group" meetings for family
           members and friends of the patient
       The importance of and all aspects of effective skin care regimens to
           prevent breakdown, including the need for frequent position
           changes, proper body alignment, pressure pads or mattresses, and
           other measures for prevention
       Anticipated disease progression
       Other information based on the patient's unique medical and other needs

8. **Specific tips for quality and reimbursement**
   Document any variances to expected outcomes. Often the diagnosis of
   CVA indicates multiple identifiable nursing needs. There are many
   models of hospice programs.
       The Medicare hospice benefit does not require that the patient be
   homebound or have identified skilled needs. For further information on
   this benefit, please refer to CMS Hospice Manual 21.
       Should the patient's status deteriorate and increased personal care
   be needed, obtain a telephone order for the increased service, noting
   frequency and estimating the duration.
       Obtain a telephone order for all medication and treatment changes of
   the medical regimen, and document these in the clinical record. Document
   coordination of services and consultation with other members of
   the IDG.
       Unless the patient is in a hospice insurance program, some insurers
   will not pay for a skilled clinician visit that is made at death if the patient is

dead when the clinician arrives at the home. From a Medicare home care perspective, the visit at the time of death may be covered when the orders and clinical record document assessment of the patient's status or signs of death/life or state law allows pronouncement of death by an RN.

Document patient deterioration

Document dehydration, dehydrating

Document patient change or instability

Document pain, other symptoms not controlled

Document status after acute episode of _____ (specify)

Document positive urine, sputum, etc. culture; patient started on _____ (specify ordered antibiotic therapy)

Document patient impacted; impaction removed manually

Document RN in frequent communication with physician regarding _____ (specify)

Document febrile at _____, pulse change at _____, irr., irr.

Document change noted in _____

Document bony prominences red, opening

Document RN contacted physician regarding _____ (specify)

Document marked SOB

Document alteration in mental status

Document medications being adjusted, regulated, or monitored

Document unable to perform own ADLs, personal care

Document all interdisciplinary team meetings and communications in the POC and in the progress notes of the clinical record

All hospice team members involved should have input into the POC and document their interventions and goals

Document in the clinical notes the clear progression and symptomatology and interventions that demonstrate the interventions and overall management of the patient with the stroke and attendant needs for hospice support

Document when/if the patient has respiratory changes, shortness of breath, exacerbation of conditions, dysphagia, changes in pain, and other symptoms and that they are identified and resolved

Remember that the clinical documentation is key to measuring compliance for quality and reimbursement purposes. Care coordination, timely verbal and initial physician orders, and assessment and addressing of spiritual and psychosocial needs should be ongoing and documented in the patient's clinical record

The documentation should support that all hospice care supports comfort and dignity while meeting patient/family needs

The documentation should include ongoing assessment and management of pain and other symptoms and the anticipation and prevention of secondary symptoms such as constipation

It is important to note that all team members, including nurses and social workers, should assess, identify, and "hear" spiritual needs that the patient/family want to be addressed. These spiritual issues are key to the provision of quality hospice care and cannot be addressed effectively and promptly by the spiritual counselor only

Document clearly symptoms, clinical changes, and assessment findings related to pain and patient care

Document patient changes, symptoms, and clinical information identified from visits and team conferences that support hospice care and a limited life expectancy

Clearly support in the documentation the rationale that supports/explains the progression of the illness from the chronic to terminal stages

Document patient changes, symptoms, psychosocial issues impacting the care, and information gathered at patient/family visits and during team meetings

The documentation should reflect ongoing effects of the terminal condition, the patient's/family's difficulty with care or coping, and the continued desire for hospice care

Document mentation, behavioral, and/or cognitive changes

Document dysphagia, weight loss, increased shortness of breath, dyspnea, infection, sepsis, new or changed medications, etc.

Document any skin changes (e.g., inflamed, painful, weeping skin site[s])

Document when the patient is actively dying, deteriorating, and progressing toward death

Remember that the "litmus test" of care coordination rests on the quality of the clinical documentation by all team members. Review one of your patient's clinical records and ask yourself the following: "If I was unable to give a verbal report/update on this patient, would a peer be able to pick up and provide the same level of care and know (from the documentation) the current orders, medications, and other details that contribute to effective hospice care?"

This patient population usually has many clinical changes that should be documented

Your assessments, observations, and clinical findings assist in painting a picture to support coverage and documentation requirements for hospice care

Document any hospitalizations and changed clinical findings

4

9. Queries for quality

Cerebral Vascular Accident (CVA) Care
- *Is patient's pain managed adequately?*
- *Is patient's anxiety managed adequately?*
- *Is patient's functional ability/status clearly documented?*
- *Have you documented to the interdisciplinary POC?*
- *Have patient's self-care deficit needs been managed?*

Stroke Care
- *Is patient's pain managed adequately?*
- *Is patient's anxiety managed adequately?*
- *Is patient's functional ability/status clearly documented?*

- *Have you documented to the interdisciplinary POC?*
- *Have patient's self-care deficit needs been managed?*

10. Resources for hospice care and practice

A helpful resource is the National Hospice on Palliative Care Organization's NHCPO latest edition of *Medical Guidelines for Determining Prognoses in Selected Non-Cancer Disease.* Call NHPCO at 1-800-646-6460

For more information, contact the Amercian Heart Association at 1-214-373-6300 or 1-800-AHAUSAI to connect with your local affiliate. The National Stroke Association also has information and can be reached at 1-800-STROKES.

4

CONSTIPATION CARE

1. General considerations

Constipation is one of the most common secondary symptoms that cause distress for hospice patients and concern of their family. Dame Cicely Saunders, considered by many to be the founder of the modern hospice movement, is reported to have given a lecture in which every fourth slide read, "Nothing matters more than the bowels." Consequently, effective bowel management is a contributor to quality hospice care. Every patient should be evaluated on admission and monitored every visit for this problem, and the entire team should be aware of this problematic area because prevention is the best cure. Many hospices use a flow chart method to identify/prevent constipation problems in the course of care. Constipation can lead to other pain problems, including hemorrhoidal pain and bleeding, anorexia, nausea, diarrhea, and impactions. See Table 4-1 for a bowel regimen to prevent narcotic-induced constipation.

2. Needs for visit

Physician order for hospice care, specific to the hospice program's admission criteria and policies

Standard precautions supplies

Vital signs equipment for baseline assessment

Other supplies or equipment, based on physician orders

3. Safety considerations

Infection control/standard precautions

Night-light

Extra caution on slippery surfaces

Removal of scatter rugs

Tub rail, grab bars for bathroom safety

Supportive and nonskid shoes

Handrail on stairs

Fall precautions

Protective skin measures

Identification and report of any skin problems

Smoke detector and fire evacuation plan

Assistance with ambulation

Others, based on the patient's unique condition and environment

4. Potential diagnoses and codes

Bowel impaction	560.30
Cancer, colon	153.9
Cancer, rectosigmoid	154.0
Constipation	564.00
Dehydration	276.5
Failure to thrive, adult	783.7
Ileus	560.1
Impaction, fecal	560.39

TABLE 4-1

BOWEL REGIMEN TO PREVENT NARCOTIC-INDUCED CONSTIPATION

Medication	Suggested Beginning Dose	Usual Range of Dosage
1. Begin with *one* of the combined stool softener and mild peristaltic stimulants:		
Dioctyl sodium sulfosuccinate 100 mg plus casanthranol 30 mg (Peri-Colace) *or*	1 capsule tid	1 capsule qd to 2 capsules tid
Docusate sodium 50 mg plus senna 187 mg (Senokot-S) *or*	1 tablet tid	1 tablet qd to 4 tablets tid
Docusate calcium 60 mg plus danthron 50 mg (Doxidan)	1 capsule bid	1 capsule qd to 2 capsules tid
2. If no bowel movement occurs in any 48 hr period, add *one* to *two* of the following: Senna 187 mg (Senokot)	2–3 tablets at bedtime	2 tablets hs to 4 tablets tid
Bisacodyl (Dulcolax)	10–15 mg PO at bedtime	5 mg PO hs to 15 mg PO tid
Milk of Magnesia	30–60 ml at bedtime	30–60 ml qd or bid
Lactulose (Chronulac: 10 g/15 ml)	30–45 ml at bedtime	15–60 ml qd or bid
Perdiem (avoid if fluid intake is reduced)	2 teaspoons at bedtime	1 teaspoon to 2 tablespoons qd
3. If no bowel movement occurs within 72 hr, perform rectal examination to rule out impaction. If not impacted, go to #4. If imapcted, go to #5.		
4. If not impacted, try *one* of the following:		
Bisacodyl (Dulcolax) suppository	10 mg	
Magnesium Citrate	8 oz PO	

Modified from Levy MH: Pain management in advanced cancer, *Semin Oncol* 12:404, 1985.

TABLE 4-1		
BOWEL REGIMEN TO PREVENT NARCOTIC-INDUCED CONSTIPATION—cont'd		
Medication	**Suggested Beginning Dose**	**Usual Range of Dosage**
Senna extract (X-prep liquid)	2½ oz PO	
Mineral oil	30–60 ml PO	
Milk of Magnesia 25 ml *and* Cascara 5 ml suspension		
Fleet enema		
5. If impacted:		
Manually disempact if stool is soft enough		
If not, soften with glycerin suppository or oil retention enema, then disempact manually		
Follow up with enema (tap water, soapsuds) until clear		
Increase daily bowel regimen		

5. Skills and services identified

- *Hospice nursing*

a. *Comfort and symptom control*
   Skilled observation and assessment of the patient with impaction/ constipation
   Observation and assessment of patient with _____ on multiple medications, admitted to hospice with _____ (e.g., restrictive lung disease)
   Presentation of hospice philosophy and services
   Explain patient rights and responsibilities
   Assess patient, family, and caregiver wishes and expectations regarding care
   Assess patient, family, and caregiver resources available for care
   Provision of volunteer support to patient and family

4

Teach family or caregiver physical care of patient

Assess pain and other symptoms, including site, duration, characteristics, and relief measures

RN to provide and teach effective oral care and comfort measures

Pain assessment and management q visit

Teach caregiver/patient use of pain assessment tool/scale and reporting mechanism(s)

Effective management of pain and prevention of secondary symptoms

Interventions of symptoms directed toward comfort and palliation

Observation and assessment, communication with physician related to signs and symptoms of continuing decompensation and increased symptoms, pain, discomfort, shortness of breath, and measures to alleviate and control

Teach patient and family about realistic expectations for the disease process

Teach care of dying and signs/symptoms of impending death

Presence and support

Other interventions, based on patient/family needs

b. *Safety and mobility considerations*

Provide patient with home safety information and instruction related to _____ and documented in the clinical record

Rehabilitation management related to safe bed mobility and transfers

Teach family about safety of patient in home

Teach patient and family about energy conservation techniques

Teach caregiver to observe for increased secretions and teach safe suctioning, when needed

Other interventions, based on patient/family needs

c. *Emotional/Spiritual considerations*

Psychosocial assessment of patient and family regarding disease and prognosis

Psychosocial aspects of pain control (e.g., depression) assessed and acknowledged with team support/intervention

Inform patient/family/caregiver of available volunteer support

Ongoing acknowledgment of spirituality and related concerns of patient/family

Other interventions, based on patient/family needs

d. *Skin care*

Pressure ulcer care as indicated

Assess skin integrity

Observation and evaluation of wound and surrounding skin

Evaluate patient's need for equipment, including supplies to decrease pressure, alternating pressure mattress, gel foam seat cushion, and heel and elbow protectors

Teach family to perform dressing changes between RN visits, specifically _____

Teach patient and family or caregiver about proper body alignment and positioning in bed to prevent skin tears from shearing skin

4

Observe and apply skilled assessment of areas for possible breakdown, including heels, hips, elbows, ankles, and other pressure-prone areas

Teach caregiver about skin care needs, including the need for frequent position changes, appropriate pressure pads and mattresses, and the prevention of breakdown

Other interventions, based on patient/family needs

e. *Elimination considerations*

Assess bowel regimen and implement program as needed

Evaluation and examination for, and manual removal of, fecal impaction (per orders)

Teach new bowel training regimen

Administer enema per order

Teach suppository administration

Assess bowel sounds, all four quadrants

Digital rectal examination per physician orders

Implement bowel and bladder training regimen

Teach patient/family and aide the importance of observing and noting bowel movements between scheduled nursing visits

Obtain patient history related to norms for bowel movements to date (e.g., "All my life I go only every other day")

Consider stool softeners and offer laxative of choice, Fleet's enemas prn, and other methods per patient wishes and physician orders

Other interventions, based on patient/family needs

f. *Hydration/Nutrition*

Assess nutrition/hydration status

Teach about need for increased fiber, fruit, and fluid diet, as appropriate

Other interventions, based on patient/family needs

g. *Other considerations*

Assess progression of disease process

RN to assess the patient's response to treatments and interventions and to report to the physician changes, unfavorable responses, or reactions

Other interventions, based on patient/family needs

• ***Home health aide or certified nursing assistant***

Effective and safe personal care

Safe ADL assistance and support

Respect for privacy while supporting patient safety

Observation and reporting

Respite care and active listening skills

Meal preparation

Homemaker services

Assistance with toileting activities and support of patient habits

Comfort care

Other duties

- *Social worker*
  Psychosocial assessment of patient and family/caregiver, including
      adjustment to long-term illness and its implications
  Identification of optimal coping strategies
  Financial assessment and counseling regarding food acquisition, ability
      to prepare, and costs of needed medications
  Intervention/support related to terminal illness and loss
  Emotional/spiritual support
  Identification of caregiver role strain necessitating respite/relief
      measures/support
  Depression/fear assessed and addressed
  Facilitate communication among patient, family, and hospice team
  Referral/linkage to community services and resources as indicated
  Grief counseling and intervention/support related to illness/loss
  Patient/caregiver counseling and support
  For patient who lives alone with no support system (e.g., able,
      available, willing caregiver[s]), obtain linkage with necessary
      community resources to allow patient to remain at home
  Identification of illness-related psychiatric condition necessitating care
  Funeral and burial planning assistance

- *Volunteer(s)*
  Support, friendship, companionship, presence, and respite care
  Comfort and dignity maintained/provided for patient and family
  Errands and transportation
  Other services, based on interdisciplinary team recommendations and
      patient/caregiver needs

- *Spiritual counselor*
  Spiritual assessment and care
  Counseling, intervention, and support related to that dimension of life
      related to life's meaning (consistent with patient's beliefs)
  Pray with or for the patient/family, using prayers familiar to patient's
      religious background (per their wishes)
  Support, listening, and presence
  Participation in sacred or spiritual rituals or practices
  Other supportive care, based on patient's/family's needs and belief
      systems

- *Dietitian/Nutritional counseling*
  Assessment of patient with decreased intake, weight loss, anorexia, and
      increased shortness of breath (e.g., "I don't feel like eating")
  Supportive counseling with patient/family indicating that patient will
      have a decreased appetite and usually at some point may not eat/drink
  Assessment and recommendations for swallowing difficulties
  Teaching and support of family members and caregivers
  Increased fluid intake as tolerated, especially fruit juices (e.g., prune,
      apple)
  Support and care with food and nourishment as desired by patient

4

Evaluation/management of nutritional deficits and needs

Encourage nutritional supplements and snacks to increase protein and caloric intake

Suggest foods high in fiber (e.g., bran, whole grains, and fruits, especially pineapple, prunes, raisins, vegetables, nuts, and legumes). Avoid increased fiber if patient is dehydrated or if severe constipation or obstruction/ileus is anticipated

- *Bereavement counselor*

  Assessment of the needs of the bereaved family and friends

  Support and intervention, based on assessment and ongoing findings

  Presence and counseling

  Supportive visits and follow-up, other interventions (e.g., mailings, calls)

  Other services related to bereavement work and support

- *Pharmacist*

  Evaluation of hospice patient with constipation on cathartics, stool softeners, and other medications for possible food/drug, drug/drug interactions

  Medication monitoring regarding therapeutic levels and dosages

  Pain consult and input into interdisciplinary POC related to pain control, palliation, and symptom management

  Assessment of medication regimen and plan for safety and compliance

- *Music, massage, art, or other therapies or services*

  Evaluation and intervention based on patient's and caregiver's unique wishes and needs that support care, comfort, and death in the setting of the patient's choice

  Assessment plan to engage patient and support comfort, quality, enjoyment, and dignity

  Pet therapy (including patient's pet, if available) and therapeutic intervention

6. Outcomes for care

- *Hospice nursing*

  Planned and effective bowel program, as evidenced by regular bowel movements and patient/family report of comfort

  Death with dignity, and symptoms controlled in setting of patient/family choice

  Optimal comfort, support, and dignity provided throughout illness

  Death with maximum comfort through effective symptom control with specialized hospice support

  Patient and caregiver able to list adverse drug reactions/problems with medication regimen and whom to call for follow-up and resolution

  Pain and symptoms managed/controlled in setting of patient/family choice (e.g., patient/family report ability to eat, sleep, speak clearer with pacing)

  Patient's/family's privacy, independence, and choices supported with respect and maintained through death

4

Enhancement and support of quality of life

Effective symptom relief and control (e.g., a peaceful and comfortable death at home, some enjoyment of life)

Maximizing the patient's quality of life (e.g., alert and pain free or as patient wishes)

Pharmacological and nonpharmacological interventions, such as localized heat application, positioning, relaxation methods, and music

Patient cared for and family supported through death, with physical, psychosocial, spiritual, and other concerns/needs acknowledged/addressed

Patient- and family-centered hospice care provided based on the patient's/family's unique situation and needs

Infection control and palliation

Grief/bereavement expression and support provided

Patient is pain free by next _____ visit

Caregiver demonstrates ability to manage pain, where applicable

Patient maintains comfort and dignity throughout illness

- *Home health aide or certified nursing assistant*
  Effective hygiene, personal care, and comfort
  ADL assistance
  Safe environment maintained

- *Social worker*
  Problem identified and addressed, with patient/caregiver and linked with appropriate support services and plan of care successfully implemented
  Patient and caregiver cope adaptively with illness and death
  Adaptive adjustment to changed body and body image
  Psychosocial support and counseling offered to patient/caregivers experiencing loss and grief
  Resources identified, community linkage as appropriate for patient and family
  Funeral and burial planning assistance

- *Volunteer(s)*
  Comfort, companionship, and friendship extended to patient/family
  Support and respite provided as defined by the needs of the patient/caregiver
  Patient and family supported by team with care, comfort, and companionship

- *Spiritual counselor*
  Spiritual support, listening, and presence offered and provided as defined by needs of patient/caregiver
  Provision of spiritual support and care as based on the assessed and ongoing needs of the patient and family
  Spiritual support offered, and patient and family needs met
  Patient and family express relief of symptoms of spiritual suffering
  Pray with or for the patient/family, using prayers familiar to the patient's religious background (per their wishes)

- *Dietitian/Nutritional counseling*
  Family and caregiver integrate dietary recommendations into nutrition
    teaching (where appropriate)
  Patient and caregiver know whom to call for nutrition- and hydration-
    related questions/concerns
  Nutrition/hydration per patient's choices
  Caregiver integrates dietary recommendations into daily meal planning

- *Bereavement counselor*
  Grief support services provided to patient and family
  Well-being and resolution process of grief initiated and followed
    through bereavement services

- *Pharmacist*
  Multiple drug regimen reviewed for food/drug and drug/drug
    interactions in patient on multiple medications
  Stability and safety in complex medication regimen with maximum
    benefit to patient
  Effective pain and symptom control and symptom management as
    reported by patient/caregiver (e.g., constipation)
  Lab reports reviewed for therapeutic dosages and effective patient
    response

- *Music, massage, art or other therapies or services*
  Therapeutic massage/touch effective for patient as self-reported or
    observed by caregivers/family
  Improved muscle tone, relaxation, and/or sleep
  Patient comfortable and relaxed (e.g., sleeping) after massage
  Music therapy intervention based on assessment to decrease pain
    perception and provide emotional expression and support
  Maintenance of comfort and physical, psychosocial, and spiritual health
  Holistic health maintained and comfort achieved through
    _____ (specify modality)
  Patient has pet's presence as desired—in all care sites, when possible

7. **Patient, family, and caregiver educational needs**
   Educational needs are the care regimens that contribute to safe and effective care at home between the hospice team's visits. These include the
   following:
     The basic tenets of hospice and the availability of support 24 hours a
       day, 7 days a week
     Home safety assessment and counseling
     Patient's medication regimen
     Safe and proper body mechanics to promote patient comfort and
       prevent caregiver safety problems
     Other teaching specific to the patient's and family's unique needs
     Support groups available to patient's family, such as the hospice
       program's "Caregiver Support Group" meetings for family
       members and friends of the patient
     Bowel training regimen and schedule

The need to call the hospice program should the patient experience discomfort (and need to be disimpacted)

The importance of prevention, where possible

Anticipated disease progression

Any other information, based on the patient's unique medical condition and needs

8. Specific tips for reimbursement and quality

Document any variances to expected outcomes. There are many models of hospice programs.

The Medicare hospice benefit does not require that the patient be homebound or have identified skilled needs. For further information on this benefit, please refer to CMS Hospice Manual 21.

Should the patient's status deteriorate and increased personal care be needed, obtain a telephone order for the increased service, noting frequency and estimating the duration.

Obtain a telephone order for all medication and treatment changes of the medical regimen and document these in the clinical record.

Unless the patient is in a hospice insurance program, some insurers will not pay for a skilled clinician visit that is made at death if the patient is dead when the clinician arrives at the home. From a Medicare home care perspective, the visit at the time of death may be covered when the orders and clinical record document assessment of the patient's status or signs of death/life or state law allows pronouncement of death by an RN.

Document the last bowel movement (if known) before RN visit

Document distention noted, as indicated

Document actual removal of fecal material

Document family and caregiver teaching regarding bowel training program

Document family and caregiver teaching regarding new diet regimen

Document patient deterioration

Document dehydration, dehydrating

Document patient change or instability

Document pain, other symptoms not controlled

Document status after acute episode of _____ (specify)

Document positive urine, sputum, etc. culture; patient started on _____ (specify ordered antibiotic therapy)

Document any impaction; impaction removed manually

Document RN in frequent communication with physician regarding _____ (specify)

Document febrile at _____, pulse change at _____, irr., irr.

Document change noted in _____

Document bony prominences red, opening

Document RN contacted physician regarding _____ (specify)

Document marked SOB

Document alteration in mental status

Document medications being adjusted, regulated, or monitored

Document unable to perform own ADLs, personal care

Document all IDT meetings and communications in the POC and in the progress notes of the clinical record

All hospice team members should have input into the POC and document their interventions and goals

Remember that clinical documentation is key to measuring compliance for quality and reimbursement purposes. Care coordination, timely verbal and initial physician orders, and assessment and addressing of spiritual and psychosocial needs should be ongoing and documented in the patient's clinical record

The documentation should support that all hospice care supports comfort and dignity while meeting patient/family needs

The documentation should include ongoing assessment and management of pain and other symptoms and the anticipation and prevention of secondary symptoms such as constipation

It is important to note that all team members, including clinicians and social workers, should assess, identify, and "hear" spiritual needs that the patient/family want to be addressed. These spiritual issues are key to the provision of quality hospice care and cannot be addressed effectively and promptly by the spiritual counselor only

Document clearly symptoms, clinical changes, and assessment findings related to pain and patient care

Document weight loss, increased shortness of breath, dyspnea, infection, sepsis, new or changed medications, etc.

Document any skin changes (e.g., inflamed, painful, weeping skin site[s])

Remember that the "litmus test" of care coordination rests on the quality of the clinical documentation by all team members. Review one of your patient's clinical records and ask yourself the following; "If I was unable to give a verbal report/update on this child/family's course of care, would a peer be able to pick up and provide the same level of care and know (from the documentation) the current orders, medications, and other details that contribute to effective hospice care?"

This patient population usually has many clinical changes that should be documented. These include weight loss, multiple and changed medication regimens with varying routes. Side effects to the drug regimen should be observed, noted, documented, and reported

Your assessments, observations, and clinical findings assist in painting a picture to support coverage and documentation requirements for hospice care

Document any hospitalizations and changed clinical findings

Document coordination of services and consultation with other members of the IDG

Document coordination with other team members at SNR nursing home, etc.

4

9. Queries for quality

Constipation care
- *Is patient's pain managed adequately?*
- *Has patient's bowel regimen been established?*
- *Is patient's anxiety managed adequately?*
- *Is patient's functional ability/status clearly documented?*
- *Have you documented to the interdisciplinary POC?*

Impaction care
- *Is patient's pain managed adequately?*
- *Is patient's anxiety managed adequately?*
- *Is the patient's functional ability/status clearly documented?*
- *What is the condition of the patient's skin?*
- *Have you documented to the interdisciplinary POC?*

10. Resources for hospice care and practice
The National Digestive Diseases Information Clearinghouse has a pamphlet entitled "Constipation" that can be obtained by calling (301) 654-3810. They can also be accessed via their web site at www.niddk.nitch.gov.

4

DEPRESSION AND PSYCHIATRIC CARE

1. General considerations

Though usually not a primary reason for admission to hospice, the hospice patient's and family's depression and psychiatric problems can present challenges to the hospice team. See also "Cancer Care," "Pain Care," or other sections that may pertain to your hospice patient.

2. Needs for visit

Physician order for hospice care, specific to the hospice program's admission criteria and policies

Standard precautions supplies

Vital signs equipment for baseline assessment

Other supplies or equipment, based on physician orders

3. Safety considerations

Infection control/standard precautions

Depression/confusion precautions

Disposal of sharps and related supplies

Supervised medication administration

Night-light

The phone number and name of the person to call with a care problem

Extra caution on slippery surfaces

Removal of scatter rugs

Tub rail, grab bars for bathroom safety

Supportive and nonskid shoes

Handrail on stairs

Fall precautions

Protective skin measures

Identification and report of any skin problems

Smoke detector and fire evacuation plan

Assistance with ambulation

Others, based on the patient's unique condition and environment

4. Potential diagnoses and codes

Agoraphobia	300.22
AIDS dementia	042 and 294.10
Alcoholism	303.90
Alzheimer's disease	331.0
Anemia	285.9
Anorexia nervosa	307.1
Anxiety state	300.00
Bipolar disorder, depressed	296.50
Bulimia	783.6
Constipation	564.00
Creutzfeldt-Jakob disease and dementia	046.1 and 294.10

CVA	436
Dementia	294.8
Depression, reactive	300.4
Depressive disorder	311
Depressive psychosis	296.20
Drug addiction	304.90
Electroshock therapy (surgical)	94.27
Failure to thrive, adult	783.7
Hypochondriasis	300.7
Korsakoff's dementia	294.0
Malaise and fatigue	780.79
Mania	296.00
Nonpsychotic brain syndrome	310.9
Obesity	278.00
Obsessive-compulsive disorder	300.3
Organic brain syndrome	310.9
Panic disorder	300.01
Panic disorder with agoraphobia	300.21
Personality disorder	301.9
Polyaddiction	304.80
Post traumatic stress disorder	309.81
Presenile dementia	290.13
Psychosis, depressive	296.20
Schizophrenia, simple	295.00
Schizophrenia, undifferentiated	295.80
Senile dementia	290.0
Traumatic stress disorder	308.3
Unipolar affective disorder	296.90

5. Skills and services identified

- *Hospice nursing*

a. *Comfort and symptom control*

Skilled assessment of the patient with _____ (specify the psychiatric disorder) admitted for hospice care

Observation and assessment of patient with _____ (specify) on multiple medications, admitted to hospice with increasing shortness of breath and pain

Psychotherapeutic interventions, including _____ (specify)

Assessment and observation of cognitive/affective behaviors

Skilled observation and assessment of all systems

Teach family or caregiver care of patient

Assess pain and other symptoms, including site, duration, characteristics, and relief measures

Assess pain, and evaluate pain management's effectiveness

RN to instruct in pain control measures and medications

Presentation of hospice philosophy and services

Explain patient rights and responsibilities

Assess patient, family, and caregiver wishes and expectations regarding care

Assess patient, family, and caregiver resources available for care

Provision of volunteer support to patient and family

Clinician to provide and teach effective oral care and comfort measures

RN to assess patient's pain or other symptoms q visit to identify need for change, addition, or other dose adjustment(s)

Teach caregiver or family care of weak, terminally ill patient

Comfort measures of backrub, hand, and other therapeutic massage

Teach patient and caregiver about disease and management

Observe for sleeping, eating, and other changes in patterns

RN to observe and assess patient's hygiene, personal care, independence with disease

RN to evaluate behavior medication plan, including support, teaching, and evaluation of compliance

Teach patient/family about depression and signs/symptoms of exacerbation that require more intervention

Teach patient/family use of standardized form/tool to use between hospice team members' visits (and for care coordination between team members)

Teach patient/family principles of effective pain management

Effective management of pain and prevention of secondary symptoms

Interventions of symptoms directed toward comfort and palliation

Observation and assessment, communication with physician related to signs and symptoms of continuing decompensation and increased symptoms, pain, discomfort, shortness of breath, and measures to alleviate and control

Teach caregiver/patient use of pain assessment tool/scale and reporting mechanism(s)

Pain assessment and management q visit, including source of pain (e.g., cancer pain, infection, pathological fracture, other medical problems, such as cardiac or arthritis pain)

Teach patient and family about realistic expectations of disease process

Teach care of dying and signs/symptoms of impending death

Presence and support

Other interventions, based on patient/family needs

b. *Safety and mobility considerations*

Provide caregiver with home safety information and instruction related to _____ and documented in the clinical record

Home safety evaluation and plan to help ensure safety

Other interventions, based on patient/family needs

c. *Emotional/Spiritual considerations*

Psychosocial assessment of patient and family regarding disease and prognosis

RN to provide emotional support to patient with severe grief reaction

RN to provide emotional support to patient and family

Inform patient/family/caregiver of available volunteer support

Assess mental status and sleep disturbance changes

RN to monitor patient's mental status for signs and symptoms of depression or _____ (specify)

Active, nonjudgmental listening to patient expression of a desire to "end it all" and referral to other team members for counseling, intervention

Reality orientation and counseling

Crisis intervention and counseling

Observation and assessment of hospice patient mental status changes/complaints of situational/other depressions

Observation of patient for neuropsychiatric complications of illness, including confusion, depression, and anxiety

RN to provide support and intervention for depression

Active listening to patients/families related to their loss, grief, and anticipation of death

Assess for and manage plans for psychosocial and/or spiritual pain (e.g., all pain, anxiety, and interpersonal and other distress)

Ongoing acknowledgment of spirituality and related concerns of patient/family

Psychosocial aspects of pain control (e.g., depression) addressed and acknowledged with team support/intervention

Other interventions, based on patient/family needs

d. *Skin care*

Observation of skin and patient's overall physical status

Teach patient and family or caregiver about proper body alignment and positioning in bed to prevent skin tears from shearing skin

Observe and apply skilled assessment of areas for possible breakdown, including heels, hips, elbows, ankles, and other pressure-prone areas

Teach caregiver about skin care needs, including the need for frequent position changes, appropriate pressure pads and mattresses, and the prevention of breakdown

Assess skin integrity

Observation and evaluation of wound and surrounding skin

Evaluate patient's need for equipment, including supplies to decrease pressure, alternating pressure mattress, gel foam seat cushion, and heel and elbow protectors

Teach family to perform dressing changes between RN visits, specifically _____

Other interventions, based on patient/family needs

e. *Elimination considerations*

RN to evaluate the patient's bowel patterns and need for stool softeners, laxatives, and dietary adjustments, and to develop bowel management plan

Initiate bowel management program per hospice physician

Teaching and ongoing assessment regarding early prevention and identification of constipation and its correction/resolution

Implement bowel assessment and management program

Teach patient/family and aide the importance of observing and noting bowel movements between scheduled nursing visits

Obtain patient history related to norms for bowel movements to date (e.g., "all my life I go only every other day")

Consider stool softeners and offer laxative of choice, Fleet's enemas prn, and other methods per patient wishes and physician orders

Other interventions, based on patient/family needs

f. *Hydration/Nutrition*

Instruct patient about specified diet _____ (specify physician orders)

Nutrition/hydration supported by offering patient's choice of favorite or desired foods or liquids

Monitor hydration and nutrition intake

Assessment and plan related to anorexia/cachexia, tube feedings, difficult/painful swallowing, and/or transitional feedings (e.g., TPN to oral)

Teach patient and family to expect decreased nutritional and fluid intake as disease progresses

Other interventions, based on patient/family needs

g. *Therapeutic/Medication regimens*

RN to teach regarding antidepressive medication and side effects

RN to monitor medication regimen and compliance with _____ therapy (specify)

Medication assessment and management q visit

Nonpharmacological interventions such as progressive muscle relaxation, imagery, positive visualization, music, massage and touch, and humor therapy of patient's choice implemented

RN to monitor/assess effectiveness of new antipsychotic drug(s) for severe agitation, psychotic behavior, and suicidal thoughts or planning

RN to monitor effectiveness of new tranquilizer regimen for severe anxiety

RN to administer injection of psychotropic medication _____ q _____ (specify orders)

RN to weigh patient (specify ordered frequency)

Medication teaching and management

Weekly venipunctures for _____ (specify)

Teach about and observe side effects of palliative chemotherapy, including constipation, anemia, and fatigue

Evaluation of medication response

Assess the patient's response to therapeutic treatments and interventions, and report any changes or unfavorable responses to the physician (i.e., extrapyramidal symptoms)

Assessment of effectiveness of new therapeutic medication regimen

Evaluate with IDT and physician the hospice patient's need for antidepressants

4

Observation and assessment of patient on tricyclic antidepressants to assist in pain relief of neuropathic origin

Evaluation/observation of patient's mood and appetite as recently started on corticosteroids

Teaching of patient/family, including information on medications and the management program (e.g., strength, type, actions, times, and compliance tips)

Encourage family/caregivers to give the patient medications on the schedule and around the clock

Medications changed using equianalgesic conversion tables/physician orders (e.g., from oral morphine to an equianalgesic dose of transdermal fentanyl)

Other interventions, based on patient/family needs

h. *Other considerations*

Assess progression of disease process

RN to assess the patient's response to treatments and interventions and to report changes, unfavorable responses, or reactions to the physician

Other interventions, based on patient/family needs

- **Home health aide or certified nursing assistant**

  Effective and safe personal care

  Safe ADL assistance and support

  Respite care and active listening skills

  Observation and reporting

  Meal preparation

  Homemaker services

  Comfort care

  Other duties

- **Social worker**

  Psychosocial assessment of patient and family/caregiver, including adjustment to long-term illness and its implications

  Identification of optimal coping strategies

  Financial assessment and counseling regarding food acquisition, ability to prepare, and costs of needed medications

  Intervention/support related to terminal illness and loss

  Emotional/spiritual support

  Depression/fear assessed and addressed

  Facilitate communication among patient, family, and hospice team

  Referral/linkage to community services and resources as indicated

  Grief counseling and intervention/support related to illness/loss

  Patient/caregiver counseling and support

  Identification of caregiver role strain necessitating respite/relief measures/support

  For patient who lives alone with no support system (e.g., able, available, willing caregiver[s]), obtain necessary resources to enable patient to remain in the home

  Identification of illness-related psychiatric condition necessitating care

Suicidal ideation assessment and evaluation, follow-up
Other interventions, based on the patient's/family's unique needs
Funeral and burial planning assistance

- **Volunteer(s)**
Support, friendship, companionship, and presence
Comfort and dignity maintained/provided for patient and family
Errands and transportation
Other services, based on interdisciplinary team recommendations and
    patient/caregiver needs

- **Spiritual counselor**
Spiritual assessment and care
Counseling, intervention, and support related to that dimension of life
    related to life's meaning (consistent with patient's beliefs)
Support, listening, and presence
Pray with or for the patient/family, using prayers familiar to patient's
    religious background (per their wishes)
Participation in sacred or spiritual rituals or practices
Other supportive care, based on patient's/family's needs and belief
    systems

- **Dietitian/Nutritional counseling**
Assessment of patient with decreased intake, weight loss, anorexia,
    and increased shortness of breath (e.g., "I don't feel like eating")
Supportive counseling with patient/family indicating that patient will
    have a decreased appetite and usually at some point may not
    eat/drink
Assessment and recommendations for swallowing difficulties
Teaching and support of family members and caregivers
Support and care with food and nourishment as desired by patient
Evaluation/management of nutritional deficits and needs
Encourage nutritional supplements and snacks to increase protein and
    caloric intake
Food and dietary recommendations incorporate patient choice and
    wishes

- **Occupational therapist**
Evaluation of ADLs, functional mobility, need for adaptive techniques
    and assistive devices
Safety assessment of patient's environment and ADLs
Assessment for energy conservation training
Instruct/supervise caregivers and volunteers in the home exercise
    program for safety/conditioning/strength

- **Bereavement counselor**
Assessment of the needs of the bereaved family and friends
Support and intervention, based on assessment and ongoing
    findings
Presence and counseling

4

Supportive visits and follow-up, other interventions (e.g., mailings, calls)
Other services related to bereavement work and support

- **Pharmacist**

    Evaluation of hospice patient with depression and constipation on cathartics, stool softeners, and other medications for possible food/drug, drug/drug interactions

    Medication monitoring regarding therapeutic levels and dosages

    Medication consult and input into interdisciplinary POC related to pain control, palliation, and symptom management

    Assessment of medication regimen and plan for safety and compliance

- **Music, massage, art, or other therapies or services**

    Evaluation and intervention based on patient's and caregivers unique wishes and needs that support care, comfort, and death in the setting of the patient's choice

    Assessment plan to engage patient and support comfort, quality, enjoyment, and dignity

    Pet therapy (including patient's pet, if available) and therapeutic intervention

6. Outcomes for care

- **Hospice nursing**

    Pharmacological and nonpharmacological interventions, such as localized heat application, positioning, relaxation methods, and music

    Mental distress, depression, and fear of dying addressed throughout care by hospice team

    Patient and family able to care for and support patient

    Patient and caregiver can verbalize symptoms, changes, or accelerations that necessitate call to physician

    Patient and family demonstrate compliance with medication regimen and other therapeutic interventions

    Patient demonstrates stabilization and increased or enhanced coping skills related to functioning and depression

    Pain and symptoms managed/controlled in setting of patient/family choice (e.g., patient and family report ability to eat, sleep, speak with pacing)

    Planned and effective bowel program, as evidenced by regular bowel movements and patient/family report of comfort

    Death with dignity, and pain/symptoms controlled in setting of patient/family choice

    Optimal comfort, support, and dignity provided throughout illness

    Death with maximum comfort through effective symptom control with specialized hospice support

    Patient verbalizes feelings in a safe environment

    Patient and caregiver demonstrate compliance with instructions related to medications, positive coping skills and other behaviors, and decision making

Lab values (i.e., lithium) will be within normal limits for patient by _____ (date)

Symptoms stabilized as evidenced by _____ (define) by _____ (date)

Caregiver effective in care management and knows whom to call for questions/concerns

Patient verbalizes understanding of and adheres to medication regimens

Anxiety decreased as noted by behaviors and self-report by patient/caregiver

Patient self-reports decreased episodes of panic and is able to leave home without spouse by _____ (specify)

Compliance with and adherence to interdisciplinary POC as demonstrated by observation and reporting by caregiver/patient

Other goals/outcomes based on the patient's unique needs and problems

Educational tools/plans incorporated in daily care, and patient/caregiver verbalizes understanding of safe, needed care

Adherence to POC as demonstrated and verbalized by caregiver and demonstrated by patient findings by _____ (specify date)

Patient states that pain is _____ on 0–10 scale by next visit

Patient/caregiver demonstrates appropriate backup or "rescue" therapies for breakthrough pain or other symptoms (e.g., dyspnea)

Patient will decide on care, interventions, and evaluation

Patient will express satisfaction with hospice support received and will experience increased comfort

Patient will be made comfortable at home through death in accordance with the patient's wishes

Effective pain control and symptom control verbalized by patient

Patient and caregiver supported through patient's death

Comfort maintained through course of care

Patient and family receive hospice support and care, and family members and friends are able to spend quality time with the patient

Caregiver able and verbalizes comfort with role and lists when to call hospice team members

Patient supported through and receives the maximum benefit from palliative chemotherapy and radiation with minimal complications

Patient/caregiver lists adverse reactions, potential complications, signs/symptoms of infection (e.g., sputum change, chest congestion)

Comfort maintained through death with dignity

Pain effectively managed, and patient verbalizes comfort

Patient/caregiver able to list adverse drug reactions/problems with medication regimen and whom to call for follow-up and resolution

Patient's/family's privacy, independence, and choices supported with respect and maintained through death

Enhancement and support of quality of life

Effective symptom relief and control (e.g., a peaceful and comfortable death at home, depression controlled, some enjoyment of life)

Maximizing the patient's quality of life (e.g., alert and pain free or as patient wishes)

Pharmacological and nonpharmacological interventions, such as localized heat application, biofeedback, massage, positioning, relaxation methods, and music

Patient cared for and family supported through death with physical, psychosocial, spiritual, and other concerns/needs acknowledged/addressed

Patient- and family-centered hospice care provided based on the patient's/family's unique situation and needs

Infection control and palliation

Grief/bereavement expression and support provided

Patient is pain free by next _____ visit

Caregiver demonstrates ability to manage pain, where applicable

Patient maintains comfort and dignity throughout illness

- ***Home health aide or certified nursing assistant***
  Effective hygiene, personal care, and comfort
  ADL assistance
  Safe environment maintained

- ***Social worker***
  Problem identified and addressed, with patient and caregiver linked with appropriate community support services and plan of care successfully implemented

  Patient and caregiver cope adaptively with illness and death

  Psychosocial support and counseling offered to patient/caregivers experiencing loss and grief

  Counseling/support related to ideation of suicide

  Caregiver system assessed, and development of stable caregiver plan facilitated

  Funeral and burial planning assistance

- ***Volunteer(s)***
  Comfort, companionship, and friendship extended to patient/family
  Support and respite provided as defined by the needs of the patient/caregiver
  Patient and family supported by team with care, comfort, and companionship

- ***Spiritual counselor***
  Intervention/support provided related to that dimension of life related to life's meaning

  Spiritual support offered and provided as defined by needs of patient/caregiver

  Participation in sacred or spiritual rituals or practices

  Provision of spiritual support and care based on the assessed and ongoing needs of the patient and family

  Spiritual support offered, and patient and family needs met

  Patient and family express relief of symptoms of spiritual suffering

  Support, listening, and presence

  Pray with or for the patient/family, using prayers familiar to the patient's religious background (per their wishes)

- *Dietitian/Nutritional counseling*
  Patient and family verbalize comprehension of changing nutritional needs
  Family and caregiver integrate recommendations into nutrition teaching (where appropriate)
  Patient and caregiver know whom to call for nutrition- and hydration-related questions/concerns
  Nutrition/hydration per patient's choices
  Caregiver integrates recommendations into daily meal planning

- *Occupational therapy*
  Patient and caregiver demonstrate maximum independence with ADLs
  Patient and caregiver demonstrate maximum safety in ADLs and functional mobility
  Patient and caregiver demonstrate effective use of energy conservation to improve quality of life

- *Bereavement counselor*
  Bereavement support provided

- *Pharmacist*
  Regimen for bowel regimen successful as self-reported by patient and in update at team meeting
  Multiple drug regimen reviewed for food/drug and drug/drug interactions in patient on multiple medications
  Stability and safety in complex medication regimen, with maximum benefit to patient
  Effective symptom control and symptom management as reported by patient/caregiver
  Laboratory reports reviewed for therapeutic dosages and effective patient response

- *Music, massage, art, or other therapies or services*
  Therapeutic massage/touch effective for patient as self-reported or observed by caregivers/family
  Improved muscle tone, relaxation, and/or sleep
  Patient comfortable and relaxed (e.g., sleeping) after massage
  Music therapy intervention based on assessment to decrease pain perception and provide emotional expression and support
  Maintenance of comfort and physical, psychosocial, and spiritual health
  Holistic health maintained and comfort achieved through _____ (specify modality)
  Patient has pet's presence as desired—in all care sites, when possible

4

7. **Patient, family, and caregiver educational needs**
   Educational needs are the care regimens that contribute to safe and effective care at home between the hospice team's visits. These include the following:
   The basic tenets of hospice and the availability of support 24 hours a day, 7 days a week

Home safety assessment and counseling

Patient's medication regimen

Safe and proper body mechanics to promote patient comfort and prevent caregiver safety problems

Other teaching specific to the patient's and family's unique needs

Support groups available to patient's family, such as the hospice program's "Caregiver Support Group" meetings for family members and friends of the patient

Anticipated disease progression

Safety concerns, medication compliance, and importance of keeping psychotherapeutic appointments at the mental health center

Importance of adequate hydration and nutrition

Signs and symptoms of recurring depression or other behaviors; side effects related to drugs that necessitate seeking medical follow-up

Home safety concerns and issues

The importance of medical follow-up, including drug levels if indicated, and family therapy

8. Specific tips for quality and reimbursement

Document any variances to expected outcomes. There are many models of hospice programs.

The Medicare hospice benefit does not require that the patient be homebound or have identified skilled needs. For further information on this benefit, please refer to CMS Hospice Manual 21.

Should the patient's status deteriorate and increased personal care be needed, obtain a telephone order for the increased service, noting frequency and estimating the duration.

Obtain a telephone order for all medication and treatment changes of the medical regimen, and document these in the clinical record.

Unless the patient is in a hospice insurance program, some insurers will not pay for a skilled clinician visit that is made at death if the patient is dead when the clinician arrives at the home. From a Medicare home care perspective, the visit at the time of death may be covered when the orders and clinical record document assessment of the patient's status or signs of death/life or state law allows pronouncement of death by an RN.

Document patient deterioration

Document dehydration, dehydrating

Document patient change or instability

Document pain, other symptoms not controlled

Document status after acute episode of _____ (specify)

Document positive urine, sputum, etc. culture; patient started on _____ (specify ordered antibiotic therapy)

Document any impaction; removed manually

Document RN in frequent communication with physician regarding _____ (specify)

Document febrile at _____, pulse change at _____, irr., irr.

Document change noted in _____

Document bony prominences red, opening

Document RN contacted physician regarding _____ (specify)

Document marked SOB

Document alteration in mental status

Document medications being adjusted, regulated, or monitored

Document that patient is unable to perform own ADLs, personal care

Document all IDT meetings and communications in the POC and in the progress notes of the clinical record

All disciplines involved should have input into the POC and document their interventions and goals

Document in the clinical notes the clear progression, symptom and interventions that demonstrate the need for interventions and overall management of pain in the clinical notes

Document when/if the patient has respiratory changes, shortness of breath, exacerbation of conditions, dysphagia, changes in pain, and other symptoms and that they are identified and resolved

Remember that the clinical documentation is key to measuring compliance for quality and reimbursement purposes. Care coordination, timely verbal and initial physician orders, and assessment and addressing of spiritual and psychosocial needs should be ongoing and documented in the patient's clinical record

The documentation should support that all hospice care supports comfort and dignity while meeting patient/family needs

The documentation should include ongoing assessment and management of pain and other symptoms and the anticipation and prevention of secondary symptoms such as constipation

It is important to note that all team members, including clinicians and social workers, should assess, identify, and "hear" spiritual needs that the patient/family want to be addressed. These spiritual issues are key to the provision of quality hospice care and cannot be addressed effectively and promptly by the spiritual counselor only

Document clearly symptoms, clinical changes, and assessment findings related to pain and patient care

Document patient changes, symptoms, and clinical information identified from visits and team conferences that support hospice care and a limited life expectancy

Document coordination of services or consultation of the other members of the IDT

Document changes to the plan of care, such as medications, services, frequency, communication, and concurrence of other team members

Clearly document the rationale that supports/explains the progression of the illness from the chronic to terminal stages

Document mentation, behavioral, and/or cognitive changes

Document dysphagia, weight loss, increased shortness of breath, dyspnea, infection, sepsis, new or changed medications, etc.

Document any skin changes (e.g., inflamed, painful, weeping skin site[s])

Document when the patient is actively dying, deteriorating, or progressing toward death

Remember that the "litmus test" of care coordination rests on the quality of the clinical documentation by all team members. Review one of your patient's clinical records and ask yourself the following: "If I was unable to give a verbal report/update on this patient, would a peer be able to pick up and provide the same level of care and know (from the documentation) the current orders, medications, and other details that contribute to effective hospice care?"

This patient population usually has many clinical changes that should be documented. These include weight loss and multiple and changed medication regimens with varying routes. Side effects of the drug regimen should be observed, noted, documented, and reported

Your assessments, observations, and clinical findings assist in painting a picture to support coverage and documentation requirements for hospice care

Document any hospitalizations and changed clinical findings

Document patient changes, symptoms, psychosocial issues impacting the care, and information gathered at the patient/family visits and during team meetings

The documentation should reflect ongoing effects of the terminal condition, the patient's/family's difficulty with care or coping, and the continued desire for hospice care

Document communications and care coordination with other care providers, such as skilled health care facility or health care home staff, inpatient team members, and hired caregivers

9. Queries for quality

Depression and psychiatric care
- *Is patient's pain managed adequately?*
- *Is patient's anxiety managed adequately?*
- *Is the patient's functional ability/status clearly documented?*
- *What are the patient's symptoms?*
- *Have you documented to the interdisciplinary POC?*

Psychiatric care
- *Is patient's pain managed adequately?*
- *Is patient's anxiety managed adequately?*
- *Is the patient's functional ability/status clearly documented?*
- *What are the patient's symptoms?*
- *Have you documented to the interdisciplinary POC?*

10. Resources for hospice care and practice

The National Institute of Mental Health offers many resources for clinicians and patient education. They can be reached by calling 1-800-421-4211 or via their web site, www.nih.gov.

DIABETES MELLITUS AND OTHER VASCULAR CONDITIONS CARE

1. General considerations

The care for diabetes mellitus and comorbid conditions such as peripheral vascular disease, cellulitis, and amputation present challenges to the hospice team. All of these patient problems usually indicate a long-term chronic disease process for the new hospice patient and family. See also "Cancer Care," "Pain Care," and other sections that may pertain to your hospice patient.

2. Needs for visit

Physician order for hospice care, specific to the hospice program's admission criteria and policies

Standard precautions/supplies

Vital signs equipment for baseline assessment

Other supplies or equipment, based on physician orders

3. Safety considerations

Infection control/standard precautions

Night-light

Extra caution on slippery surfaces

Removal of scatter rugs

Tub rail, grab bars for bathroom safety

Supportive and nonskid shoes

Handrail on stairs

Fall precautions

Protective skin measures

Identification and report of any skin problems

Smoke detector and fire evacuation plan

Assistance with ambulation

Foot care and protection

Avoidance of heating pads, electric blankets, extremes of hot/cold

Disposal of sharps and related supplies

Safety related to decreased sensation in extremities and protection from heat and cold

Disposal of soiled dressings and related supplies

Anticoagulant precautions

Supervised medication administration

Multiple medications (e.g., side effects, needles, safe storage)

Safety for home medical equipment

Supportive and well-fitting shoes and socks

Emergency symptoms and actions to take

The phone number and name of person to call with a care problem

Others, based on the patient's unique condition and environment

4. Potential diagnoses and codes

AKA right or left	V49.76
AMI	410.90
Amputee, bilateral	V49.70
Amputation, infected right or left BKA, AKA	997.62
Amputation, transmetatarsal (right or left) (surgical)	84.12
Angina	413.9
Arterial graft (surgical)	39.58
Arterial insufficiency	447.1
Arterial occlusive disease	447.1
Atherosclerosis	440.9
Bilateral amputee	V49.70
BKA, right or left (surgical)	84.15
Bullous pemphigoid	694.5
Cellulitis of the arm	682.3
Cellulitis of the trunk	682.2
Cellulitis RLE, LLE	682.6
Cellulitis and abscess (legs)	682.6
Cellulitis of the trunk	682.2
CHF	428.0
Chronic ischemic heart disease	414.9
Chronic renal failure	585
Circulatory disease	459.9
COPD	496
Coronary artery disease	414.00
CVA	436
Decubitus ulcer (pressure ulcer)	707.0
Diabetes glaucoma	250.50 and 365.44
Diabetes mellitus, with complications (NIDDM)	250.90
Diabetes mellitus, with complications (IDDM)	250.91
Diabetic neuropathy	250.60 and 357.2
Diabetic retinopathy (insulin dependent)	250.51 and 362.01
Diabetic retinopathy (non–insulin dependent)	250.50 and 362.01
Electrolyte/fluid imbalance	276.9
Excoriation of skin	919.8
Failure to thrive, adult	783.7
Femoral-popliteal bypass (surgical)	39.29
Foot abscess	682.7
Gangrene, foot, due to DM	250.70 and 785.4
Gangrene toe	785.4
Hyperglycemia	790.6
Hypertension and diabetes	401.9 and 250.80
Hypoglycemia, diabetic	250.80
Ketoacidosis, insulin dependent	250.11
Ketoacidosis, non–insulin dependent	250.10
Left heart failure	428.1
Obesity	278.00
Pain in limb	729.5

4

Peripheral vascular disease and diabetes	443.9 and 250.00
Pressure (decubitus) ulcer	707.0
Staph infection	041.10
Stasis ulcer	454.2
Thrombophlebitis	451.9
Toe amputation (surgical)	84.11
Ulcer, right or left, lower extremity	707.10
Urinary tract infection	599.0
Vascular insufficiency	459.9
Vasculitis and diabetes	447.6 and 250.70

5. Skills and services identified

- *Hospice nursing*

a. *Comfort and symptom control*

Complete initial systems assessment of the patient with
_____ (specify) admitted to hospice for _____
(specify problem necessitating care)

Skilled observation and all systems assessment of patient with diabetes
mellitus

Presentation of hospice philosophy and services

Explain patient rights and responsibilities

Assess patient, family, and caregiver wishes and expectations
regarding care

Assess patient, family, and caregiver resources available
for care

Provision of volunteer support to patient and family

Teach family or caregiver physical care of patient

Assess pain and other symptoms, including site, duration, characteristics,
and relief measures

Assess pain and evaluate the pain management's effectiveness

Teach care of bedridden patient

Measure vital signs and pain, q visit

Assess cardiovascular, pulmonary, and respiratory status

Teach patient/family principles of effective pain management

Teach caregivers symptom control and relief measures

Identify and monitor pain, symptoms, and relief measures

Teach patient and family about use of home glucose monitoring

Teach insulin administration and other DM care regimens including
foot care, skin care, and emergency measures for signs and
symptoms of hyper/hypoglycemia

RN to assess patient's pain or other symptoms q visit to identify need
for change, addition, or other plan or dose adjustment

Assess peripheral circulation

Check pedal pulses for equality, rate, and strength

Assess amount, site(s) of edema

Pain management and relief interventions

Teach patient correct application of compression stockings

Assess pain, site, frequency, and duration

Teach effective personal hygiene and proper handwashing techniques

Teach signs and symptoms of (further) infection

Teach signs/symptom of hyperglycemia and hypoglycemia and emergency measures to patient and family

Assess for long-term ability of patient and family to comply with regimen

Teaching and training, observation and assessment related to diabetes care and management

Ongoing monitoring and assessment of blood glucose readings and patient's management of compliance with new DM regimen

Instruct patient in equipment and use of blood glucose monitoring program

Assess for signs of decreased circulation and report to physician

Teach patient's family care regimen

Teach patent/family use of standardized form/tool to use between hospice team members' visits (and for care coordination among team members)

RN to teach patient and family on all aspects of care of the patient with diabetes, including foot care, signs/care of hypoglycemia or hyperglycemia, and the importance of medical follow-up

Observation and assessment, communication with physician related to signs and symptoms of continuing decompensation and increased symptoms, pain, discomfort, shortness of breath, and measures to alleviate and control

Pain assessment and management q visit, including source of pain (e.g., neuropathy, phantom pain, claudification, infection, and other problems, such as cardiac or arthritis pain)

Effective management of pain and prevention of secondary symptoms

RN to provide and teach effective oral care and comfort measures

Teach patient/family about realistic expectations of disease process

Teach care of dying and signs/symptoms of impending death

Presence and support

Other interventions, based on patient/family needs

b. *Safety and mobility considerations*

Patient provided with home safety information and instruction related to _____ and documented in the clinical record

Teach patient or family member safe home blood glucose monitoring process

Teach patient all aspects of safe care with new SQ insulin infusion pump at home

Teach family about safety of patient in home

Teach family about energy conservation techniques

Assess safety related to amputation and balance/mobility

Other interventions, based on patient/family needs

c. *Emotional/Spiritual considerations*

Psychosocial assessment of patient and family regarding disease and prognosis

RN to provide emotional support to patient and family

Assess patient's and caregiver's coping skills

Interventions of symptoms directed toward comfort and palliation

Observation and assessment of mental status changes/complaints of depression in new hospice patient with pain and wound

Observation of patient for neuropsychiatric complications of illness, including confusion, depression, and anxiety

Clinician to provide support and intervention for depression

Teach patient/family about depression and signs/symptoms of exacerbation that require more intervention

Inform patient/family/caregiver of available volunteer support

Assess for and manage plans for psychosocial and/or spiritual pain (e.g., all pain, anxiety, interpersonal and other distress)

Psychosocial aspects of pain control (e.g., depression) assessed and acknowledged with team support/intervention

Ongoing acknowledgment of spirituality and related concerns of patient/family

Other interventions, based on patient/family needs

d. *Skin care*

Pressure ulcer care as indicated

Assess skin integrity

Evaluate patient's need for equipment, including supplies to decrease pressure, alternating pressure mattress, gel foam seat cushion, and heel and elbow protectors

Observation and evaluation of wound and surrounding skin

Teach patient, family, or caregiver about proper body alignment and positioning in bed to prevent skin tears from shearing skin

Observation and skilled assessment of areas for possible breakdown, including heels, hips, elbows, and ankles

Teach family to perform dressing changes between RN visits, specifically _____

Teach caregiver about skin care needs, including the need for frequent position changes, appropriate pressure pads and mattresses, and the prevention of breakdown

Pre-medicate patient with pain medication before dressing change

Dressing change _____ site (specify physician orders)

Gently wash and dry site

Evaluate temperature, redness of site, and amount of swelling

Culture open wound as ordered, and send for culture and sensitivity test

Instruct patient or caregiver on dressing change procedure

Apply occlusive (or other ordered) dressing to wound

Assess and objectively document wound progress

Obtain specific wound dressing orders, including sterile or nonsterile procedure(s)

Specify dressing regimen and frequency of wound changes q visit

Observation, assessment, and supportive care related to vascular problems, including diabetes and cellulitis with weeping skin sites

4

Comprehensive management of diabetes and wound care regimens
Other interventions, based on patient/family needs

e. *Elimination considerations*
   Assess bowel regimen, and implement program as needed
   Check for and remove impaction as needed
   Condom catheter or indwelling catheter as indicated
   Assess amount and frequency of urinary output
   RN to teach caregiver daily catheter care
   RN to evaluate the patient's bowel patterns and need for stool
       softeners, laxatives, and dietary adjustments, and to develop bowel
       management plan
   Teach patient or family urine check procedures, as ordered
   Teaching and ongoing assessment related to early prevention and
       identification of constipation and its correction/resolution
   Initiate bowel management program per hospice physician
   Implement bowel assessment and management program
   Teach patient/family and aide the importance of observing and noting
       bowel movements between scheduled nursing visits
   Obtain patient history related to norms for bowel movements to date
       (e.g., "All my life I go only every other day")
   Consider stool softeners and offer laxative of choice, Fleet's enemas
       prn, and other methods per patient wishes and physician orders
   Other interventions, based on patient/family needs

f. *Hydration/Nutrition*
   Detailed nutritional assessment related to diabetes, weight,
       constipation, and immobility
   Assess nutrition and hydration statuses
   Diet counseling for patient with anorexia
   Teach feeding-tube care to family
   Nutrition/hydration supported by offering patient's choice of favorite or
       desired foods or liquids
   Nutrition/hydration maintained by offering patient high-protein diet and
       foods of choice as tolerated
   Teach patient and family to expect decreased nutritional and fluid
       intake as disease progresses
   Other interventions, based on patient/family needs

g. *Therapeutic/Medication regimens*
   Comprehensive management of medications, including antibiotics and
       those for pain and diabetes
   Teaching of patient/family, including medications and the management
       program (e.g., strength, type, actions, times, and compliance tips)
   Encourage family/caregivers to give patient medications on the
       schedule and around the clock
   Monitor patient for side effects of drugs and drug/food and drug/drug
       interactions
   Teach new pain and symptom control medication regimen

RN to assess the patient's unique response to treatments or interventions, and to report changes, unfavorable responses, or reactions to the physician

Medication assessment and management

Teach patient and caregiver use of PCA pump

Assess for electrolyte imbalance

Nonpharmacological interventions such as progressive muscle relaxation, imagery, positive visualization, music, massage and touch, and humor therapy of patient's choice implemented

Teach new antibiotic regimen of _____ (specify)

Teaching and training related to IV antibiotic therapy (e.g., infusion hook-up and discontinuance, signs and symptoms of infiltration, reaction)

Teach new medication regimen

Teach patient or family to mix insulin(s)

Venipuncture for FBS as indicated

Teach about new insulin and medication regimen

Teach action of ordered insulin(s)

Teach use of single-site rotations for injections or other ordered rotation method

Medications changed using equianalgesic conversion tables/physician orders (e.g., from oral morphine to an equianalgesic dose of transdermal fentanyl)

Other interventions, based on patient/family needs

h. *Other considerations*

Administer or teach foot care regimen

Assess need for podiatrist to provide needed foot care

Assess progression of disease process

RN to assess the patient's response to treatments and interventions and to report to the physician changes, unfavorable responses, or reactions

Other interventions, based an patient/family needs

- *Home health aide or certified nursing assistant*

Effective and safe personal care

Safe ADL assistance and support

Respite care and active listening skills

Observation and reporting

Meal preparation

Homemaker services

Comfort care

Other duties

- *Social worker*

Psychosocial assessment of patient and family/caregiver, including adjustment to long-term illness and its implications

Identification of optimal coping strategies

Identification of caregiver role strain necessitating respite/relief measures/support

Financial assessment and counseling regarding food acquisition, ability
to prepare, and costs of needed medications
Intervention/support related to terminal illness and loss
Emotional/spiritual support
Depression/fear assessed and addressed
Facilitate communication among patient, family, and hospice team
Referral/linkage to community services and resources as indicated
Grief counseling and intervention/support related to illness/loss
Patient/caregiver counseling and support
For patient who lives alone with no support system (e.g., able,
available, willing caregiver[s]), obtain resources that enable patient
to remain in the home
Identification of illness-related psychiatric condition necessitating care
Funeral and burial planning assistance

- *Volunteer(s)*
Support, friendship, companionship, and presence
Comfort and dignity maintained/provided for patient and family
Errands and transportation
Other services, based on IDT recommendations and patient/caregiver
needs

- *Spiritual counselor*
Spiritual assessment and care
Counseling, intervention, and support related to that dimension of life
related to life's meaning (consistent with patient's beliefs)
Pray with or for the patient/family, using prayers familiar to patient's
religious background (per their wishes)
Support, listening, and presence
Participation in sacred or spiritual rituals or practices
Funeral planning and assistance
Other supportive care, based on patient/family needs and belief systems

- *Dietitian/Nutritional counseling*
Assessment of patient with decreased intake, weight loss, anorexia, and
increased shortness of breath (e.g., "I don't feel like eating")
Supportive counseling with patient/family indicating that patient will
have a decreased appetite and usually at some point may not
eat/drink
Assessment and recommendations for swallowing difficulties
Teaching and support of family members and caregivers
Support and care with food and nourishment as desired by patient
Evaluation/management of nutritional deficits and needs
Encourage nutritional supplements and snacks to increase protein and
caloric intake
Food and dietary recommendations incorporate patient choice and wishes

- *Occupational therapist*
Evaluation of ADLs and functional mobility
Assess for need for adaptive equipment and assistive devices

4

Safety assessment of patient's environment and ADLs
Assessment for energy conservation training
Assessment of upper-extremity function, retraining motor skills

- *Physical therapist*
  Evaluation
  Safety assessment of patient's environment
  Safe transfer training or bed mobility exercises
  Pain assessment/reduction factors
  Strengthening exercises/program
  Assessment of gait safety and home safety measures
  Instruct/supervise caregiver and volunteers on home exercise program
      for conditioning and strength
  Assistive, adaptive devices and evaluation of equipment and teaching

- *Speech-language pathologist*
  Evaluation for speech/swallowing problems
  Food texture recommendations
  Alternate functional communication

- *Bereavement counselor*
  Assessment of the needs of the bereaved family and friends
  Support and intervention, based on assessment and ongoing findings
  Presence and counseling
  Supportive visits and follow-up, other interventions (e.g., mailings,
      calls)
  Other services related to bereavement work and support

- *Pharmacist*
  Evaluation of hospice patient with constipation on cathartics, stool
      softeners, and other medications for possible food/drug, drug/drug
      interactions
  Medication monitoring regarding therapeutic levels and dosages
  Pain consult and input into interdisciplinary POC related to pain
      control, palliation, and symptom management
  Assessment of medication regimen and plan for safety and compliance

- *Music, massage, art, or other therapies or services*
  Evaluation and intervention based on patient's and caregiver's unique
      wishes and needs that support care, comfort, and death in the setting
      of the patient's choice
  Assessment plan to engage patient and support comfort, quality,
      enjoyment, and dignity
  Pet therapy (including patient's pet, if available) and therapeutic
      intervention

6. Outcomes for care

- *Hospice nursing*
  Death with dignity, and symptoms controlled in setting of patient/family
      choice

Mental distress, depression, and fear of dying addressed throughout care by hospice team

Patient and family able to care for and support patient

Patient and caregiver can verbalize symptoms, changes, or accelerations that necessitate call to physician

Patient and family demonstrate compliance with medication regimen and other therapeutic interventions

Patient demonstrates stabilization and increased or enhanced coping skills related to functioning and depression

Pain and symptoms managed/controlled in setting of patient/family choice (e.g., patient/family report ability to eat, sleep, speak with pacing)

Planned and effective bowel program, as evidenced by regular bowel movements and patient/family report of comfort

Optimal comfort, support, and dignity provided throughout illness

Death with maximum comfort through effective symptom control with specialized hospice support

Patient and caregiver able to list adverse drug reactions/problems with medication regimen and whom to call for follow-up and resolution

Patient's and family's privacy, independence, and choices supported with respect and maintained through death

Enhancement and support of quality of life

Effective symptom relief and control (e.g., a peaceful and comfortable death at home, depression controlled, some enjoyment of life)

Maximizing the patient's quality of life (e.g., alert and pain free or as patient wishes)

Pharmacological and nonpharmacological interventions such as localized heat application, biofeedback, massage, positioning, relaxation methods, and music

Patient cared for and family supported through death with physical, psychosocial, spiritual, and other concerns/needs acknowledged/addressed

Patient- and family-centered hospice care provided based on the patient/family's unique situation and needs

Patient states pain is _____ on 0–10 scale by next visit

Patient and caregiver demonstrate appropriate backup or "rescue" therapies for breakthrough pain or other symptoms (e.g., dyspnea)

Patient and family verbalize satisfaction with care

Compliance with wound care and associated regimen by _____ (specify date)

Pain control/comfort achieved as verbalized by patient

Teaching program related to the prevention of infection and injuries demonstrated by caregivers

Wound healed and site infection free (e.g., no redness, swelling)

Patient/caregiver will demonstrate _____ % (specify) compliance with instructions related to care

Patient and caregiver demonstrate and practice effective handwashing and other infection control measures (specify, e.g., disposal of dressings)

Adherence to POC by patient and caregivers and ability to demonstrate safe and supportive care

Symptoms stabilized as evidenced by _____ (define) by _____ (date)

Caregiver effective in care management and knows whom to call for questions/concerns

Patient verbalizes understanding of and adheres to medication regimens

Patient compliant with self-care regarding DM and aspects of regimen by _____ (date)

Blood sugar in normal patient range, and patient verbalizes understanding of factors that contribute to prevention of complications

Patient/caregiver will demonstrate _____ % behavioral compliance with instructions related to medications, leg elevation, diet, and care

Adherence to POC by patient and caregivers and ability to demonstrate safe and supportive care

Optimal circulation for patient

Educational tools/plans incorporated in daily care, and patient/caregiver verbalizes understanding of safe, needed care

Patient will decide on care, interventions, and evaluation

Caregiver effective in care management and knows whom to call for questions/concerns

Patient will express satisfaction with hospice support received and will experience increased comfort

Patient will be made comfortable at home through death in accordance with the patient's wishes

Effective pain control and symptom control verbalized by patient

Patient verbalizes understanding of and adheres to care and medication regimens

Patient and caregiver supported through patient's death

Comfort maintained through course of care

Patient and family receive hospice support and care, and family members and friends are able to spend quality time with the patient

Caregiver able and verbalizes comfort with role and understands when to call hospice team members

Patient supported through and receives the maximum benefit from palliative chemotherapy and radiation with minimal complications

Patient/caregiver lists adverse reactions, potential complications, signs/symptoms of infection (e.g., sputum change, chest congestion)

Comfort maintained through death with dignity

Pain effectively managed, and patient verbalizes comfort

Patient is protected from injury, has stable respiratory status, and is compliant with medication, safety, and care regimens

Comfort and individualized intervention of patient with immobility/bedbound status (e.g., skin, urinary, musculature, vascular)

Spiritual and psychosocial needs met (specify) as defined by patient and caregiver throughout course of care

Infection control and palliation of wound site

Grief/bereavement expression and support provided

4

Caregiver demonstrates ability to manage pain, where applicable
Patient maintains comfort and dignity throughout illness
Other goals/outcomes, based on the patient's unique needs and problems

- ***Home health aide or certified nursing assistant***
Effective hygiene, personal care, and comfort
ADL assistance
Safe environment maintained

- ***Social worker***
Problem identified and addressed, with patient/caregiver linked with
    appropriate support services and plan of care successfully implemented
Patient and caregiver cope adaptively with illness and death
Adaptive adjustment to changed body and body image
Psychosocial support and counseling offered to patient/caregivers
    experiencing loss and grief
Resources identified, community linkage as appropriate for patient/family
Caregiver system assessed, and development of stable caregiver plan
    facilitated
Funeral and burial planning assistance

- ***Volunteer(s)***
Comfort, companionship, and friendship extended to patient/family
Support and respite provided as defined by the needs of the
    patient/caregiver
Patient and family supported by team with care, comfort, and
    companionship

- ***Spiritual counseling***
Spiritual support offered and provided as defined by needs of
    patient/caregiver
Provision of spiritual support and care based on the assessed and
    ongoing needs of the patient and family
Spiritual support offered, and patient and family needs met
Patient and family express relief of symptoms of spiritual suffering
Support, listening, and presence
Intervention and support provided related to that dimension of life
    related to life's meaning (consistent with patient's beliefs)
Participation in sacred or spiritual rituals or practices
Pray with or for the patient/family, using prayers familiar to the
    patient's religious background (per their wishes)

- ***Dietitian/Nutritional counseling***
Family and caregiver integrate recommendations into nutrition teaching
    (where appropriate)
Patient and caregiver know whom to call for nutrition- and
    hydration-related questions/concerns
Nutrition/hydration per patient's choices
Caregiver integrates recommendations into daily meal planning
Patient and family verbalize comprehension of changing nutritional needs

- *Occupational therapist*
  Patient and caregiver demonstrate maximum independence with ADLs, adaptive techniques, and assistive devices
  Patient and caregiver demonstrate maximum safety in ADLs and functional mobility
  Patient and caregiver demonstrate effective use of energy conservation
  Verbalization/demonstration of improved functional activity level and enhanced quality of life
  Patient and caregiver demonstrate effective use of diaphragmatic breathing to reduce shortness of breath and relaxation techniques to help in pain/symptom management
  Patient and caregiver demonstrate correct use of exercise and splints

- *Physical therapist*
  Prevention of complications
  Home exercise and upper-extremity program taught to caregiver
  Optimal strength, mobility, function maintained/achieved
  Compliance with home exercise program by _____ (specify date)

- *Speech-language pathologist*
  Communication method implemented, and patient able to be understood as self-reported or reported by family/caregivers
  Safe swallowing and functional communication
  Recommended lists of foods/textures for safety and patient choice

- *Bereavement counselor*
  Support services related to grief provided to patient and family
  Well-being and resolution process of grief initiated and followed through bereavement services

- *Pharmacist*
  Regimen for bowel/other regimen successful as self-reported by patient and in update at team meeting
  Multiple drug regimen reviewed for food/drug and drug/drug interactions in patient on multiple medications
  Stability and safety in complex medication regimen, with maximum benefit to patient
  Effective pain and symptom control and symptom management as reported by patient/caregiver

- *Music, massage, art, or other therapies or services*
  Therapeutic massage/touch effective for patient as self-reported or observed by caregivers/family
  Improved muscle tone, relaxation, and/or sleep
  Patient comfortable and relaxed (e.g., sleeping) after massage
  Pet therapy (including patient's pet, if available) and therapeutic intervention
  Music therapy intervention based on assessment to decrease pain perception and provide emotional expression and support

4

Maintenance of comfort and physical, psychosocial, and spiritual health
Holistic health maintained and comfort achieved through
_____ (specify modality)

7. Patient, family, and caregiver educational needs

Educational needs are the care regimens that contribute to safe and effective care at home between the hospice team's visits. These include the following:

The basic tenets of hospice and the availability of support 24 hours a day, 7 days a week

Home safety assessment and counseling

The patient's medication regimen

Safe and proper body mechanics to promote patient comfort and prevent caregiver safety problems

Anticipated disease progression

Other teaching specific to the patient's and family's unique needs

Support groups available to patient's family, such as the hospice program's "Caregiver Support Group" meetings for family members and friends of the patient

8. Specific tips for quality and reimbursement

Document any variances to expected outcomes. There are many models of hospice programs.

The Medicare hospice benefit does not require that the patient be homebound or have identified skilled needs. For further information on this benefit, please refer to CMS Hospice Manual 21.

Should the patient's status deteriorate and increased personal care be needed, obtain a telephone order for the increased service, noting frequency and estimating the duration.

Obtain a telephone order for all medication and treatment changes of the medical regimen, and document these in the clinical record.

Unless the patient is in a hospice insurance program, some insurers will not pay for a skilled clinician visit that is made at death if the patient is dead when the clinician arrives at the home. From a Medicare home care perspective, the visit at the time of death may be covered when the orders and clinical record document assessment of the patient's status or signs of death/life or state law allows pronouncement of death by an RN.

Document patient deterioration

Document dehydration, dehydrating

Document patient change or instability

Document pain, other symptoms not controlled

Document status after acute episode of _____ (specify)

Document positive urine, sputum, etc. culture; patient started on _____ (specify ordered antibiotic therapy)

Document patient impacted; impaction removed manually

Document RN in frequent communication with physician regarding _____ (specify)

Document febrile at _____, pulse change at _____, irr., irr.

Document change noted in _____

Document bony prominences red, opening

Document RN contacted physician regarding _____ (specify)

Document marked SOB

Document alteration in mental status

Document medications being adjusted, regulated, or monitored

Document unable to perform own ADLs, personal care

Document all IDT meetings and communications in the POC and in the progress notes of the clinical record

All hospice team members involved should have input into the POC and document their interventions and goals

Document the wound, indicate stage, drainage, color, amount, and the specific care provided

Communicate any POC changes in your documentation

Document progress in wound healing or deterioration in wound status and measure in progress notes at least 1 time a week, noting other pertinent diagnoses that impede progress

Decrease visit frequency as appropriate

If wound culture is obtained, document the results

Document if patient or family member unable to do dressing (retinopathy, severity of wound, etc.)

Document any other learning barriers

Document the specific teaching accomplished and the behavioral outcomes of that teaching

Document patient's level of independence in care

Document the care coordination between disciplines and interdisciplinary care planning

Wound care is an area in which some managed-care companies and other payors are attempting to decrease the allowed numbers of visits. It is the professional clinician's responsibility to remember that it is not just the dressing change that occurs. When a clinician makes the home visit, an assessment of the wound healing or deterioration and teaching occur. These skills usually require the skills of a nurse. All these components contribute to safer, effective wound care

Remember that the clinical documentation is key to measuring compliance for quality and reimbursement purposes. Care coordination, timely verbal and initial physician orders, and assessment and addressing of spiritual and psychosocial needs should be ongoing and documented in the patient's clinical record

The documentation should support that all hospice care supports comfort and dignity while meeting patient/family needs

The documentation should include ongoing assessment and management of pain and other symptoms and the anticipation and prevention of secondary symptoms such as constipation

It is important to note that all team members, including clinician and social workers, should assess, identify, and "hear" spiritual needs that the patient/family want to be addressed. These spiritual issues

4

are key to the provision of quality hospice care and cannot be addressed effectively and promptly by the spiritual counselor only

Document clearly symptoms, clinical changes, and assessment findings related to pain and patient care

Document weight loss, increased shortness of breath, dyspnea, infection, sepsis, new or changed medications, etc.

Document any skin changes (e.g., inflamed, painful, weeping skin site[s])

Remember that the "litmus test" of care coordination rests on the quality of the clinical documentation by all team members. Review one of your patient's clinical records and ask yourself the following: "If I was unable to give a verbal report/update on this patient's/family's course of care, would a peer be able to pick up and provide the same level of care and know (from the documentation) the current orders, medications, and other details that contribute to effective hospice care?"

This patient population usually has many clinical changes that should be documented. These include weight loss and multiple and changed medication regimens with varying routes. Side effects to the drug regimen should be observed, noted, documented, and reported

Your assessments, observations, and clinical findings assist in painting a picture to support coverage and documentation requirements for hospice care

Document any hospitalizations and changed clinical findings

Document patient changes, symptoms, and psychosocial issues impacting the patient, family, and plan of care

Document changes to the POC such as medications, services, frequency, communication, and concurrence of other team members

Document coordination of services or consultation of the other members of the IDT

Document communications and care coordination with other care providers, such as skilled health care facility or nursing home staff, inpatient team members, and hired caregivers

9. Queries for quality

Diabetes mellitus and other vascular conditions care
- Is patient's pain managed adequately?
- Is patient's anxiety managed adequately?
- Is patient's functional ability/status clearly documented?
- What are the patient's symptoms?
- Have you documented to the interdisciplinary POC?

Peripheral vascular disease care
- Is patient's pain managed adequately?
- Is patient's anxiety managed adequately?
- Is patient's functional ability/status clearly documented?
- What are the patient's symptoms?
- Have you documented to the interdisciplinary POC?

10. Resources for hospice care and practice

The American Diabetes Association (ADA) has resources available for patients and their families. It can be reached at 1-800-342-2383. It offers literature, meal planning, videos, weight planning and management services, and patient advocates. It also has a monthly magazine entitled *Forecast* for all ADA members.

The Department of Health & Human Services National Diabetes Information Clearinghouse can be reached at 1-301-654-3327 for a listing of professional and patient education publications.

Another helpful resource is the NHPC's latest edition of *Medical Guidelines for Determining Prognoses in Selected Non-Cancer Diseases*. Call the NHPCO at 1-800-646-6460 for more information.

4

HEAD AND NECK CANCER CARE

1. General considerations

Patients and their families often seek or are referred to hospice care after a long battle with cancer and surgeries and resulting **tracheostomies** and **laryngectomies**. This patient population may be on alternative feeding mechanisms and have feeding tubes or be on total parenteral nutrition (TPN). Hospice can positively impact the symptoms and side effects of the surgeries and disease processes for patients and families. Body image adjustments with depression, pain, dyspnea, bleeding, and food intolerance with nutritional depletion may be seen in this patient population. See also "Cancer Care," "Constipation Care," "Brain Tumor Care," and "Pain Care" should these sections pertain to your hospice patients and families.

2. Needs for visit

Physician order for hospice care, specific to the hospice program's
     admission criteria and policies
Standard precautions supplies
Vital signs equipment for baseline assessment
Other supplies or equipment, based on physician orders

3. Safety considerations

Infection control/standard precautions
Avoid respiratory irritants (e.g., powder), and keep site covered during
     activities (e.g., shaving) that may lead to inhalation
Importance of shielding the stoma site
Avoid swimming or any contact with water near stoma site
A working phone
Supportive and well-fitting nonslip shoes
Night-light
Tub rail, grab bars, shower seat for bathroom safety
Fall precautions/protocol
Protective skin measures and skin site care
Medication safety (e.g., side effects, storage)
Safety related to home medical equipment
Emergency symptoms that necessitate immediate reporting/assistance
     and actions to take
The phone number and name of person to call with a care problem
Identification and report of any skin problems
Smoke detector and fire evacuation plan
Others, based on the patient's unique condition and environment

4. Potential diagnoses and codes

Airway obstruction, chronic	496
Attention to tracheostomy	V55.0

Brain cancer	198.3
Bronchitis, acute	466.0
Cancer of the esophagus	150.9
Cancer of the head or neck	195.0
Cancer of the larynx	161.9
Cancer of the pharynx	149.0
Cancer of the tongue	141.9
Cancer of the trachea	162.0
Candidiasis, esophageal	112.84
Candidiasis, oral	112.0
Dysphagia	787.2
Esophagus, cancer of the	150.9
Gastrostomy, percutaneous (surgical)	43.11
Gastrostomy (other) (surgical)	4319
Head and neck cancer	195.0
Laryngeal cancer	161.9
Laryngectomy (surgical)	30.4
Metastases, general	199.1
Nasogastric tube feeding (surgical)	96.6
Nasogastric tube insertion (surgical)	96.07
Nasopharyngeal cancer	147.9
Oropharyngeal cancer	146.9
Pharynx, cancer of the	149.0
Pneumonia	486
Pneumonia, aspiration	50.70
Respirator, dependence on	V46.1
Respiratory failure, acute	518.81
Respiratory insufficiency (acute)	518.82
Seizure disorder	780.39
Tongue, cancer of the	141.9
Trachea, cancer of the	162.0
Tracheitis, acute	464.10
Tracheostomy, attention to	V55.0
Tracheostomy closure (surgical)	31.72
Tracheostomy permanent (surgical)	31.29

4

5. Skills and services identified

- *Hospice nursing*

a. *Comfort and symptom control*

Skilled observation and complete system assessment of the patient with head and neck cancer/tracheostomy admitted to hospice

Skilled observation and assessment of the patient with a laryngectomy resulting from _____ (specify)

Presentation of hospice philosophy and services

Explain patient rights and responsibilities

Assess patient, family, and caregiver wishes and expectations regarding care

Assess patient, family, and caregiver resources available for care

Provision of volunteer support to patient and family

Teach family or caregiver physical care of patient

Assess pain and other symptoms, including site, duration, characteristics, and relief measures

RN to provide and teach effective oral care and comfort measures

Comfort measures of backrub and hand or other therapeutic massage

Assess pulmonary status in patient with new tracheostomy

Pain assessment and management

Suction per physician orders

Teach patient and caregiver infection control measures (e.g., cleaning cannula)

Implement and teach respiratory therapy program

Teach care of tracheostomy

Provide care of tracheostomy

Teach signs and symptoms of URI and infection at site

Assess pulmonary status

Assessment of respiratory status, including the amount and character of secretions

Assess vital signs

Teach patient, family, and caregiver suction procedure(s) with return demonstration

Measure weight

RN to instruct in pain control measures and medication

RN to assess patient's pain or other symptoms q visit to identify need for change, addition, or other plan or dose adjustment

Provide and teach daily tracheostomy management, including tube changes and stoma site care

Teach patient, family, and caregiver regimen for inner cannula care

Assessment of breath sounds and rate and rhythm of respiration

Teach signs and symptoms of respiratory infections

Review back-up ventilator support system and compressor system back-up

Effective management of pain and prevention of secondary symptoms

Interventions of symptoms directed toward comfort and palliation

Observation and assessment, communication with physician related to signs and symptoms of oncological emergencies (e.g., spinal cord compression, superior vena cava syndrome, hypercalcemia) and measures and symptom treatment

Teach caregiver/patient use of pain assessment tool/scale and reporting mechanism(s)

Observation and assessment of patient with nausea and vomiting who is receiving palliative radiation and chemotherapy

Assessment and relief/comfort measures related to dry mouth due to radiation therapy (e.g., mouth wetting product or medications to stimulate salivary glands, if appropriate per physician)

Comfort measures of "artificial saliva, spit" through frequent use of squirt bottle and mouth rinses and chewing of sugarless gum or candy

Avoidance of antihistamines and other drying products that exacerbate the mouth dryness, if possible

Teach caregiver or family care of weak, terminally ill patient

Teach patient/family about realistic expectations of disease process

Teach care of dying, signs/symptoms of impending death

Presence and support

Other interventions, based on patient/family needs

b. *Safety and mobility considerations*

Provide caregiver with home safety information and instruction related to _____ and documented in the clinical record

Teach patient, family, and caregiver oxygen utilization and safety concerns

Teach patient, family, and caregiver environmental safety concerns

Teach patient, family, or caregiver environmental safety concerns regarding airway aspiration

Teach family regarding safety of patient in home

Teach family regarding energy conservation techniques

Other interventions, based on patient/family needs

c. *Emotional/Spiritual considerations*

Psychosocial assessment of patient and family regarding disease and prognosis

RN to provide emotional support to patient and family

Emotional support of patient/family during radiation and chemotherapy in regards to loss, grief, and isolation

Provide support to patient during chemotherapy/radiation for cancer treatment

Psychosocial aspects of pain control (e.g., depression) assessed and acknowledged with team support/intervention

Ongoing acknowledgment of spirituality and related concerns of patient/family

Inform patient/family/caregiver of available volunteer support

Assessment and care/support related to depression, changed body image concerns, fever, mouth sores/ulcers, complaints of extreme tiredness, and dry/cracking skin in patient receiving palliative chemotherapy

Other interventions, based on patient/family needs

4

d. *Skin care*

RN to teach patient care of irradiated skin sites

Observation and evaluation of wound and surrounding skin

Evaluate patient's need for equipment, including supplies to decrease pressure, alternating pressure mattress, gel foam seat cushion, and heel and elbow protectors

Teach family to perform dressing changes between RN visits, specifically _____

Teach patient, family, or caregiver about proper body alignment and positioning in bed to prevent skin tears from shearing skin

Observe and apply skilled assessment of areas for possible breakdown including heels, hips, elbows, ankles, and other pressure-prone areas

Teach caregiver about skin care needs, including the need for frequent position changes, appropriate pressure pads and mattresses, and the prevention of breakdown

Teach patient, family, and caregiver site care

Other interventions, based on patient/family needs

e. *Elimination considerations*

Assess bowel regimen, and implement program as needed

Observation and complete systems assessment of the patient with an indwelling catheter

RN to change catheter every 4 weeks and prn for catheter problems, including patient complaints, signs and symptoms of infection, and other factors necessitating evaluation and possible catheter change

RN to teach caregiver daily care of catheter

RN to evaluate the patient's bowel patterns and need for stool softeners, laxatives, dietary adjustments, and develop bowel management plan

Other interventions, based on patient/family needs

f. *Hydration/Nutrition*

Instruct patient/caregiver about specific diet _____ (specify physician orders)

Assess nutrition/hydration statuses

Nutrition/hydration supported by offering patient's choice of favorite or desired foods or liquids

Nutrition/hydration maintained by offering patient high-protein diet and foods of choice as tolerated

Encourage optimal nutrition through high-calorie, high-protein snacks

Assessment and plan related to anorexia/cachexia, tube feedings, difficulty swallowing, and/or transitional feedings (e.g., TPN to oral)

Assessments and interventions/plan related to patient/family complaints of dry mouth, with painful chewing, difficulty speaking, and denture fit concerns after radiation and surgery

Teach patient and family to expect decreased nutritional and fluid intake as disease progresses

Other interventions, based on patient/family needs

g. *Therapeutic/Medication regimens*

Teach and observe regarding side effects of palliative chemotherapy, including constipation, anemia, and fatigue

RN to assess the patient's unique response to treatments or interventions, and to report changes or unfavorable responses or reactions to the physician

Medication information and instruction regarding drug/drug and drug/food interactions

Nonpharmacological interventions such as progressive muscle relaxation, imagery, positive visualization, music, massage and touch, and humor therapy of patient's choice implemented

Medication teaching and management

Teach patient and caregiver use of PCA pump

Other interventions, based on patient/family needs

h. *Other considerations*

Assess progression of disease process

RN to assess the patient's response to treatments and interventions and to report to physician changes, unfavorable responses, or reactions

Other interventions, based on patient/family needs

- *Home health aide or certified nursing assistant*

Effective and safe personal care

Safe ADL assistance and support

Respite care and active listening skills

Observation and reporting

Meal preparation

Homemaker services

Comfort care

Other duties

- *Social worker*

Psychosocial assessment of patient and family/caregiver, including adjustment to illness and its implications

Identification of optimal coping strategies

Financial assessment and counseling regarding food acquisition, ability to prepare, and costs of needed medications

Intervention/support related to terminal illness and loss

Emotional/spiritual support

Depression/fear assessed and addressed

Facilitate communication among patient, family, and hospice team

Referral/linkage to community services and resources as indicated

Grief counseling and intervention/support related to illness/loss

Patient/caregiver counseling and support

For patients who live alone with no support system (e.g., able, available, willing caregiver[s]), obtain resources to enable patient to remain in home setting

Identification of caregiver role strain necessitating respite/relief measures/support

Identification of illness-related psychiatric condition necessitating care

Funeral and burial planning assistance

- *Volunteer(s)*

Support, friendship, companionship, and presence

Advocacy and respite

Comfort and dignity maintained/provided for patient and family

Errands and transportation

Other services, based on IDT recommendations and patient/caregiver needs

4

- *Spiritual counselor*
  Spiritual assessment and care
  Counseling, intervention, and support related to that dimension of life
     related to life's meaning (consistent with patient's beliefs)
  Support, listening, and presence
  Participation in sacred or spiritual rituals or practices
  Other supportive care, based on patient's/family's needs and belief system
  Pray with or for the patient/family, using prayers familiar to patient's
     religious background (per their wishes)

- *Dietitian/Nutritional counseling*
  Assessment of patient with decreased intake, weight loss, anorexia, and
     increased shortness of breath (e.g., "don't feel like eating")
  Supportive counseling with patient/family indicating that patient will
     have a decreased appetite and usually at some point may not
     eat/drink
  Assessment and recommendations for safety and swallowing
     difficulties
  Teaching and support of family members and caregivers
  Support and care with food and nourishment as desired by patient
  Evaluation/management of nutritional deficits and needs
  Encourage nutritional supplements and snacks to increase protein and
     caloric intake
  Food and textural dietary recommendations to incorporate patient
     choice and wishes
  Tube-feeding considerations/counseling related to swallowing, other
     problems

- *Occupational therapist*
  Evaluation of ADLs and functional mobility
  Assess for need for adaptive equipment and assistive devices
  Safety assessment of patient's environment and ADLs
  Assessment for energy conservation training
  Assessment of upper-extremity function, retraining motor skills

- *Physical therapist*
  Evaluation
  Safety assessment of patient's environment
  Safe transfer training or bed mobility exercises
  Pain assessment/reduction factors
  Strengthening exercises/program
  Assessment of gait safety and home safety measures
  Instruct/supervise caregiver and volunteers on home exercise program
     for conditioning and strength
  Assistive, adaptive devices evaluation of equipment and teaching

- *Speech-language pathologist*
  Evaluation for speech/swallowing problems
  Food texture recommendations
  Alternate functional communication/alaryngeal speech

- *Bereavement counselor*
  Assessment of the needs of the bereaved family and friends
  Support and intervention, based on assessment and ongoing findings
  Presence and counseling
  Supportive visits and follow-up, other interventions (e.g., mailings, calls)
  Other services related to bereavement work and support

- *Pharmacist*
  Evaluation of hospice patient with constipation on cathartics, stool
    softeners, and other medications for possible food/drug, drug/drug
    interactions
  Medication monitoring regarding therapeutic levels and dosages
  Pain consult and input into interdisciplinary POC related to pain
    control, palliation, and symptom management
  Assessment of medication regimen and plan for safety and compliance
  Assessment for need for liquid medications

- *Music, massage, art, or other therapies or services*
  Evaluation and intervention based on patient's and caregiver's unique
    wishes and needs that support care, comfort, and death in the setting
    of the patient's choice
  Assessment plan to engage patient and support comfort, quality,
    enjoyment, and dignity
  Pet therapy (including patient's pet, if available) and therapeutic
    intervention

6. Outcomes for care

- *Hospice nursing*
  Planned and effective bowel program, as evidenced by regular bowel
    movements and patient/family report of comfort
  Death with dignity, and symptoms controlled in setting of patient/
    family choice
  Optimal comfort, support, and dignity provided throughout illness
  Death with maximum comfort through effective symptom control with
    specialized hospice support
  Patient/caregiver able to list adverse drug reactions/problems with
    medication regimen and whom to call for follow-up and
    resolution
  Pain and symptoms managed/controlled in setting of patient/family
    choice (e.g., patient/family report ability to eat, sleep, speak clearer
    with pacing)
  Patient's/family's privacy, independence, and choices supported with
    respect and maintained through death
  Enhancement and support of quality of life
  Effective symptom relief and control (e.g., a peaceful and comfortable
    death at home, some enjoyment of life)
  Maximizing the patient's quality of life (e.g., alert and pain free or
    as patient wishes)

4

Pharmacological and nonpharmacological interventions, such as localized heat application, positioning, relaxation methods, and music

Patient cared for and family supported through death, with physical, psychosocial, spiritual, and other concerns/needs acknowledged/addressed

Patient- and family-centered hospice care provided based on the patient's/family's unique situation and needs

Infection control and palliation

Grief/bereavement expression and support provided

Patient is pain free by next visit _____

Caregiver demonstrates ability to manage pain, where applicable

Patient maintains comfort and dignity throughout illness

Patient and caregiver verbalize satisfaction with care

Educational tools/plans incorporated in daily care, and patient and caregiver verbalize understanding of safe, needed care

Patient will decide on care, interventions, and evaluation

Caregiver effective in care management and knows whom to call for questions/concerns

Patient will express satisfaction with hospice support received and will experience increased comfort

Patient will be made comfortable at home through death in accordance with the patient's wishes

Effective pain control and symptom control verbalized by patient

Patient verbalizes understanding of and adheres to care and medication regimens

Patient and caregiver supported through patient's death

Comfort maintained through course of care

The patient and family receive hospice support and care, and family members and friends are able to spend quality time with the patient

Caregiver able and verbalizes comfort with role and lists when to call hospice team members

Patient supported through and receives the maximum benefit from palliative chemotherapy and radiation with minimal complications

Patient and caregiver list adverse reactions, potential complications, signs/symptoms of infection (e.g., sputum change, chest congestion)

Comfort maintained through death with dignity

Pain effectively managed, and patient verbalizes comfort

Patient has stable respiratory status with patent airway

Comfort and individualized intervention of patient with immobility/bedbound status (e.g., skin, urinary, musculature, vascular)

Spiritual and psychosocial needs met (specify) as defined by patient and caregiver throughout course of care

Patient is protected from injury, has stable respiratory status, and is compliant with medication, safety, and care regimens

Patient self-care related to daily trach care

Early detection and intervention regarding problems of patients with immobility/bedbound status (e.g., skin, urinary, musculature, vascular)

Patient states pain is _____ on 0–10 scale by next visit

Patient and caregiver demonstrate appropriate back-up or "rescue" therapies for breakthrough pain or other symptoms (e.g., dyspnea)

- *Home health aide or certified nursing assistant*
  Effective hygiene, personal care, and comfort
  ADL assistance
  Safe environment maintained

- *Social worker*
  Problem identified and addressed, with patient/caregiver linked with appropriate support services and plan of care successfully implemented
  Patient and caregiver cope adaptively with illness and death
  Adaptive adjustment to changed body and body image
  Psychosocial support and counseling offered to patient/caregivers experiencing loss and grief
  Caregiver system assessed, and development of stable caregiver plan facilitated
  Funeral and burial planning assistance

- *Volunteer(s)*
  Comfort, companionship, and friendship extended to patient/family
  Support and respite provided as defined by the needs of the patient/caregiver
  Patient and family supported by team with care, comfort, and companionship

- *Spiritual counselor*
  Support, listening, and presence
  Spiritual support offered and provided as defined by needs of patient/caregiver
  Pray with or for the patient/family, using prayers familiar to patient's religious background (per their wishes)
  Provision of spiritual support and care as based on the assessed and ongoing needs of the patient and family
  Spiritual support offered, and patient and family needs met
  Patient and family express relief of symptoms of spiritual suffering

- *Dietitian/Nutritional counseling*
  Patient and family verbalize comprehension of changing nutritional needs
  Family and caregiver integrate recommendations into nutrition teaching (where appropriate)
  Patient and caregiver know whom to call for nutrition- and hydration-related questions/concerns
  Nutrition/hydration per patient's choices
  Caregiver integrates dietary recommendations into daily meal planning

- *Occupational therapist*
  Patient and caregiver demonstrate maximum independence with ADLs, adaptive techniques, and assistive devices

4

Patient and caregiver demonstrate maximum safety in ADLs and functional mobility

Patient and caregiver demonstrate effective use of energy conservation Verbalization/demonstration of improved functional activity level and enhanced quality of life

Patient and caregiver demonstrate effective use of diaphragmatic breathing to reduce shortness of breath and relaxation techniques to help in pain/symptom management

Patient and caregiver demonstrate correct use of exercises

- *Physical therapist*
  Prevention of complications
  Home exercise and upper-extremity program taught to caregiver
  Optimal strength, mobility, function maintained/achieved
  Compliance with home exercise program by _____ (date)

- *Speech-language pathologist*
  Communication method implemented, and patient able to be understood as self-reported or reported by family/caregivers
  Safe swallowing and functional communication
  Recommended lists of foods/textures for safety and patient choice

- *Bereavement counselor*
  Grief support services provided to patient and family
  Well-being and resolution process of grief initiated and followed through bereavement services

- *Pharmacist*
  Regimen for bowel regimen successful as self-reported by patient and in update at team meeting
  Multiple drug regimen reviewed for food/drug and drug/drug interactions in patient on multiple medications
  Stability and safety in complex medication regimen with maximum benefit to patient
  Effective pain and symptom control and symptom management as reported by patient/caregiver
  Laboratory reports reviewed for therapeutic dosages and effective patient response

- *Music, massage, art, or other therapies or services*
  Therapeutic massage/touch effective for patient as self-reported or observed by caregivers/family
  Improved muscle tone, relaxation, and/or sleep
  Patient comfortable and relaxed (e.g., sleeping) after massage
  Patient has pet's presence as desired—in all care sites, when possible
  Music therapy intervention based on assessment to decrease pain perception and provide emotional expression and support
  Maintenance of comfort and physical, psychosocial, and spiritual health

Holistic health maintained and comfort achieved through
_____ (specify modality)

7. **Patient, family, and caregiver educational needs**
   Educational needs are the regimens that the caregiver will be managing
   with or for the patient. These include the following:
   The basic tenets of hospice and the availability of support 24 hours a
   day, 7 days a week
   Home safety assessment and counseling
   The patient's medication regimen
   Safe and proper body mechanics to promote patient comfort and
   prevent caregiver safety problems
   Other teaching specific to the patient's and family's unique needs
   Support groups available to patient's family, such as the hospice
   program's "Caregiver Support Group" meetings for family
   members and friends of the patient
   Importance of adequate hydration, optimal nutrition, and rest for
   healing and recovery
   Effective handwashing techniques, prevention of infections, and
   avoidance of respiratory irritants such as cigarette smoke
   All aspects of stoma site care, including self-observational skills,
   cleansing routines, need for humidity, hygiene measures, and
   safety care related to stoma
   Anticipated disease progression
   Other information based on the patient's unique medical history and
   other identified needs

8. **Specific tips for quality and reimbursement**
   Unless the patient is in a hospice insurance program, some insurers will
   not pay for a skilled clinician visit that is made at death if the patient is
   dead when the clinician arrives at the home. From a Medicare home
   care perspective, the visit at the time of death may be covered when the
   orders and clinical record document assessment of the patient's status
   or signs of death/life or state law allows pronouncement of death by
   an RN.
   Document patient deterioration
   Document dehydration, dehydrating
   Document patient change or instability
   Document pain, other symptoms not controlled
   Document status after acute episode of _____ (specify)
   Document positive urine, sputum, etc. culture; patient started
   on _____ (specify ordered antibiotic therapy)
   Document patient impacted; impaction removed manually
   Document RN in frequent communication with physician
   regarding _____ (specify)
   Document febrile at _____, pulse change at _____, irr., irr.
   Document change noted in _____
   Document bony prominences red, opening

4

Document RN contacted physician regarding —— (specify)

Document marked SOB

Document alteration in mental status

Document medications being adjusted, regulated, or monitored as well as patient response

Document unable to perform own ADLs, personal care

Document all interdisciplinary team meetings and communications in the POC and in the progress notes of the clinical record

All hospice team members involved should have input into the POC and document their interventions and goals

Document changes to the plan of care, such as medications, services, frequency, communication, and concurrence of other team members

Document coordination of services or consultation of the other members of the IDT

Document communications and care coordination with other care providers, such as skilled health care facility or nursing home staff, inpatient team members, hired caregivers, and others

Document any variances to expected outcomes. There are many models of hospice programs.

The Medicare hospice benefit does not require that the patient be homebound or have identified skilled needs. For further information on this benefit, please refer to CMS Hospice Manual 21.

Should the patient's status deteriorate and increased personal care be needed, obtain a telephone order for the increased service, noting frequency and estimating the duration.

Obtain a telephone order for all medication and treatment changes of the medical regimen, and document these in the clinical record.

Document the clear progression of symptoms and interventions that provide evidence of caring for a patient with terminal cancer in the clinical notes.

Document when/if the patient has respiratory changes, shortness of breath, exacerbation of conditions, dysphagia, pain, and other symptoms and that they are identified and resolved

Remember that the clinical documentation is key to measuring compliance for quality and reimbursement purposes. Care coordination, timely verbal and initial physician orders, and assessment and addressing of spiritual and psychosocial needs should be clearly documented in the patient's clinical record

The documentation should support that all hospice care supports comfort and dignity while meeting patient/family needs

The documentation should include the ongoing assessment and management of pain and other symptoms and the anticipation and prevention of secondary symptoms such as constipation

It is important to note that all team members, including clinicians and social workers, should assess, identify, and "hear" spiritual needs that the patient/family want to be addressed. These spiritual issues are key to the provision of quality hospice care and cannot

be addressed effectively and promptly by the spiritual
counselor only

Document clearly symptoms, clinical changes, and assessment findings
that constitute evidence of the end stage of cancer

Document patient changes, symptoms, and clinical information identified
from visits and team conferences that support hospice care and a
limited life expectancy

Clearly document the rationale that supports/explains the progression of
the illness from the chronic to terminal stages

Document mentation, behavioral, and/or cognitive changes

Document dysphagia, weight loss, increased shortness of breath,
dyspnea, infection, sepsis, new or changed medications, etc.

Document any skin changes (e.g., inflamed, painful, weeping skin
site[s])

Document when the patient is actively dying, deteriorating, or progressing
toward death

Remember that the "litmus test" of care coordination rests within the
quality of the clinical documentation by all team members. Review
one of your patient's clinical records and ask yourself the following:
"If I was unable to give a verbal report/update on this patient, would
a peer be able to pick up and provide the same level of care and
know (from the documentation) the current orders, medications, and
other details that contribute to effective hospice care?"

9. Queries for quality

Head and neck cancer care
- *Is patient's pain managed adequately?*
- *Is patient's anxiety managed adequately?*
- *What are the patient's symptoms?*
- *Does patient/family have access to appropriate community resources,
  and are they documented in the record?*
- *Have you documented to the interdisciplinary POC?*

Laryngectomy care
- *Is patient's pain managed adequately?*
- *Is patient's anxiety managed adequately?*
- *Is patient's functional ability/status clearly documented?*
- *Have the patient's respiratory and communication needs been identi-
  fied and documented?*
- *Have you documented to the interdisciplinary POC?*

Tracheostomy care
- *Is patient's pain managed adequately?*
- *Is patient's anxiety managed adequately?*
- *Is patient's functional ability/status clearly documented?*
- *Have the patient's respiratory and communication needs been identi-
  fied and documented?*
- *Have you documented to the interdisciplinary POC?*

4

10. Resources for hospice care and practice

Reference Guide for Clinicians: Management of Cancer Pain: Adults and Consumer's Guide: Management of Cancer Pain can be ordered by calling 1-800-358-9295. The patient guides are available in English and Spanish. The National Cancer Institute can be accessed online at www.nci.nih.gov

The American Cancer Society has a resource entitled *Speech after Laryngectomy* that addresses the kinds of speech and artificial devices for patients. This resource can be obtained by calling 1-800-ACS-2345 (www.cancer.org).

The Oral Cancer Foundation's web site is at http://www.oralcancer.org. Oncolink is at http://www.oncolink.upenn.edu. Oncolink is a service provided by the University of Pennsylvania Cancer Center that includes general information about cancer, head and neck cancers, and radiation oncology.

Support for People with Oral and Head and Neck Cancer (SPOHNC) (pronounced "spunk") is dedicated to meeting the needs of oral and head and neck cancer patients. They offer a "News from SPOHNC" newsletter and offer support and encouragement. They call be reached at (516) 759-5333 or at www.spohnc.org.

4

INFUSION CARE

1. General considerations

The reasons for infusion therapy vary depending on the hospice's policies and the unique problems of the patient and family and may include medications for pain control and improvement of cardiac symptoms, transfusions to maintain function and quality of life, and parenteral hydration and palliative chemotherapy in some cases. **IV care, enteral parenteral care, parenteral therapy,** and **vascular access device care** are also addressed in this section.

Please refer to "AIDS Care," "Breast Cancer and Mastectomy Care," "Cardiac Care (End Stage)" and "Pain Care," should these sections also pertain to your patients and families.

2. Needs for visit

Physician order for hospice care, specific to the hospice program's admission criteria and policies
Standard precautions supplies
Vital signs equipment for baseline assessment
Specific initial and ongoing physician orders, including solution ordered, rate, site change, frequency
Solution
Tubing
Catheter(s)
Pump
Tape
Tourniquet
2×2s
Alcohol swabs
Anaphylaxis kit
Other equipment as directed per organizational protocol(s)

3. Safety considerations

Infection control/standard precautions
Night-light
Chemical spill kit at the home
Clean area for storage of infusion supplies
Access to running water and electricity
Multiple medications (e.g., side effects, safe storage)
Safety for home medical equipment (pump)
Emergency symptoms and actions to take
The phone number and name of person to call with a care problem
Smoke detector and fire evacuation plan
Others, based on the patient's unique condition and environment
Medical equipment safety and storage (e.g., infusion pump)
A working phone, running water, and refrigerator

4

Infusion protocol precautions
Reactions or other symptoms that necessitate immediate
   reporting/assistance

4. Potential diagnoses and codes

AIDS (general)	042
Amputation, site infection	997.62
Appendix abscess	540.1
Bacteremia	790.7
Bone, aseptic necrosis	733.40
Bone marrow transplant (surgical)	41.00
Bone metastases	198.5
Breast cancer	174.9
Cancer of the head/neck	195.0
Cardiomyopathy	425.4
Cellulitis, right or left lower leg	682.6
Cervix, cancer of	180.9
Colon cancer	153.9
Congestive heart failure	428.0
COPD	496
CVA	436
Cytomegalovirus and colitis	078.5 and 558.9
Cytomegalovirus and esophagitis	078.5 and 530.10
Cytomegalovirus and kidney	078.5 and 593.9
Cytomegalovirus and retinitis	078.5 and 363.20
Dehydration	276.5
Diabetes mellitus, with complications, adult	250.90
Diabetes mellitus, with complications, juv.	250.91
Dysphagia	787.2
Endocarditis	424.90
Esophagus, cancer of	150.9
Failure to thrive, adult	783.7
Fluid and electrolyte imbalance	276.9
Foot abscess	682.7
Fracture, pathological	733.10
Gastric cancer, metastatic	197.8
Head or neck, cancer of the	195.0
Heart disease, end stage	429.9
Heart transplant (surgical)	37.51
Hickman catheter insertion (surgical)	38.93
Hyperemesis gravidarum, antepartum	643.03
Hypertension	401.9
Hypovolemia	276.5
Liver, end stage disease	571.8
Lung transplant (surgical)	33.50
Lyme disease	088.81
Metastases, general	199.1
Osteomyelitis	730.20

4

Osteomyelitis, ankle	730.27
Osteomyelitis, leg	730.26
Osteomyelitis (foot, ankle)	730.27
Osteomyelitis (lower leg, knee)	730.26
Osteomyelitis (pelvic region and thighs)	730.25
Osteomyelitis (site unspecified) acute	730.20
Ovarian cancer	183.0
Pancreatic cancer	157.9
Pelvic inflammatory disease (acute)	614.9
Pericarditis, acute	420.90
Pneumonia	486
Pneumonia, aspiration	507.0
Retinitis	363.20
Seizure disorder	780.39
Sinusitis	473.9
Spinal cord tumor	239.7
Staph infection	041.10
Syphilis	097.9
Urinary tract infection	599.0
Venous thrombosis	453.9
Viral meningitis	047.9
Wound infection, postoperative	998.59

5. Skills and services identified

- ***Hospice nursing***

a. *Comfort and symptom control*

    Observation and complete systems assessment of the patient needing infusion therapy for _____ (specify)

    Presentation of hospice philosophy and services

    Explain patient rights and responsibilities

    Assess patient, family, and caregiver wishes and expectations regarding care

    Assess patient, family, and caregiver resources available for care

    Provision of volunteer support to patient and family

    Teach family or caregiver physical care of patient

    RN to provide and teach effective oral care and comfort measures

    Assess pain and other symptoms, including site, duration, characteristics, and relief measures

    Provide site care and implement therapy program

    Assess needle, supplies, and site for contamination

    Teach patient, family, and caregiver effective handwashing techniques

    Teach signs and symptoms of impeded or rapid flow of medication solution

    Comfort measures of backrub and hand or other therapeutic massage

    RN to change tubing and filter q _____ per hospice protocol

    Teach family or caregiver to document date and time for all infusions started and completed

4

Teach patient, family, and caregiver about position of site with IV

Teach patient, family, and caregiver signs and symptoms of infection, phlebitis

Teach patient, family, and caregiver when to contact on-call RN or physician

Teach patient and family signs and symptoms of phlebitis, occlusion, displacement, infection, and other possible problems

RN to monitor patient for evidence of infection, metabolic problems, or other complications in patient on TPN

Teach self-observational and record-keeping skills to patient and care-giver for documenting response to _____ therapy

Pain assessment and ongoing management

PICC line flushed per organizational policy

Teaching and training related to the operation and troubleshooting of access device and pump (e.g., alarms, 800 numbers, whom to call)

Patient and caregiver provided with information and instruction about care and maintenance of the line, insertion site, and dressing changes

Teaching provided regarding the meticulous care that must be provided to prevent contamination and possible infection

Dressing change q heparin lock change, flush at end of therapy with _____ (specify); cap change q heparin lock change per organizational policy

Change battery q _____ (per protocol)

Perform sterile dressing change and site care q _____ (specify)

RN to restart peripheral IV or subcutaneous site q _____ (specify orders)

Assess pain, and evaluate the pain management's effectiveness

Teach care of bedridden

Measure vital signs, including pain, q visit

Assess cardiovascular, pulmonary, and respiratory status

Teach new pain- or symptom-control medication regimen

Teach caregivers symptom control and relief measures

Oxygen on at _____ liter per _____ (specify physician orders)

Identify and monitor pain, symptoms, and relief measures

RN to assess patient's pain or other symptoms q visit to identify need for change, addition, or other plan or dose adjustment

Observation and assessment, communication with physicians related to signs and symptoms of continuing decompensation and increased symptoms, pain, discomfort, shortness of breath, and measures to alleviate and control

Effective management of pain and prevention of secondary symptoms

Interventions of symptoms directed toward comfort and palliation

Teach caregiver/patient use of pain assessment tool/scale and reporting mechanism(s)

Teach patient and family about realistic expectations of disease process

Teach care of dying, and signs/symptoms of impending death

Presence and support

Other interventions, based on patient/family needs

b. *Safety and mobility considerations*

Provide caregiver with home safety information and instruction related to _____ and documented in the clinical record

Teach signs and symptoms of infiltration and home safety

RN to teach patient and caregiver in correct operation and care related to safe use of PCA pump for pain management

Teach family about safety of patient in home

Teach family about energy conservation techniques

Other interventions, based on patient/family needs

c. *Emotional/Spiritual considerations*

Psychosocial assessment of patient and family regarding disease and prognosis

RN to provide emotional support to patient and family

Assess mental status and sleep disturbance changes

Assessment and care/support related to depression, changed body image concerns, fever, mouth sores/ulcers, complaints of extreme tiredness and dry/cracking skin in patient receiving palliative chemotherapy

Psychosocial aspects of pain control (e.g., depression) assessed and acknowledged with team support/intervention

Ongoing acknowledgment of spirituality and related concerns of patient/family

Other interventions, based on patient/family needs

d. *Skin care*

Pressure ulcer care as indicated

Assess skin integrity

RN to teach patient about care of irradiated skin sites

Provide site care per protocols

Observation and evaluation of wound and surrounding skin

Evaluate patient's need for equipment, including supplies to decrease pressure, alternating pressure mattress, gel foam seat cushion, and heel and elbow protectors

Teach family to perform dressing changes between RN visits, specifically _____

Teach patient, family, or caregiver about proper body alignment and positioning in bed to prevent skin tears from shearing skin

Observe and apply skilled assessment of areas for possible breakdown, including heels, hips, elbows, ankles, and other pressure-prone areas

Teach caregiver about skin care needs, including the need for frequent position changes, appropriate pressure pads and mattresses, and the prevention of breakdown

Other interventions, based on patient/family needs

e. *Elimination considerations*

Assess bowel regimen, and implement program as needed

Assess urinary elimination changes related to hydration, change, status

Observation and assessment of patient with a peripherally inserted central catheter (PICC) for long-term therapy

Check for and remove impaction as needed

Condom catheter or indwelling catheter as indicated

Assess amount and frequency of urinary output

RN to teach caregiver daily care of catheter

RN to evaluate the patient's bowel patterns and need for stool softeners, laxatives, and dietary adjustments and to develop bowel management plan

Implement bowel assessment and management program

Teach patient/family and aide the importance of observing and noting bowel movements between scheduled nursing visits

Obtain patient history related to norms for bowel movements to date (e.g., "All my life I go only every other day")

Consider stool softeners, and offer laxative of choice, Fleet's enemas PRN, and other methods per patient wishes and physician orders

Other interventions, based on patient/family needs

f. *Hydration/Nutrition*

Assess nutrition/hydration status

Diet counseling for patient with anorexia

Teach family or caregiver about feeding tubes or pumps

Nutrition/hydration supported by offering patient's choice of favorite or desired foods or liquids

Nutrition/hydration maintained by offering patient high-protein diet and foods of choice as tolerated

Assessment and plan related to anorexia/cachexia, tube feedings, difficult/painful swallowing, and/or transitional feedings (e.g., TPN to oral)

Assessment and interventions/plan related to patient/family complaints of dry mouth, with painful chewing, difficulty speaking, and denture fit concerns after radiation and surgery

Teach patient and family to expect decreased nutritional and fluid intake as disease progresses

Other interventions, based on patient/family needs

g. *Therapeutic/Medication regimens*

RN to assess the patient's response to therapeutic treatments and interventions and to report any changes or unfavorable responses to the physician

Teach and observe regarding side effects of palliative chemotherapy, including constipation, anemia, and fatigue

Venipuncture q _____ (specify ordered frequency) for monitoring plate let and other counts

Teach flush of heparin with NS solution techniques to ensure patency of heparin lock and use of line for ordered medications

RN to instruct patient and caregiver regarding multiple medications, including schedule, route, functions, and possible side effects

RN to obtain blood for _____ (specify test and frequency) from central venous catheter per protocol

Medication assessment and management

4

Teach new pain and symptom control medication regimen

Morphine pump (specify pump, doses, etc.) for increased comfort

Obtain venipuncture as ordered q _____ (ordered frequency)

Teach about new medications and effects

Assess for electrolyte imbalance

Teach patient and caregiver use of PCA pump

RN to instruct in pain control measures and medications

Nonpharmacological interventions, such as progressive muscle relaxation, imagery, positive visualization, music, massage and touch, and humor therapy of patient's choice implemented

Other interventions, based on patient/family needs

h. *Other considerations*

Assess progression of disease process

RN to assess the patient's response to treatments and interventions and to report to the physician changes, unfavorable responses, or reactions

Other interventions, based on patient/family needs

- *Home health aide or certified nursing assistant*

Effective and safe personal care

Safe ADL assistance and support

Active listening skills

Observation and reporting

Meal preparation

Homemaker services

Comfort care

Other duties

- *Social worker*

Psychosocial assessment of patient and family/caregiver, including adjustment to long-term illness and its implications

Identification of optimal coping strategies

Identification of caregiver role strain necessitating respite/relief/support measures

Financial assessment and counseling regarding food acquisition, ability to prepare, and costs of needed medications

Intervention/support related to terminal illness and loss

Emotional/spiritual support

Depression/fear assessed and addressed

Facilitate communication among patient, family, and hospice team

Referral/linkage to community services and resources as indicated

Grief counseling and intervention/support related to illness/loss

Patient/caregiver counseling and support

For patients who live alone with no support system (e.g., able, available, willing caregiver[s]), obtain resources to enable patient to remain in home

Identification of illness-related psychiatric condition necessitating care

Funeral and burial planning assistance

4

- *Volunteer(s)*
  Support, friendship, companionship, and presence
  Comfort and dignity maintained/provided for patient and family
  Advocacy and respite
  Errands and transportation
  Other services, based on interdisciplinary team recommendations and
    patient/caregiver needs

- *Spiritual counselor*
  Spiritual assessment and care
  Counseling, intervention, and support related to that dimension of life
    related to life's meaning (consistent with patient's beliefs)
  Support, listening, and presence
  Pray with or for the patient/family, using prayers familiar to patient's
    religious background (per their wishes)
  Participation in sacred or spiritual rituals or practices
  Other supportive care, based on patient's/family's needs and belief
    systems

- *Dietitian/Nutritional counseling*
  Assessment of patient with decreased intake, weight loss, anorexia, and
    increased shortness of breath (e.g., "don't feel like eating")
  Supportive counseling with patient/family indicating that patient will
    have a decreased appetite and usually at some point may not
    eat/drink
  Assessment and recommendations for swallowing difficulties
  Teaching and support of family members and caregivers
  Support and care with food and nourishment as desired by patient
  Evaluation/management of nutritional deficits and needs
  Encourage nutritional supplements and snacks to increase protein and
    caloric intake
  Food and dietary recommendations incorporate patient choice and
    wishes
  Assist care team related to fluid needs and prevention of overhydration,
    overfeeding, and other problems
  Counseling related to infusion therapy

- *Occupational therapist*
  Evaluation of ADLs and functional mobility
  Assessment of need for adaptive equipment and assistive devices
  Safety assessment of patient's environment and ADLs
  Assessment for energy conservation training
  Assessment of upper-extremity function, retraining motor skills

- *Physical therapist*
  Evaluation
  Safety assessment of patient's environment
  Safe transfer training or bed mobility exercises
  Pain assessment/reduction factors
  Strengthening exercises/program

4

Assessment of gait safety and home safety measures
Instruct/supervise caregiver and volunteers on home exercise program
for safety conditioning and strength
Assistive, adaptive devices and evaluation of equipment and teaching

- *Speech-language pathologist*
Evaluation for speech/swallowing problems
Food texture recommendations
Alternate functional communication

- *Bereavement counselor*
Assessment of the needs of the bereaved family and friends
Support and intervention, based on assessment and ongoing findings
Presence and counseling
Supportive visits, follow-up, and other interventions (e.g., mailings,
calls)
Other services related to bereavement work and support

- *Pharmacist*
Evaluation of hospice patient with constipation on cathartics, stool
softeners, and other medications for possible food/drug, drug/drug
interactions
Medication monitoring regarding therapeutic levels and dosages
Pain consult and input into interdisciplinary plan of care related to pain
control, palliation, and symptom management
Assessment of medication regimen and plan for safety and compliance

- *Music, massage, art, or other therapies or services*
Evaluation and intervention based on patient's and caregiver's unique
wishes and needs that support care, comfort, and death in the setting
of the patient's choice
Assessment plan to engage patient and support comfort, quality,
enjoyment, and dignity
Pet therapy (including patient's pet, if available) and therapeutic
intervention

6. Outcomes for care

- *Hospice nursing*
Patient cared for and family supported through death, with physical,
psychosocial, spiritual, and other needs acknowledged/addressed
Mental distress, depression, and fear of dying addressed throughout
care by hospice team
Patient and family able to care for and support patient
Patient and caregiver can verbalize symptoms, changes, or accelerations
that necessitate call to physician
Patient and family demonstrate compliance with medication regimen
and other therapeutic interventions
Patient demonstrates stabilization and increased or enhanced coping
skills related to functioning and depression

Pain and symptoms managed/controlled in setting of patient/family choice (e.g., patient/family report ability to eat, sleep, speak with pacing)

Planned and effective bowel program, as evidenced by regular bowel movements and patient/family report of comfort

Death with dignity, and pain/symptoms controlled in setting of patient/family choice

Optimal comfort, support, and dignity provided throughout illness

Death with maximum comfort through effective symptom control with specialized hospice support

Patient and caregiver able to list adverse drug reactions/problems with medication regimen and whom to call for follow-up and resolution

Patient's/family's privacy, independence, and choices supported with respect and maintained through death

Enhancement and support of quality of life

Effective symptom relief and control (e.g., a peaceful and comfortable death at home, depression controlled, some enjoyment of life)

Maximizing the patient's quality of life (e.g., alert and pain free or as patient wishes)

Pharmacological and nonpharmacological interventions, such as localized heat application, biofeedback, massage, positioning, relaxation methods, and music

Patient- and family-centered hospice care provided based on the patient's/family's unique situation and needs

Patient verbalizes understanding of and adheres to medication regimens

Patient receives the maximum benefit from infusion therapy, with no evidence of complications (specify)

Patient and caregiver list adverse reactions, potential complications, signs/symptoms of infection

Infusion therapy catheter or port will remain patent and infection free through course of therapy

Patient and caregiver demonstrate understanding of care and associated regimens

Pain effectively managed (or other goal of infusion therapy, e.g., hydration achieved, infection controlled) as patient's pain is controlled and patient verbalizes comfort

Other goals/outcomes based on the patient's unique needs and problems

Effective and safe personal care

Completion of ADLs

Patient and caregiver will cope adaptively with stress and illness

Caregiver or patient demonstrates safe and supportive care and coping skills related to the successful implementation of the POC

Linkage to community resources accomplished by _____ (specify date)

Patient and caregiver will verbalize/demonstrate activities related to plan for accessing community resources and ongoing support by _____ (specify date)

Nutrition optimal for patient on infusion therapy for _____

Patient reports understanding and compliance as evidenced in food diary reviewed with dietitian

Patient and caregiver know whom to call for nutrition-related questions/concerns

Medication regimen evaluated for drug/drug and drug/food interactions and problems

Laboratory reports reviewed for therapeutic dosages and safe, effective patient response

Stability and safety in complex multiple medication regimens

Patient is protected from injury, has stable respiratory status, and is compliant with medication, safety, and care regimens

Comfort and individualized intervention of patient with immobility/bedbound status (e.g., skin, urinary, musculature, vascular)

Spiritual and psychosocial needs met (specify) as defined by patient and caregiver throughout course of care

Patient states pain is _____ on 0–10 scale by next visit

Patient/caregiver demonstrates appropriate back-up or "rescue" therapies for breakthrough pain or other symptoms (e.g., dyspnea)

Patient and caregiver verbalize satisfaction with care

Educational tools/plans incorporated in daily care, and patient and caregiver verbalize understanding of safe, needed care

Patient will decide on care, interventions, and evaluation

Caregiver effective in care management and knows whom to call for questions/concerns

Patient will express satisfaction with hospice support received and will experience increased comfort

Patient will be made comfortable at home through death in accordance with the patient's wishes

Effective pain control and symptom control verbalized by patient

Patient verbalizes understanding of and adheres to care and medication regimens

Patient and caregiver supported through patient's death

Comfort maintained through course of care

Patient and family receive hospice support and care, and family members and friends are able to spend quality time with the patient

Caregiver able and verbalizes comfort with role and understands when to call hospice team members

Patient supported through and receives the maximum benefit from palliative chemotherapy and radiation with minimal complications

Patient and caregiver list adverse reactions, potential complications, signs/symptoms of infection (e.g., sputum change, chest congestion)

Comfort maintained through death with dignity

Pain effectively managed and patient verbalizes comfort

Patient and family demonstrate compliance with self-observational and other care regimen skills taught

Patient's wound site shows evidence of healing as demonstrated by _____ (specify factors that identify improvement for this patient)

Patient and family verbalize troubleshooting for IV line care and when to call for assistance

IV line is patent, skin site is without problems (e.g., pain, infection), and patient receives course of IV therapy without problems

Infection control and palliation

Grief/bereavement expression and support provided

Patient is pain free by next _____ visit

Caregiver demonstrates ability to manage pain, where applicable

Patient maintains comfort and dignity throughout illness

- *Home health aide or certified nursing assistant*
  Effective hygiene, personal care, and comfort
  ADL assistance
  Safe environment maintained

- *Social worker*
  Problem identified and addressed, with patient and caregiver linked with appropriate support services and plan of care successfully implemented
  Patient and caregiver cope adaptively with illness and death
  Psychosocial support and counseling offered to patient/caregivers experiencing loss and grief
  Resources identified, community linkage as appropriate for patient/family
  Identification of effective coping strategies
  Caregiver system assessed, and development of stable caregiver plans facilitated
  Funeral and burial planning assistance

- *Volunteer(s)*
  Comfort, companionship, and friendship extended to patient/family
  Support provided as defined by the needs of the patient/caregiver
  Patient and family supported by team with care, comfort, and companionship
  Funeral and burial planning assistance

- *Spiritual counselor*
  Spiritual support offered and provided as defined by needs of patient/caregiver
  Provision of spiritual support and care based on the assessed and ongoing needs of the patient and family
  Support, listening, and presence
  Participation in sacred or spiritual rituals or practices
  Intervention and support related to that dimension of life related to life's meaning (consistent with patient's beliefs)
  Spiritual support offered, and patient and family needs met
  Pray with or for the patient/family, using prayers familiar to the patient's religious background (per their wishes)

- *Dietitian/Nutritional counseling*
  Family and caregiver integrate recommendations into nutrition teaching (where appropriate)
  Patient and caregiver know whom to call for nutrition- and hydration-related questions/concerns
  Nutrition/hydration per patient's choices

Caregiver integrates recommendations into daily meal planning

Patient and family verbalize comprehension of changing nutritional needs

Patient and caregiver know whom to call for nutrition- and hydration-related questions and concerns

- *Occupational therapist*

  Patient and caregiver demonstrate maximum independence with ADLs, adaptive techniques, and assistive devices

  Patient and caregiver demonstrate maximum safety in ADLs and functional mobility

  Patient and caregiver demonstrate effective use of energy conservation techniques

  Verbalization/demonstration of improved functional activity level and enhanced quality of life

  Patient and caregiver demonstrate effective use of diaphragmatic breathing to reduce shortness of breath and relaxation techniques to help in pain/ symptom management

  Patient and caregiver demonstrate correct use of exercise and splints for maximum upper extremity function and joint position

- *Physical therapist*

  Prevention of complications

  Home exercise and upper-extremity program taught to caregiver

  Optimal strength, mobility, and function maintained/achieved

  Compliance with home exercise program by _____ (specify date)

  Safety in mobility and transfers

- *Speech-language pathologist*

  Communication method implemented, and patient able to be understood as self-reported or reported by family/caregivers

  Safe swallowing and functional communication

  Recommended lists of foods/textures for safety and patient choice

- *Bereavement counselor*

  Support services related to grief provided to patient and family

  Well-being and resolution process of grief initiated and followed through bereavement services

- *Pharmacist*

  Regimen for bowel regimen successful as self-reported by patient and in update at team meeting

  Multiple drug regimen reviewed for food/drug and drug/drug interactions in patient on multiple medications

  Stability and safety in complex medication regimen, with maximum benefit to patient

  Infusion medication(s) and blood level laboratory report reviewed for therapeutic dosage and safe, effective patient response and results reported to physician

  Effective pain and symptom control and symptom management as reported by patient/caregiver

- *Music, massage, art, or other therapies or services*
  Therapeutic massage/touch effective for patient as self-reported or
      observed by caregivers/family
  Improved muscle tone, relaxation, and/or sleep
  Patient comfortable and relaxed (e.g., sleeping) after massage
  Music therapy intervention based on assessment to decrease pain
      perception and provide emotional expression and support
  Maintenance of comfort and physical, psychosocial, and spiritual health
  Patient has pet's presence as desired—in all care sites, when possible
  Holistic health maintained and comfort achieved through
      _____ (specify modality)

7. **Patient, family, and caregiver educational needs**
   Educational needs are the care regimens that contribute to safe and
   effective care at home between the hospice team's visits.
   These include the following:
   > The basic tenets of hospice and the availability of support 24 hours a
   >   day, 7 days a week
   > Home safety assessment and counseling
   > Anticipated disease progression
   > Patient's medication regimen
   > Safe and proper body mechanics to promote patient comfort and
   >   prevent caregiver safety problems
   > Teach safe needle disposal, and provide container
   > Support groups available to patient's family, such as the hospice
   >   program's "Caregiver Support Group" meetings for family
   >   members and friends of the patient
   > Signs and symptoms that necessitate calling the physician
   > Teach patient and caregiver all aspects of care related to wound,
   >   including effective hand washing, disposal of soiled dressings,
   >   and other infection-control measures
   > The importance of nutrition in the healing process
   > Teach patient about all medications, including schedule, route,
   >   functions, and possible side effects
   > The patient's medications and their relationship to each other
   > Simple IV troubleshooting techniques and problem resolution
   > Care of the infusion access site and device and all aspects of care
   >   related to the safe delivery of the therapy, including teaching
   >   device function, potential problems, self-observational skills,
   >   safety, and site care
   > The importance of compliance to the regimen
   > The importance of medical follow-up
   > Effective handwashing techniques and other infection-control
   >   measures
   > Safe disposal of needles and other sharps in the home
   > The symptoms that would necessitate calling emergency services
   > Other teaching specific to the patient and caregiver's needs based on
   >   the patient's unique medical condition

4

8. Specific tips for quality and reimbursement

Document any variances to expected outcomes. Many models of hospice programs exist.

The Medicare hospice benefit does not require that the patient be homebound or have identified skilled needs. For further information on this benefit, please refer to CMS Hospice Manual 21.

Should the patient's status deteriorate and increased personal care be needed, obtain a telephone order for the increased service, noting frequency and estimating the duration.

Obtain a telephone order for all medication and treatment changes of the medical regimen and document these in the clinical record.

Unless the patient is in a hospice insurance program, some insurers will not pay for a skilled clinician visit made at death if the patient is dead when the clinician arrives at the home. From a Medicare home care perspective, the visit at the time of death may be covered when the orders and clinical record document assessment of the patient's status or signs of death/life or state law allows pronouncement of death by an RN.

Document patient deterioration

Document dehydration, dehydrating

Document patient change or instability

Document pain, other symptoms not controlled

Document status after acute episode of _____ (specify)

Document positive urine, sputum, etc. culture; patient started on _____ (specify ordered antibiotic therapy)

Document patient impacted; impaction removed manually per physician's orders

Document RN in frequent communication with physician regarding _____ (specify)

Document febrile at _____, pulse change at _____, irr., irr.

Document change noted in _____

Document bony prominences red, opening

Document RN contacted physician regarding _____ (specify)

Document marked SOB

Document alteration in mental status

Document medications being adjusted, regulated, or monitored as well as patient response

Document unable to perform own ADL, personal care

Document all IDT meetings and communications in the POC and in the progress notes of the clinical record

All hospice team members should have input into the POC and document their interventions and goals

Document the clear progression of symptoms and interventions that demonstrate the overall management of pain in the clinical notes

Document when/if the patient has respiratory changes, shortness of breath, exacerbation of conditions, dysphagia, changes in pain, and other symptoms and that they are identified and resolved

Remember that the clinical documentation is key to measuring compliance for quality and reimbursement purposes. Care coordination, timely verbal and initial physician orders, and assessment and addressing of spiritual and psychosocial needs should be ongoing and documented in the patient's clinical record

The documentation should support that all hospice care supports comfort and dignity while meeting patient/family needs

The documentation should include ongoing assessment and management of pain and other symptoms and the anticipation and prevention of secondary symptoms such as constipation

It is important to note that all team members, including clinicians and social workers, should assess, identify, and "hear" spiritual needs that the patient/family want to be addressed. These spiritual issues are key to the provision of quality hospice care and cannot be addressed effectively and promptly by the spiritual counselor only

Document clearly symptoms, clinical changes, and assessment findings related to pain and patient care

Document patient changes, symptoms, and clinical information identified from visits and team conferences that support hospice care and a limited life expectancy

Clearly support in the documentation the rationale that supports/explains the progression of the illness from the chronic to terminal stages

Document mentation, behavioral, and/or cognitive changes

Document dysphagia, weight loss, increased shortness of breath, dyspnea, infection, sepsis, new or changed medications, etc.

Document any skin changes (e.g., inflamed, painful, weeping skin or infusion site[s])

Document when the patient is actively dying, deteriorating, progressing toward death

Remember that the "litmus test" of care coordination rests on the quality of the clinical documentation by all team members. Review one of your patient's clinical records and ask yourself the following: "If I was unable to give a verbal report/update on this patient, would a peer be able to pick up and provide the same level of care and know (from the documentation) the current orders, medications, and other details that contribute to effective hospice care?"

Side effects to the drug regimen should be observed, noted, documented, and reported

Document coordination of services or consultation of the other members of the IDT

Document communications and care coordination with other care providers, such as skilled health care facility or health care home staff, inpatient team members, and hired caregivers

Your assessments, observations, and clinical findings assist in painting a picture to support coverage and documentation requirements for hospice care

Document any hospitalizations and changed clinical findings

Document patient changes, symptoms, psychosocial issues impacting
the care, information gathered at the patient/family visits and during
team meetings

The documentation should reflect ongoing effects of the terminal
condition, the patient's/family's difficulty with care or coping,
and the continued desire for hospice care

9. **Queries for quality**

Infusion care
- *Is patient's pain managed adequately?*
- *Is patient's anxiety managed adequately?*
- *Is patient's functional ability/status clearly documented?*
- *Does patient/family have access to appropriate medical supplies,
  and are the sources documented in the record?*
- *Have you documented to the interdisciplinary POC?*

IV care
- *Is patient's pain managed adequately?*
- *Is patient's anxiety managed adequately?*
- *Is patient's functional ability/status clearly documented?*
- *Does patient/family have access to appropriate medical supplies,
  and are the sources documented in the record?*
- *Have you documented to the interdisciplinary POC?*

Enternal-Parenteral care
- *Is patient's pain managed adequately?*
- *Is patient's anxiety managed adequately?*
- *Is patient's functional ability/status clearly documented?*
- *Does patient/family have access to appropriate medical supplies,
  and are the sources documented in the record?*
- *Have you documented to the interdisciplinary POC?*

Parenteral therapy
- *Is patient's pain managed adequately?*
- *Is patient's anxiety managed adequately?*
- *Is patient's functional ability/status clearly documented?*
- *Does patient/family have access to appropriate medical supplies,
  and are the sources documented in the record?*
- *Have you documented to the interdisciplinary POC?*

Vascular access device care
- *Is patient's pain managed adequately?*
- *Is patient's anxiety managed adequately?*
- *Is patient's functional ability/status clearly documented?*
- *Does patient/family have access to appropriate medical
  supplies, and are the sources documented in the
  record?*
- *Have you documented to the interdisciplinary POC?*

4

10. Resources for hospice care and practice
Infusion Nurses Society
220 Norwood Park South
Norwood, MA 02062
(782)-440-9408
(781)-440-9409 (fax)
www.ins1.org

Intravenous Nurses Certification Corporation (INCC)
220 Norwood Park S
Norwood, MA 02062, 1-800-434-INCC

National Home Infusion Association
205 Daingerfield Rd.
Alexandria, VA 22314
(703) 549-3740
(703) 683-1484 (fax)
www.nhia.org

4

LUNG CARE (END STAGE)

1. General considerations

Patients and their family members may be referred to hospice care after long battles with **chronic obstructive pulmonary diseases (COPD)** such as asthma, bronchitis, and tuberculosis. Care is directed toward controlling and reducing the symptoms of the specific lung pathology. Supportive and skillful care is directed toward comfort and relief of coughing, shortness of breath, feelings of tightness and dyspnea, and other complaints and problems.

2. Needs for visit

Physician order for hospice care, specific to the hospice program's admission criteria and policies

Standard precautions supplies

Vital signs equipment for baseline assessment

Other supplies or equipment, based on physician orders

3. Safety considerations

Infection control/standard precautions

Night-light

Disposal of soiled tissues and used respiratory supplies

Avoidance of environmental respiratory irritants

Oxygen safety precautions

Bathroom safety supports, including shower bench, tub rails

Activity pacing

Protective skin measures

Identification and report of any skin problems

Fall precautions/protocol

Multiple medications (e.g., side effects, interactions, safe storage)

Stairway precautions/handrail on stairs

Pacing considerations

Symptoms that necessitate immediate reporting/assistance

The phone number of whom to call with a care problem

Supportive and well-fitting, nonslip shoes

Safety for home medical equipment (e.g., wheelchair, walker)

Smoke detector and fire evacuation plan

Others, based on the patient's unique condition and environment

4. Potential diagnoses and codes

Airway obstruction, chronic	496
Asthma	493.90
Bronchiolitis	466.19
Bronchitis, acute	466.0
Bronchitis	490
Chronic ischemic heart disease	414.9

Congestive heart failure	428.0
COPD	496
Cor pulmonale	416.9
Dehydration	276.5
Emphysema	492.8
Failure to thrive, adult	783.7
Hemoptysis	786.3
Hypertension	401.9
Influenza with pneumonia	487.0
Interstitial emphysema	518.1
Left heart failure	428.1
Lung cancer	162.9
Lung disease	518.89
Metastases, general	199.1
Orthostatic hypotension	458.0
Peripheral vascular disease	443.9
Pleural effusion	511.9
Pneumonia	486
Pneumonia aspiration	507.0
Pneumonia, *Pneumocystis carinii* and AIDS	042 and 136.3
Pneumonia with influenza	487.0
Protein-caloric malnutrition	263.9
Pulmonary edema	514
Pulmonary fibrosis	515
Respirator, dependence	V46.1
Respiratory failure, acute	518.81
Tracheal bronchus disease	519.1
Tuberculosis (lung)	011.90
Tuberculosis, bronchial	011.30
Tuberculosis, bronchus	011.30
Ventilator, dependence on	V46.1

4

5. Skills and services identified

- *Hospice nursing*

a. *Comfort and symptom control*

Complete initial assessment of all systems of patient with
_____ admitted to hospice for _____ (specify)

Presentation of hospice philosophy and services

Explain patient rights and responsibilities

Observation and assessment of patient with TB for presence/absence of
productive cough, fever, night sweats, weight loss, chest pain,
cough, and other symptoms

Comprehensive assessment of patient with COPD admitted
for _____ (specify)

Skilled evaluation and all systems assessment of the patient with COPD

Observation and complete systems assessment of the patient with
asthma

Observation and assessment of patient with end stage lung disease on multiple medications, admitted to hospice with increasing shortness of breath, complaints of dyspnea, poor activity tolerance, and on oxygen therapy _____ hours a day (specify)

Observation and assessment of patient with restrictive lung disease admitted to hospice with significant weight loss, on steroids and multiple bronchodilators

Assess patient, family, and caregiver wishes and expectations regarding care

Assess patient, family, and caregiver resources available for care

Arrange of volunteer support to patient and family

Teach family or caregiver physical care of patient

Assess pain and other symptoms, including site, duration, characteristics, and relief measures

Observation and assessment of pain and other symptoms to be managed within parameters of disease process

Teaching and training of family caregivers related to disease and infection-control procedures

Monitoring of respiratory and other systems

Evaluate lung sounds, and assess amount, site(s), wheezing, rhonchi, etc.

Teach patient or caregiver to identify and avoid specific factors that precipitate an exacerbation (asthma attack)

Teach patient or caregiver how to use aerosol inhalers or treatments at home

Assess signs and symptoms of CHF

Assess vital signs, including pain, q visit

Evaluate sites and amount of edema

Assess respiratory and cardiovascular statuses

Assess need for chest PT

Pain assessment and management q visit

Teach patient effective coughing, deep breathing, and pursed lip or diaphragmatic breathing

Teach other pulmonary treatment as indicated

Assess breath and lung sounds

Teach patient, family, and caregiver use of nebulizer therapy

Postural drainage as ordered

Pain assessment and management for cough and chest pain

Respiratory rate and lung sounds assessed for improvement or deterioration

Evaluate sites and amount of edema

Teach patient correct use and techniques of inhalers

RN to monitor respiratory rate and pattern

RN to evaluate for presence or absence of cough and its frequency, character, and sputum production

Teach use of home peak flow meter

RN to assess patient's pain or other symptoms q visit to identify need for change, addition, or other plan or dose adjustment

Ongoing skilled observation and assessment of wheezing, cough, dyspnea, shortness of breath, and other symptoms

Effective management of pain and prevention of secondary symptoms

RN to provide and teach effective oral care and comfort measures

Teaching and training regarding the home environment and care needed

Intervention of symptoms directed toward comfort and palliation

Observation and assessment, communication with physician related to signs and symptoms of continuing decompensation, increased symptoms, pain, discomfort, and shortness of breath and measures to alleviate and control

Teach caregiver/patient use of pain assessment tool/scale and reporting mechanism(s)

Teach patient/family about realistic expectations of disease process

Teach care of dying and signs/symptoms of impending death

Presence and support

Other interventions, based on patient/family needs

b. *Safety and mobility considerations*

Patient provided with home safety information and instruction related to _____ and documented in the clinical record

Teach about safe oxygen or nebulizer therapy use in the home setting

Teach family about safety of patient in home

Teach energy conservation techniques

Clinician to teach energy conservation techniques and controlled breathing exercises

Teach patient, family, and caregiver safe, effective oxygen therapy at home

Teach about copious secretions and their safe disposal

Other interventions, based an patient/family needs

c. *Emotional/Spiritual considerations*

Psychosocial assessment of patient and family regarding disease and prognosis

Provide emotional support to patient and family

Assess patient and family coping skills

Provide emotional support to patient and family

Psychosocial aspects of pain control (e.g., depression) assessed and acknowledged with team support/intervention

Ongoing acknowledgment of spirituality and related concerns of patient/family

Other interventions, based on patient/family needs

d. *Skin care*

Teach patient, family, or caregiver about proper body alignment and positioning in bed to prevent skin tears from shearing skin

Observation and skilled assessment of areas for possible breakdown, including heels, hips, elbows, ankles, and other pressure-prone areas

Teach caregiver about patient's skin care needs, including the need for frequent position changes, appropriate pressure pads and mattresses, and the prevention of breakdown

Other interventions, based on patient/family needs

e. *Elimination considerations*

RN to teach caregiver daily care of catheter

RN to evaluate the patient's bowel patterns and need for stool softeners, laxatives, and dietary adjustments and to develop bowel management plan

Other interventions, based on patient/family needs

f. *Hydration/Nutrition*

Assessment of nutrition and hydration status of patient at risk for poor nutritional status with severe lung disease

Assess nutrition/hydration status

Teach ordered diet regimen of _____ (specify)

Nutrition/hydration supported by offering patient's choice of favorite or desired foods or liquids

Nutrition/hydration maintained by offering patient high-protein diet and foods of choice as tolerated

Teach patient and family to expect decreased nutritional and fluid intake as disease progresses

Other interventions, based on patient/family needs

g. *Therapeutic/Medication regimens*

Medication management of patient on multiple medications; assess for side effects and compliance

Teach patient or caregiver new medication regimen

Obtain sputum culture as indicated q _____

Venipuncture as ordered q _____

RN to assess the patient's response to treatments and interventions and report changes, unfavorable responses, or reactions to the physician

Medication management and response to medications and side effects

Teach about and observe for steroid side effects

Nonpharmacological interventions, such as progressive muscle relaxation, imagery, positive visualization, music, massage and touch, and humor therapy of patient's choice implemented

Medication review and management including drug/drug and drug/food interactions

RN to instruct in pain-control measures and medications

Teach patient and caregiver use of PCA pump

Other interventions, based on patient/family needs

h. *Other considerations*

Assess progression of disease process

RN to assess the patient's response to treatments and interventions and to report to the physician changes, unfavorable responses, or reactions

Other interventions, based on patient/family needs

4

- *Home health aide or certified nursing assistant*
  Effective and safe personal care
  Safe ADL assistance and support
  Observation and reporting
  Respite care and active listening skills
  Meal preparation
  Homemaker services
  Comfort care
  Other duties

- *Social worker*
  Psychosocial assessment of patient and family/caregiver, including
      adjustment to long-term illness and its implications
  Identification of optimal coping strategies
  Financial assessment and counseling regarding food acquisition, ability
      to prepare, and costs of needed medications
  Intervention/support related to terminal illness and loss
  Emotional/spiritual support
  Depression/fear assessed
  Facilitate communication among patient, family, and hospice team
  Referral/linkage to community services and resources as indicated
  Grief counseling and intervention/support related to illness/loss
  Patient/caregiver counseling and support
  Identification of caregiver role strain necessitating respite/relief
      measures/support
  Obtain resources to enable patient to remain in the home
  Identification of illness-related psychiatric condition necessitating care
  Funeral and burial planning assistance

- *Volunteer(s)*
  Support, friendship, companionship, and presence
  Comfort and dignity maintained/provided for patient and family
  Errands and transportation
  Advocacy and respite
  Other services, based on interdisciplinary team recommendations and
      patient/caregiver needs

- *Spiritual counselor*
  Spiritual assessment and care
  Counseling, intervention, and support related to that dimension of life
      related to life's meaning (consistent with patient's beliefs)
  Support, listening, and presence
  Pray with or for the patient/family, using prayers familiar to patient's
      religious background (per their wishes)
  Participation in sacred or spiritual rituals or practices
  Other supportive care, based on patient's/family's needs and belief

- *Dietitian/Nutritional counseling*
  Assessment of patient with decreased intake, weight loss, anorexia, and
      increased shortness of breath (e.g., "I don't feel like eating")

Supportive counseling with patient/family indicating that patient will have a decreased appetite and usually at some point may not eat/drink

Assessment and recommendations for swallowing difficulties

Teaching and support of family members and caregivers

Support and care with food and nourishment as desired by patient

Evaluation/management of nutritional deficits and needs

Encourage nutritional supplements and snacks to increase protein and fat intake with moderate/low carbohydrate intake

Food and dietary recommendations incorporate patient choice and wishes

- *Occupational therapist*

  Evaluation of ADLs, functional mobility

  Assess for need for adaptive equipment and assistive devices

  Safety assessment of patient's environment and ADLs

  Assessment for energy conservation training

  Assessment of upper-extremity function, retraining motor skills

- *Physical therapist*

  Evaluation

  Safety assessment of patient's environment

  Safe transfer training or bed mobility exercises

  Pain assessment/reduction factors

  Strengthening exercises/program

  Assessment of gait safety and home safety measures

  Instruct/supervise caregiver and volunteers with regard to home exercise program for conditioning and strength

  Assistive, adaptive devices and evaluation of equipment and teaching

- *Bereavement counselor*

  Assessment of the needs of the bereaved family and friends

  Support and intervention, based on assessment and ongoing findings

  Presence and counseling

  Supportive visits, follow-up, and other interventions (e.g., mailings, calls)

  Other services related to bereavement work and support

- *Pharmacist*

  Evaluation of hospice patient on multiple medications (nebulizer, inhalers, antibiotics, steroids, aminophylline, etc.) for possible food/drug and drug/drug interactions

  Medication monitoring regarding therapeutic levels and dosages

  Pain consult and input into interdisciplinary POC related to pain control, dyspnea, and need for palliation and symptom management

  Assessment of medication regimen and plan for safety and compliance

- *Music, massage, art, or other therapies or services*

  Evaluation and intervention based on patient's and caregiver's unique wishes and needs that support care, comfort, and death in the setting of the patient's choice

4

Assessment plan to engage patient and support comfort, quality, enjoyment, and dignity

6. Outcomes for care

* ***Hospice nursing***

Death with dignity, and symptoms controlled in setting of patient/ family choice

Optimal comfort, support, and dignity provided throughout illness

Planned and effective bowel program, as evidenced by regular bowel movements and patient/family report of no problems

Death with maximum comfort through effective symptom control with specialized hospice support

Patient and caregiver able to list adverse drug reactions/problems with medication regimen and whom to call for follow-up and resolution

Dyspnea, pain, and other symptoms managed/controlled in setting of patient/family choice (e.g., patient/family report ability to eat, sleep, speak more clearly with pacing)

Patient's/family's privacy, independence, and choices supported with respect and maintained through death

Enhancement and support of quality of life

Effective symptom relief and control (e.g., a peaceful and comfortable death at home, some enjoyment of life)

Maximizing the patient's quality of life (e.g., alert and pain free or as patient wishes)

Pharmacological and nonpharmacological interventions, such as localized heat application, positioning, use of fan for dyspnea (if desired), relaxation methods, and music

Patient cared for and family supported through death with physical, psychosocial, spiritual, and other concerns/needs acknowledged/addressed

Patient- and family-centered hospice care provided based on the patient's/family's unique situation and needs

Infection control and palliation

Grief/bereavement expression and support provided

Patient is pain free by next _____ visit

Caregiver demonstrates ability to manage pain, where applicable

Patient maintains comfort and dignity throughout illness

Patient and caregiver verbalize satisfaction with care

Educational tools/plans incorporated in daily care, and patient/caregiver verbalizes understanding of safe, needed care

Patient and family will decide on care, interventions, and evaluation

Caregiver effective in care management and knows whom to call for questions/concerns

Patient will express satisfaction with hospice support received and will experience increased comfort

Patient will be made comfortable at home through death in accordance with the patient's wishes

Effective pain control and symptom control verbalized by patient

Patient and family verbalize understanding of and adhere to care and medication regimens

Patient and caregiver supported through patient's death

Comfort maintained through course of care

Patient and family receive hospice support and care, and family members and friends are able to spend quality time with the patient

Caregiver able and verbalizes comfort with role and understands when to call hospice team members

Patient supported through and receives the maximum benefit from palliative chemotherapy and radiation with minimal complications

Patient and caregiver list adverse reactions, potential complications, signs/symptoms of infection (e.g,, sputum change, chest congestion)

Comfort maintained through death with dignity

Pain effectively managed, and patient verbalizes comfort

Patient has stable respiratory status with patent airway and decreased dyspnea

Patient is protected from injury, has stable respiratory status, and is compliant with medication, safety, and care regimens

Comfort and individualized intervention of patient with immobility/bedbound status (e.g., skin, urinary, musculature, vascular)

Spiritual and psychosocial needs met (specify) as defined by patient and caregiver throughout course of care

Patient and caregiver demonstrate necessary disposal of secretions using infection-control procedure taught

Compliance to care program as evidenced by observation and demonstration during nurse's and other team members' visits

Patient states pain is _____ on 0–10 scale by next visit

Patient and caregiver demonstrate appropriate back-up or "rescue" therapies for breakthrough pain or other symptoms (e.g,, dyspnea)

- ***Home health aide or certified nursing assistant***
  Effective hygiene, personal care and comfort
  ADL assistance and ambulation
  Safe environment maintained

- ***Social worker***
  Problem identified and addressed, with patient/caregiver linked with appropriate support services and plan of care successfully implemented
  Patient and caregiver cope adaptively with illness and death
  Adaptive adjustment to changed body and body image
  Psychosocial support and counseling offered to patient/caregivers experiencing loss and grief
  Caregiver system assessed, and development of stable caregiver plan facilitated

- ***Volunteer(s)***
  Comfort, respite, companionship, and friendship extended to patient/family

Support provided as defined by the needs of the patient/caregiver

Patient and family supported by team with care, comfort, and companionship

- *Spiritual counseling*

 Spiritual support offered and provided as defined by needs of patient/caregiver

 Provision of spiritual support and care based on the assessed and ongoing needs of the patient and family

 Spiritual support offered, and patient and family needs met

 Patient and family express relief of symptoms of spiritual suffering

 Pray with or for the patient/family, using prayers familiar to the patient's religious background (per their wishes)

- *Dietitian/Nutritional counseling*

 Family and caregiver integrate recommendations into nutrition teaching (where appropriate)

 Patient and caregiver know whom to call for nutrition- and hydration-related questions/concerns

 Nutrition/hydration per patient's choices

 Caregiver integrates recommendations into daily meal planning

 Patient and family verbalize comprehension of changing nutritional needs

- *Occupational therapist*

 Maximize independence in ADLs for patient/caregiver

 Optimal function maintained/attained

 Patient and caregiver demonstrate ADL program for maximum safety

 Patient and caregiver demonstrate energy conservation techniques

 Splints used to maintain functional joint position

 Patient and caregiver demonstrate ADL program for maximum safety and independence

 Patient and caregiver demonstrate maximum independence with ADLs, adaptive techniques, and assistive devices

 Patient and caregiver demonstrate maximum safety in ADLs and functional mobility

 Patient and caregiver demonstrate effective use of energy conservation techniques

 Verbalization/demonstration of improved functional activity level and enhanced quality of life

 Patient and caregiver demonstrate effective use of diaphragmatic breathing to reduce shortness of breath and relaxation techniques to help in pain/symptom management

- *Physical therapist*

 Prevention of complications

 Home exercise and upper-extremity program taught to caregiver

 Optimal strength, mobility, and function maintained/achieved

 Compliance with home exercise program by _____ (specify date)

- *Bereavement counselor*

 Grief support services provided to patient and family

Well-being and resolution process of grief initiated and followed
   through bereavement services

- *Pharmacist*
   Multiple drug regimen reviewed for food/drug and drug/drug
      interactions in patient on multiple medications
   Stability and safety in complex medication regimen with maximum
      benefit to patient
   Effective pain, dyspnea, and symptom control and symptom
      management as reported by patient/caregiver
   Lab reports reviewed for therapeutic dosages and effective patient
      response

- *Music, massage, art, or other therapies or services*
   Therapeutic massage/touch effective for patient as self-reported or
      observed by caregivers/family
   Improved muscle tone, relaxation, and/or sleep
   Patient comfortable and relaxed (e.g., sleeping) after massage
   Music therapy intervention based on assessment to decrease pain
      perception and provide emotional expression and support
   Maintenance of comfort and physical, psychosocial, and spiritual health
   Holistic health maintained and comfort achieved through
            _____ (specify modality)

7. **Patient, family, and caregiver educational needs**
   Educational needs are the care regimens that contribute to safe and
   effective care at home between the hospice team's visits. These include
   the following:
      The basic tenets of hospice and the availability of support 24 hours a
         day, 7 days a week
      Home safety assessment and counseling
      The patient's medication regimen
      Safe and proper body mechanics to promote patient comfort and
         prevent caregiver safety problems
      Other teaching specific to the patient's and family's unique needs
      Support groups available to patient's family, such as the hospice
         program's "Caregiver Support Group" meetings for family
         members and friends of the patient
      Anticipated disease progression
      Safe, effective inhaler or metered dose unit use
      Safe, effective oxygen therapy use at home
      The importance of diet, rest, and exercise
      Other teaching specific to the patient's and caregiver's unique
         medical and other identified needs
      The prevention of infections and avoidance of stress and other
         "triggers" for the individual patient. These can include environmen-
         tal factors such as pollens, smoke, animals, dust, and
         chemicals
      Effective handwashing techniques, tissue/sputum disposal, and other
         aspects of infection control

Other teaching specific to the patient and caregiver; based on their unique needs

8. Specific tips for quality and reimbursement

Document any variances to expected outcomes. There are many models of hospice programs.

The Medicare hospice benefit does not require that the patient be homebound or have identified skilled needs. For further information on this benefit, please refer to CMS Hospice Manual 21.

Should the patient's status deteriorate and increased personal care be needed, obtain a telephone order for the increased service, noting frequency and estimating the duration.

Obtain a telephone order for all medication and treatment changes of the medical regimen and document these in the clinical record.

Unless the patient is in a hospice insurance program, some insurers will not pay for a skilled clinician visit that is made at death if the patient is dead when the clinician arrives at the home. From a Medicare home care perspective, the visit at the time of death may be covered when the orders and clinical record document assessment of the patient's status or signs of death/life or state law allows pronouncement of death by an RN.

Document patient deterioration

Document dehydration, dehydrating

Document patient change or instability

Document pain, other symptoms not controlled

Document status after acute episode of _____ (specify)

Document positive urine, sputum, etc. culture; patient started on _____ (specify ordered antibiotic therapy)

Document any impaction; impaction removed manually

Document RN in frequent communication with physician regarding _____ (specify)

Document febrile at _____, pulse change at _____, irr., irr.

Document change noted in _____

Document bony prominences red, opening

Document RN contacted physician regarding _____ (specify)

Document marked SOB

Document alteration in mental status

Document medications being adjusted, regulated, or monitored, and patient response

Document unable to perform own ADLs, personal care

Document all interdisciplinary team meetings and communications in the POC and in the progress notes of the clinical record

All hospice team members should have input into the POC and document their interventions and goals

Document changes to the POC, such as medications, services, frequency, communication, and concurrence of other team members

Document coordination of services or consultation of the other members of the IDT

Document communications and care coordination with other care
   providers, such as skilled nursing facility or nursing home staff,
   inpatient team members, and hired caregivers

Document all abnormal breath and lung sounds heard and location.

Obtain a telephone order for any POC changes, and document these
   changes

These patients are usually sick, so be objective and document what
   the patient looks like (frail, pale, poor intake, SOB, unable to
   do ADLs, etc.)

Document patient's continued poor activity level because of SOB

Document the ordered rate of oxygen flow, mode, and specific hours
   needed

Discuss patient at case conference with physical therapy,
   occupational therapy, home health aide, and other ordered
   services

Document any increased SOB

Document any change, including medications, on the POC

Document RN contacted physician regarding _____ (specify)

Document RN in frequent communications with physician
   regarding _____ (specify)

Document febrile at _____, or tachycardia at _____, irr., irr.

New onset (any symptom)

Document dehydration, dehydrating

Document stable, unstable

Document pain uncontrolled, any other symptom not controlled

Document positive sputum culture; physician started patient
   on _____ (specify ordered medication)

Document medications being regulated

Document bony prominences, red or opening skin sites

Document care coordination among the IDT members, such as phone
   calls, case conferences, or team meetings

Phone calls to physicians for changes in the patient's condition;
   obtaining orders for a change on the plan of care or requesting an
   increase in the visit frequency needs physician orders

Document all abnormalities, such as fever, tachycardia, rales, wheezing,
   and rhonchi

Document the instability of the patient; document any edema,
   SOB, medication reaction, further acute episodes, pulse
   irregularities

Obtain a telephone order to change the visit frequency or make any
   changes to the POC

Often these patients have other medical problems, specifically
   cardiac, that impede progress; document these problems also

Document medications changed or medications being regulated on the
   daily visit note or record

Document the clear progression of symptoms and interventions that
   demonstrate the overall management of the patient with end-stage
   lung disease in the clinical notes

Document when/if the patient has respiratory changes, shortness of breath, exacerbation of conditions, dysphagia, pain, and other symptoms and that they are identified and resolved

Remember that the clinical documentation is key to measuring compliance for quality and reimbursement purposes. Care coordination, timely verbal and initial physician orders, and assessment and addressing of spiritual and psychosocial needs should be clearly documented in the patient's clinical record

The documentation should support that all hospice care supports comfort and dignity while meeting patient/family needs

The documentation should include the ongoing assessment and management of pain and other symptoms and the anticipation and prevention of secondary symptoms such as constipation

It is important to note that all team members, including clinicians and social workers, should assess, identify, and "hear" spiritual needs that the patient/family want to be addressed. These spiritual issues are key to the provision of quality hospice care and cannot be addressed effectively and promptly by the spiritual counselor only

Document clearly symptoms, clinical changes, and assessment findings that support the end stage of the lung process

Document patient changes, symptoms, and clinical information identified from visits and team conferences that support hospice care and a limited life expectancy

Clearly support in the documentation the rationale that supports/explains the progression of the illness from the chronic to terminal stages

Document mentation, behavioral, and/or cognitive changes

Document dysphagia, weight loss, increased shortness of breath, dyspnea, infection, sepsis, new or changed medications, etc.

Document any skin changes (e.g., inflamed, painful, weeping skin site[s])

Document when the patient is actively dying, deteriorating, progressing toward death

Remember that the "litmus test" of care coordination rests on the quality of the clinical documentation completed by all team members. Review one of your patient's clinical records and ask yourself the following: "If I was unable to give a verbal report/update on this patient, would a peer be able to pick up and provide the same level of care and know (from the documentation) the current orders, including specific medications and other details that contribute to effective hospice care?"

This patient population usually has many clinical changes that should be documented. These include weight loss, dyspnea, and multiple and changed medication regimens with varying routes, including nebulizer therapy, steroids, antibiotics, varying bronchodilators such as aminophylline. Some patients have cardiac side effects to the drug regimen that should be observed, noted, documented, and reported (e.g., patient has ascites, is cyanotic, has severe finger clubbing noted on admission, has peripheral edema). All these clinical findings are examples that assist in painting a picture to support coverage and documentation requirements for hospice care

Document any hospitalizations and changed clinical finding

In the clinical documentation, paint the picture of the patient with end stage lung disease. The patient may be very short of breath and have poor or no activity tolerance or energy. This is the kind of clinical documentation specificity that clearly shows why the hospice team was called in at this point along the patient's illness continuum and supports coverage and documentation requirements of an insurance provider, such as Medicare

For this and other noncancer diagnoses, document clearly the symptoms and clinical and assessment findings that constitute evidence of the end stage of the chronic illness process

Document patient changes, symptoms, and psychosocial issues affecting care, including information gathered at the patient/family visits and during team meetings

The documentation should reflect ongoing effects of the terminal condition, the patient's/family's difficulty with care or coping, and the continued desire for hospice care

9. **Queries for quality**

   Lung care (end stage)
   • *Is patient's dyspnea managed adequately?*
   • *Is patient's anxiety managed adequately?*
   • *Is patient's functional ability/status clearly documented?*
   • *What safety plans have been established?*
   • *Have you documented to the interdisciplinary POC?*

   Chronic obstructive pulmonary disease care
   • *Is patient's dyspnea managed adequately?*
   • *Is patient's anxiety managed adequately?*
   • *Is patient's functional ability/status clearly documented?*
   • *What safety plans have been established?*
   • *Have you documented to the interdisciplinary POC?*

   Pulmonary disease care
   • *Is patient's dyspnea managed adequately?*
   • *Is patient's anxiety managed adequately?*
   • *Is patient's functional ability/status clearly documented?*
   • *What safety plans have been established?*
   • *Have you documented to the interdisciplinary POC?*

10. **Resources for hospice care and practice**
   The American Lung Association publishes the *Asthma Handbook* and can be reached at 1-800-232-5864 or visit online at www.lungusa.org

Another helpful resource is the NHPCO's latest edition of *Medical Guidelines for Determining Prognoses in Selected Non-Cancer Diseases.* Call the NHPCO at (703)-243-5900 for more information or visit online at www.nhpco.org.

National Cancer Institute, www.nci.nih.gov

4

PAIN CARE

1. General considerations

It has been said that the most common nursing diagnosis or patient problem may be pain. It is important to remember that patients (and family members providing the direct care) are the experts on their pain, their histories, and often even the necessary relief measures. This information can be most easily elicited during completion of the pain assessment tool. Once asked, hospice patients will readily assess and discuss their pain perceptions.

Hospice clinicians are becoming the experts in this area, and experienced clinicians develop accepted assessment tools, protocols for medication titration, and overall pain management. For effective pain management, efforts of the entire hospice team must be directed toward comfort and validation or verbalization of relief, when possible. Part Seven provides pain assessment and management resources for your review and information. See also Box 4-1 for information on cancer-related pain.

2. Needs for visit

Physician order for hospice care, specific to the hospice program's admission criteria and policies

Standard precautions/supplies

Vital signs equipment for baseline assessment

Other supplies or equipment, based on physician orders

3. Safety considerations

Infection control/standard precautions

Night-light

Extra caution on slippery surfaces

Removal of scatter rugs

Tub rail, grab bars for bathroom safety

Supportive and nonskid shoes

Handrail on stairs

Fall precautions/protocol

Protective skin measures

Identification and report of any skin problems

Smoke detector and fire evacuation plan

Assistance with ambulation

Others, based on the patient's unique condition and environment

4

4. Potential diagnoses and codes

Pain can come from any cause, source, or diagnosis. Please refer to the other care guidelines for specific diagnosis codes such as cancer, depression, and any other section that is appropriate for your patient's pain problems.

5. Skills and services identified

- *Hospice nursing*
a. *Comfort and symptom control*

   Comprehensive initial assessment of systems in patient with pain for
   baseline information

   Presentation of hospice philosophy and services

   Explain patient rights and responsibilities

   Observation and assessment of patient with _____ (specify)
   on multiple medications, admitted to hospice with increasing
   shortness of breath and pain

   Assess patient, family, and caregiver wishes and expectations regarding
   care

   Assess patient, family, and caregiver resources available for care

   Provision of volunteer support to patient and family

   Teach family or caregiver physical care of patient

   Pain assessment and management q visit, including source/type of pain
   (e.g., cancer pain, infection, pathological fracture, and other medical
   problems such as cardiac or arthritis pain)

   RN to provide and teach effective oral care and comfort measures

   Assess pain and other symptoms, including site, duration, characteristics,
   and relief measures

   RN to assess patient's pain q visit to identify need for change, addition,
   or other plan or dose adjustment

   RN to assess all aspects of pain, including site(s), character,
   description, relation to activity or position, type of pain (constant,
   spontaneous, episodic), and other factors patient identifies

   RN to teach patient and caregivers about the importance of and
   rationale for round-the-clock schedule of analgesia for continuous
   pain management

   Teach patient how to use the standardized pain scale

   Teach patient how to rate pain using the scale of 0–10 or other scale
   specific to the patient's ability

   Assist patient in establishing goals for relief

   Evaluate pain in relation to other symptoms, including fatigue,
   confusion, constipation, depression, and SOB

   RN to evaluate need for noninvasive methods of pain control, including
   heat or cold applications and a transcutaneous electrical nerve
   stimulation (TENS) unit

   Assess pain, and evaluate pain management's effectiveness

   Teach care of bedridden patient

   Measure vital signs, including pain, q visit

   Assess cardiovascular, pulmonary, and respiratory status

   Teach caregiver care of weak, terminally ill patient

   Comfort measures of backrub and hand or other therapeutic massage

   Teach patient/family use of standardized form/tool to use between
   hospice team members' visits (and for care coordination between
   team members)

4

Teach patient/family principles of effective pain management

Observation and assessment, communication with physician related to signs and symptoms of continuing decompensation and increased symptoms, pain, discomfort, and shortness of breath, and measures to alleviate and control

Effective management of pain and prevention of secondary symptoms

Interventions of symptoms directed toward comfort and palliation

Teach caregiver/patient use of pain assessment tool/scale and reporting mechanism(s)

Teach patient and family about realistic expectations of disease process

Teach care of dying and signs/symptoms of impending death

Presence and support

Other interventions, based on patient/family needs

b. *Safety and mobility considerations*

Provide caregiver with home safety information and instruction related to _____ and documented in the clinical record

Assess relationship of pain to increased safety risks, such as falls, in the home; counsel regarding safety and precautions

Other interventions, based on patient/family needs

c. *Emotional/Spiritual considerations*

Psychosocial assessment of patient and family regarding disease and prognosis

RN to provide emotional support to patient and family

RN to evaluate for emotional distress and other factors affecting pain

Assess mental status and sleep disturbance changes

Assess for and manage plans for psychosocial and/or spiritual pain (e.g., all pain, anxiety, interpersonal distress)

Assessment and care/support related to depression, changed body image concerns, fever, mouth sores/ulcers, complaints of extreme tiredness, and dry/cracking skin in patient receiving palliative chemotherapy

Psychosocial aspects of pain control (e.g., depression, others) assessed and acknowledged with team support/intervention

Ongoing acknowledgment of spirituality and related concerns of patient/family

Other interventions, based on patient/family needs

d. *Skin care*

Assess skin integrity

Observation and evaluation of wound and surrounding skin

Evaluate patient's need for equipment, including supplies to decrease pressure, alternating pressure mattress, gel foam seat cushion, and heel and elbow protectors

RN to teach patient regarding care of irradiated skin sites

Teach patient, family, or caregiver about proper body alignment and positioning in bed to prevent skin tears from shearing skin

Observe and apply skilled assessment of areas for possible breakdown, including heels, hips, elbows, ankles, and other pressure-prone areas

4

Teach caregiver regarding skin care needs, including the need for
frequent position changes, appropriate pressure pads and mattresses,
and the prevention of breakdown

Other interventions, based on patient/family needs

e. *Elimination considerations*

RN to develop bowel management plan

Assess amount and frequency of urinary output

RN to evaluate the patient's bowel patterns and need for stool
softeners, laxatives, dietary adjustments, and to develop bowel
management plan

Teaching and ongoing assessment regarding prevention and early
identification of constipation and its correction/resolution

Initiate bowel management program per hospice physician

Implement bowel assessment and management program

Teach patient, family, and aide the importance of observing and noting
bowel movements between scheduled nursing visits

Obtain patient history related to norms for bowel movements to date
(e.g., "All my life I go only every other day")

Consider stool softeners, and offer laxative of choice, Fleet's enemas
prn, and other methods per patient wishes and physician's orders

Other interventions, based on patient/family needs

f. *Hydration/Nutrition*

Assess nutrition/hydration statuses

Nutrition/hydration supported by offering patient's choice of favorite or
desired foods or liquids

Nutrition/hydration maintained by offering patient high-protein diet and
foods of choice as tolerated

Assessment and plan related to anorexia/cachexia, tube feedings,
difficulty/painful swallowing, and/or transitional feedings
(e.g., TPN to oral)

Teach patient and family to expect decreased nutritional and fluid
intake as disease progresses

Assessment and interventions/plan related to patient/family complaints
of dry mouth, with painful chewing, difficulty speaking, and denture
fit concerns after radiation and surgery

Other interventions, based on patient/family needs

g. *Therapeutic/Medication regimens*

Monitor for signs/symptoms of narcotic overdose and treat as
appropriate (e.g., following established protocols)

RN to implement nonpharmacological interventions with medication
schedule, including therapeutic massage, hypnosis, distraction,
imagery, progressive muscle relaxation, humor, music therapies,
and biofeedback

Administer antiemetic on round-the-clock basis to control
nausea caused by narcotic analgesia ordered for continuous
pain

Patient taught about and provided with educational materials regarding pain medication and side effects

RN to titrate the dose to achieve patient pain relief with minimal side effects (per the range noted in the physician orders)

RN to assess the patient's response to therapeutic treatments and interventions and to report any changes or unfavorable responses to the physician

Medication assessment and management q visit

Teach new pain- and symptom-control medication regimen

Teach patient and caregiver use of PCA pump

Nonpharmacological interventions such as progressive muscle relaxation, imagery, positive visualization, music, massage and touch, and humor therapy of patient's choice implemented

RN to instruct in pain control measures and medications

Teach about and observe side effects of palliative chemotherapy, including constipation, anemia, and fatigue

Venipuncture q _____ (specify ordered frequency) for monitoring platelet count

Teaching of patient/family, including medications, pain management program, strength, type, actions, times, and compliance tips

Encourage family/caregivers to give the patient medications on the schedule per physician orders

Medications changed using equianalgesic conversion tables/physician orders (e.g., from oral morphine to an equianalgesic dose of transdermal fentanyl)

RN to instruct in the use of breakthrough or "rescue" dosing of pain medication

Other interventions, based on patient/family needs

h. *Other considerations*

Assess progression of disease process

RN to assess the patient's response to treatments and interventions and to report to the physician changes, unfavorable responses, or reactions

Other interventions, based on patient/family needs

4

• *Home health aide or certified nursing assistant*

Effective and safe personal care

Safe ADL assistance and support

Observation and reporting

Report patient complaints of unrelieved, new, or changed pain

Respite care and active listening skills

Meat preparation

Homemaker services

Comfort care

Other duties

• *Social worker*

Psychosocial assessment of patient and family/caregiver, including adjustment to illness, pain, and its implications

Identification of optimal coping strategies

Financial assessment and counseling regarding food acquisition, ability to prepare, and costs of needed medications

Intervention/support related to terminal illness and loss

Emotional/spiritual support

Depression/fear assessed

Facilitate communication among patient, family, and hospice team

Referral/linkage to community services and resources as indicated

Grief counseling and intervention/support related to illness/loss

Patient/caregiver counseling and support

Identification of caregiver role strain necessitating respite/relief measures/support

For patients who live alone with no support system (e.g., able, available, willing caregiver[s]), obtain resources to enable patient to remain in home setting

Identification of illness-related psychiatric condition necessitating support and care/intervention

Evaluate impact of pain on quality of life

Funeral and burial planning assistance

- *Volunteer(s)*

  Support, friendship, companionship, and presence

  Comfort and dignity maintained/provided for patient and family

  Errands and transportation

  Advocacy and respite

  Other services, based on IDT recommendations and patient/caregiver needs

- *Spiritual counselor*

  Spiritual assessment and care

  Counseling, intervention, and support related to that dimension of life related to life's meaning (consistent with patient's beliefs)

  Pray with or for the patient/family, using prayers familiar to patient's religious background (per their wishes)

  Support, listening, and presence

  Participation in sacred or spiritual rituals or practices

  Other supportive care, based on patient's/family's needs and belief systems

- *Dietitian/Nutritional counseling*

  Assessment of patient with decreased intake, weight loss, anorexia, and pain

  Supportive counseling with patient/family indicating that patient will have a decreased appetite and possible inability to eat/drink

  Assessment and recommendations for swallowing difficulties, nausea, vomiting, and constipation associated with pain medications

  Teaching and support of family members and caregivers

  Support and care with food and nourishment as desired by patient

  Evaluation/management of nutritional deficits and needs

  Encourage nutritional supplements and snacks to increase protein and caloric intake

Food and dietary recommendations incorporate patient choice and
  wishes

- *Occupational therapist*
  Evaluation of ADLs and functional mobility
  Assess for need for adaptive equipment and assistive devices
  Safety assessment of patient's environment and ADLs
  Assessment for energy conservation training
  Assessment of upper-extremity function, retraining motor skills, and/or
    splinting for contracture(s)

- *Physical therapist*
  Evaluation
  Safety assessment of patient's environment
  Safe transfer training or bed mobility in patient with pain
  Pain assessment/reduction factors
  Strengthening exercises/program
  Assessment of gait safety and home safety measures
  Instruct/supervise caregiver and volunteers on home exercise program
    for conditioning and strength
  Assistive, adaptive devices and evaluation of equipment and teaching

- *Speech-language pathologist*
  Evaluation for speech/swallowing problems
  Food texture recommendations
  Alternate functional communication

- *Bereavement counselor*
  Assessment of the needs of the bereaved family and friends
  Support and intervention, based on assessment and ongoing findings
  Presence and counseling
  Supportive visits, follow-up, and other interventions (e.g., mailings, calls)
  Other services related to bereavement work and support

- *Pharmacist*
  Evaluation of hospice patient with constipation on cathartics, stool
    softeners, and other medications for possible food/drug and
    drug/drug interactions
  Medication monitoring regarding therapeutic levels and dosages
  Pain consult and input into interdisciplinary POC related to pain
    control, palliation, and symptom management
  Assessment of medication regimen and plan for pain relief and safety

- *Music, massage, art, or other therapies or services*
  Evaluation and intervention based on patient's and caregiver's unique
    wishes and needs that support care, comfort, and death in the setting
    of the patient's choice
  Assessment plan to engage patient and support comfort, quality,
    enjoyment, dignity, and pain/symptom relief
  Pet therapy (including patient's pet, if available) and therapeutic
    intervention

4

6. Outcomes for care

- *Hospice nursing*

    Pain and symptoms managed/controlled in setting of patient/family choice (e.g., patient/family report ability to eat, sleep, speak with pacing)

    Planned and effective bowel program, as evidenced by regular bowel movements and patient/family report of comfort

    Death with dignity, and pain/symptoms controlled in setting of patient/family choice

    Optimal comfort, support, and dignity provided throughout illness

    Death with maximum comfort through effective symptom control with specialized hospice support

    Patient and caregiver able to list adverse drug reactions and problems with medication regimen and whom to call for follow-up and resolution

    Spiritual and psychosocial needs met (specify) as defined by patient and caregiver throughout course of care

    Patient's/family's privacy, independence, and choices supported with respect and maintained through death

    Enhancement and support of quality of life

    Effective pain and other symptom relief and control (e.g., a peaceful and comfortable death at home, some enjoyment of life)

    Maximizing the patient's quality of life (e.g., alert and pain free or as patient wishes)

    Pharmacological and nonpharmacological interventions, such as localized heat application, positioning, relaxation methods, and music

    Patient cared for and family supported through death, with physical, psychosocial, spiritual, and other concerns/needs acknowledged/addressed

    Patient- and family-centered hospice care provided based on the patient's/family's unique situation and needs

    Infection control and palliation

    Grief/bereavement expression and support provided

    Patient is protected from injury, has stable respiratory status, and is compliant with medication, safety, and care regimens

    Comfort and individualized intervention of patient with immobility/bedbound status (e.g., skin, urinary, musculature, vascular)

    Patient and caregiver verbalize satisfaction with care

    Educational tools/plans incorporated in daily care, and patient and caregiver verbalize understanding of safe, needed care

    Patient will decide on care, interventions, and evaluation

    Caregiver effective in care management and knows whom to call for questions/concerns

    Patient will express satisfaction with hospice support received and will experience increased comfort

Patient will be made comfortable at home through death in accordance with the patient's wishes

Effective pain control and symptom control verbalized by patient

Patient verbalizes understanding of and adheres to care and medication regimens

Patient and caregiver supported through patient's death

Comfort maintained through course of care

The patient and family receive hospice support and care, and family members and friends are able to spend quality time with the patient

Caregiver able and verbalizes comfort with role and understands when to call hospice team members

Patient supported through and receives the maximum benefit from palliative chemotherapy and radiation with minimal complications

Patient and caregiver list adverse reactions, potential complications, and signs/symptoms of infection (e.g., sputum change, chest congestion)

Comfort maintained through death with dignity

Pain effectively managed, and patient verbalizes comfort

Patient has stable respiratory status with patent airway (e.g., no dyspnea, infection free)

Patient will decide on care and pain intervention and evaluation

Patient will experience increased comfort and pain control through self-report and _____ (specify parameters)

Patient will have palliative care and comfort maintained through death

Patient and caregiver knowledgeable about side effects (e.g., constipation) and interventions needed

Control of pain and other symptoms that affect daily function, quality of life, and ability to interact with friends/family

Teaching related to safety, medications, and self-care successful as demonstrated by patient's verbalization and (specify measurable parameters)

Effective pain control and symptom relief by _____ (specify date)

Patient and caregiver knowledgeable about pain regimen, relief measures, and care for optimal relief/control

Early detection and intervention of problems related to patients with immobility/bedbound status (e.g., skin, urinary, musculature, vascular, others)

Patient/caregiver demonstrates appropriate back-up or "rescue" therapies for breakthrough pain or other symptoms (e.g., dyspnea)

Caregiver demonstrates ability to manage pain, where applicable

Patient maintains comfort and dignity throughout illness

Patient states pain is at _____ on 0–10 scale by next visit.

4

- **Home health aide or certified nursing assistant**

Effective hygiene, personal care, and comfort

ADL assistance

Safe environment maintained

- *Social worker*

  Problem identified and addressed, with patient/caregiver linked with appropriate support services and POC successfully implemented

  Patient and caregiver cope adaptively will illness and death

  Adaptive adjustment to changed body and body image

  Psychosocial support and counseling offered to patient/caregivers experiencing loss and grief

  Caregiver system assessed, and development of stable caregiver plan facilitated

- *Volunteer(s)*

  Comfort, companionship, and friendship extended to patient/family

  Support provided as defined by the needs of the patient/caregiver

  Patient and family supported by team with care, comfort, and companionship

  Advocacy and respite

  Funeral and burial planning assistance

- *Spiritual counselor*

  Spiritual support offered and provided as defined by needs of patient/caregiver

  Provision of spiritual support and care as based on the assessed and ongoing needs of the patient and family

  Spiritual support offered, and patient and family needs met

  Participation in sacred or spiritual rituals or practices

  Patient and family express relief of symptoms of spiritual suffering

  Support, listening, and presence

  Intervention and support provided related to that dimension of life related to life's meaning (consistent with patient's beliefs)

  Pray with or for the patient/family, using prayers familiar to the patient's religious background (per their wishes)

- *Dietitian/Nutritional counseling*

  Family and caregiver integrate recommendations into nutrition teaching and daily meal planning

  Patient and caregiver know whom to call for nutrition/hydration concerns

  Patient and family verbalize comprehension of changing nutritional needs

- *Occupational therapist*

  Patient and caregiver demonstrate maximum independence with ADLs, adaptive techniques, and assistive devices

  Patient and caregiver demonstrate maximum safety in ADLs and functional mobility

  Patient and caregiver demonstrate effective use of energy conservation techniques

  Verbalization/demonstration of improved functional activity level and enhanced quality of life

  Patient and caregiver demonstrate effective use of diaphragmatic breathing to reduce shortness of breath and relaxation techniques to help in pain/symptom management

Patient and caregiver demonstrate correct use of exercise and splints for maximum upper-extremity function and joint position

- *Physical therapist*
  Prevention of complications
  Home exercise and upper-extremity program taught to caregiver
  Optimal strength, mobility, function maintained/achieved
  Pain management program effective as verbalized by patient/caregiver

- *Speech-language pathologist*
  Communication method implemented, and patient able to be understood as self-reported or reported by family/caregivers
  Safe swallowing and functional communication
  Recommended lists of foods/textures for safety and patient choice

- *Bereavement counselor*
  Support services related to grief provided to patient and family
  Well-being and resolution process of grief initiated and followed through bereavement services

- *Music, massage, art, or other therapies or services*
  Therapeutic massage/touch effective for patient as self-reported or observed by caregivers/family
  Improved relaxation (relief from pain) and/or sleep
  Patient comfortable and relaxed (e.g., sleeping) after massage
  Music therapy intervention based on assessment to decrease pain perception and provide emotional expression and support
  Maintenance of comfort and physical, psychosocial, and spiritual health
  Holistic health maintained and comfort achieved through _____ (specify modality)
  Patient has pet's presence as desired—in all care sites, when possible

7. **Patient, family, and caregiver educational needs**
   Educational needs are the care regimens that contribute to safe and effective care at home between the hospice team's visits. These include the following:
   The basic tenets of hospice and the availability of support 24 hours a day, 7 days a week
   Home safety assessment and counseling
   The patient's medication regimen
   Safe and proper body mechanics to promote patient comfort and prevent caregiver safety problems
   Anticipated disease progression
   Support groups available to patient's family, such as the hospice program's "Caregiver Support Group" meetings for family members and friends of the patient
   Other teaching specific to the patient's and family's unique needs
   Importance of all aspects of the pain-control regimen (e.g., timing)

8. **Specific tips for quality and reimbursement**
   Unless the patient is in a hospice insurance program, some insurers will not pay for a skilled clinician visit made at death if the patient is dead

when the clinician arrives at the home. From a Medicare home care perspective, the visit at the time of death may be covered when the orders and clinical record document assessment of the patient's status or signs of death/life or state law allows pronouncement of death by an RN.

Document patient deterioration

Document dehydration, dehydrating

Document patient change or instability

Document pain, other symptoms not controlled

Document status after acute episode of _____ (specify)

Document positive urine, sputum, etc. culture; patient started on _____ (specify ordered antibiotic therapy)

Document patient impacted; impaction removed manually per physician's orders

Document RN in frequent communication with physician regarding _____ (specify)

Document febrile at _____, pulse change at _____, irr., irr.

Document change noted in _____

Document bony prominences red, opening

Document RN contacted physician regarding _____ (specify)

Document marked SOB

Document alteration in mental status

Document medications being adjusted, regulated, or monitored and patient response

Document unable to perform own ADLs, personal care

Document all interdisciplinary team meetings and communications in the POC and in the progress notes of the clinical record

All hospice team members involved should have input into the POC and document their interventions and goals

Document any variances to expected outcomes. There are many models of hospice programs.

The Medicare hospice benefit does not require that the patient be homebound or have identified skilled needs. For further information on this benefit, please refer to CMS Hospice Manual 21.

Should the patient's status deteriorate and increased personal care be needed, obtain a telephone order for the increased service, noting frequency and estimating the duration.

Obtain a telephone order for all medication and treatment changes of the medical regimen and document these in the clinical record.

The health care skills used primarily in the area of pain and other symptom management will be (1) observation and assessment; (2) management and evaluation of the patient's POC; (3) administration of medications, depending on the patient's unique medical condition; and (4) teaching and training activities related to the medication regimen, side effects, and safe and effective administration of medication.

Examples of teaching or training activities may be, for example, teaching the patient and family the use of the PCA pump, safe administration of medication, and care of the bedbound patient.

Document all case provided, including that related to pain management and the patient response to those interventions. Document any changes to the POC and physician communications, and obtain orders for any changes.

Document changes or alterations to the POC and the patient's response to the changed interventions. The documentation should reflect the learning accomplishments of the patient/family including side effects and adverse reaction information.

Document in the clinical notes the clear progression of symptoms and interventions that demonstrate the overall management of the patient with pain

Document when/if the patient has respiratory changes, shortness of breath, exacerbation of conditions, dysphagia, changes in pain, and other symptoms and that they are identified and resolved

Remember that the clinical documentation is key to measuring organizational compliance for quality and reimbursement purposes. Care coordination, timely verbal and initial physician orders, and assessment and addressing of spiritual and psychosocial needs should be ongoing and documented in the patient's clinical record

The documentation should support that all hospice care supports comfort and dignity while meeting patient/family needs

The documentation should include ongoing assessment and management of pain and other symptoms and the anticipation and prevention of secondary symptoms such as constipation

It is important to note that all team members, including clinicians and social workers, should assess, identify, and "hear" spiritual needs that the patient/family want to be addressed. These spiritual issues are key to the provision of quality hospice care and cannot be addressed effectively and promptly by the spiritual counselor only

Document clearly symptoms, clinical changes, and assessment findings related to pain and patient care

Document patient changes, symptoms, and clinical information identified from visits and team conferences that constitute evidence of the need for hospice care and a limited life expectancy

Clearly support in the documentation the rationale that supports/explains the progression of the illness from the chronic to terminal stages

Document mentation, behavioral, and/or cognitive changes

Document dysphagia, weight loss, increased shortness of breath, dyspnea, infection, sepsis, new or changed medications, etc.

Document any skin changes (e.g., inflamed, painful, weeping skin site[s])

Document when the patient is actively dying, deteriorating, and progressing toward death

Remember that the "litmus test" of care coordination rests on the quality of the clinical documentation by all team members. Review one of your patient's clinical records and ask yourself the following: "If I was unable to give a verbal report/update on this patient, would a peer be able to pick up and provide the same level of care and know (from the documentation) the current orders, medications, and other details that contribute to effective hospice care?"

Side effects to the drug regimen should be observed, noted, documented, and reported

Document changes to the plan of care, such as medications, services, frequency, communication, and concurrence of other team members

Document communications and care coordination with other care providers, such as skilled nursing facility or nursing home staff, inpatient team members, and hired caregivers

Your assessments, observations, and clinical findings assist in painting a picture to support coverage and documentation requirements for hospice care

Document any hospitalizations and changed clinical findings

Document patient changes, symptoms, psychosocial issues impacting the care, and information gathered at the patient/family visits and during team meetings

The documentation should reflect ongoing effects of the terminal condition, the patient's/family's difficulty with care or coping, and the continued desire for hospice care

Document coordination of services and consultations with the other members of the IDG

9. **Queries for quality**
   - *Has the patient's pain been completely and thoroughly documented?*
   - *Is the patient's anxiety managed adequately?*
   - *Is the patient's functional ability/status clearly documented?*
   - *What is the patient's bowel regimen, and has it been clearly documented?*
   - *Have you documented to the interdisciplinary POC?*

10. **Resources for hospice care and practice**
    The Mayday Pain Resource Center is a clearinghouse for information and resources to improve the quality of pain management and can be reached at (818)359-8111, ext. 3829, or visit www.cityofhope.org/prc. The Roxane Pain Institute provides informational booklets and articles on pain management and can be reached at 1-800-335-9100.

    Available free from the Agency for Health Care Policy and Research (AHCPR) are three resources: *Clinical Practice Guideline Number 9: Management of Cancer Pain, Quick Reference Guide for Clinicians: Management of Cancer Pain: Adults,* and *Consumer's Guide: Management of Cancer Pain.* The patient guides are available in English and Spanish, and all can be ordered by calling 1-800-358-9295.

    National Cancer Institute, www.nci.nih.gov.

    Many drug companies provide easily carried equianalgesic charts; contact the representatives, who are very willing to help clinicians and share resources.

PROSTATE CANCER CARE

1. General considerations

Many patients with prostate cancer have a long history of curative-focused care interventions such as surgery, radiation, and chemotherapy. The hospice team interventions focus on care and comfort, while providing support to the patient and the family.

Please refer to "Cancer Care," "Pain Care," and "Supportive Care" should these sections also pertain to your patient.

2. Needs for visit

Physician order for hospice care, specific to the hospice program's admission criteria and policies

Standard precautions supplies

Vital signs equipment for baseline assessment

Other supplies or equipment, based on physician orders

3. Safety considerations

Infection control/standard precautions

Night-light

Extra caution on slippery surfaces

Removal of scatter rugs

Tub rail, grab bars for bathroom safety

Supportive and nonskid shoes

Handrail on stairs

Fall precautions/protocol

Phone number of person to call with a care or pain problem

Supportive and well-fitting, nonslip shoes

Equipment safety for home medical equipment (e.g., wheelchair, walker)

Protective skin measures

Identification and report of any skin problems

Smoke detector and fire evacuation plan

Assistance with ambulation

Others, based on the patient's unique condition and environment

4

4. Potential diagnoses and codes

Adenocarcinoma, metastatic	199.1
Attention to other artificial opening of urinary tract	V55.6
Bladder cancer	188.9
Bone metastasis	198.5
Cancer of the prostate	185
Failure to thrive, adult	783.7
Fracture, pathological	733.10
Incontinence of feces	787.6
Incontinence of urine	788.30
Kidney, cancer of the (renal)	189.0

Pain, low back	724.2
Pressure ulcer	707.0
Prostate, cancer of	185
Prostatectomy (TURP) (surgical)	60.9
Prostatitis	601.9
Rectosigmoid, cancer of	154.0
Rectum, cancer of the	154.1
Renal cell cancer, metastatic	198.0
Urinary tract infection	599.0

5. Skills and services identified

- *Hospice nursing*

a. *Comfort and symptom control*

Skilled observation and complete systems assessment of the patient with prostate cancer admitted to hospice

Presentation of hospice philosophy and services

Explain patient rights and responsibilities

Assess patient, family, and caregiver wishes and expectations regarding care

Assess patient, family, and caregiver resources available for care

Assess pain and other symptoms, including site, duration, characteristics, and relief measures

Provision of volunteer support to patient and family

Teach family or caregiver physical care of patient

RN to provide and teach effective oral care and comfort measures

Teach care of bedridden patient

Measure vital signs and pain q visit

Assess cardiovascular, pulmonary, and respiratory statuses

Oxygen on at _____ liters per _____ (specify physician orders)

Pain assessment and management

RN to assess patient's pain or other symptoms q visit to identify need for change, addition, or other plan or dose adjustment

RN to teach patient and caregiver about disease process and management

Comfort measures of backrub and hand or other therapeutic massage

Teach caregiver or family care of weak, terminally ill patient

Observation, assessment, and supportive care to patient and family

Teach patient/family use of standardized form/tool to use between hospice team members' visits (and for care coordination between team members)

Supportive care and scopolamine patches per physician orders

Teach patient/family principles of effective pain management

Effective management of pain and prevention of secondary symptoms

Interventions of symptoms directed toward comfort and palliation

Pain assessment and management q visit, including source of pain (e.g., cancer pain, infection, pathological fracture, other medical problems such as cardiac or arthritis pain)

Observation and assessment, communication with physician related to signs and symptoms of continuing decompensation and increased symptoms, pain, discomfort, and shortness of breath, and measures to alleviate and control

Teach patient and family about realistic expectations of disease process

Teach care of dying and signs/symptoms of impending death

Presence and support

Other interventions, based on patient/family needs

b. *Safety and mobility considerations*

Provide caregiver with home safety information and instruction related to _____ (specify) and documented in the clinical record

Teach family regarding safety of patient in home

Teach family regarding energy conservation techniques

Teach family regarding home safety and fall precautions

Other interventions, based on patient/family needs

c. *Emotional/Spiritual considerations*

Psychosocial assessment of patient and family regarding disease and prognosis

RN to provide emotional support to patient and family

Assess mental status and sleep disturbance changes

Observation of patient for neuropsychiatric complications of illness, including confusion, depression, and anxiety

Clinician to provide support and intervention for depression

Teach patient/family about depression and signs/symptoms of exacerbation that necessitate more intervention

Assess for and manage plans for psychosocial and/or spiritual pain (e.g., all pain, anxiety, interpersonal and other distress)

Observation and assessment of mental status changes/complaints of depression in new hospice patient with cancer of the prostate

Psychosocial aspects of pain control (e.g., depression) assessed and acknowledged with team support/intervention

Ongoing acknowledgment of spirituality and related concerns of patient/family

Other interventions, based on patient/family needs

d. *Skin care*

RN to teach patient regarding irradiated skin sites

Teach caregiver regarding patient's skin care needs, including the need for frequent position changes, appropriate pressure pads and mattresses, and the prevention of breakdown

Pressure ulcer care as indicated

Assess skin integrity q visit

Observation and evaluation of wound and surrounding skin

Evaluate patient's need for equipment, including supplies to decrease pressure, alternating pressure mattress, gel foam seat cushion, and heel and elbow protectors

Teach family to perform dressing changes between RN visits, specifically _____

4

Teach patient, family, or caregiver about proper body alignment and positioning in bed to prevent skin tears from shearing skin

Observe and apply skilled assessment of areas for possible breakdown, including heels, hips, elbows, ankles, and other pressure-prone areas

Other interventions, based on patient/family needs

e. *Elimination considerations*

Assess bowel regimen, and implement program as needed

RN to assess patient's bowel patterns and need for stool softeners, laxatives, and dietary adjustments, and to develop bowel management plan

Assess amount and frequency of urinary output

Teach catheter care to caregiver

Check for and remove impaction as needed

Condom catheter or indwelling catheter care as ordered

Observation and complete systems assessment of patient with an indwelling catheter

RN to change catheter every 4 weeks and to make 3 PRN visits for catheter problems, including patient complaints, signs and symptoms of infection, and other factors necessitating evaluation and possible catheter change

RN to teach caregiver daily care of catheter

Teaching and ongoing assessment for prevention and early identification of constipation and its correction/resolution

Initiate bowel management program per physician

Implement bowel assessment management program

Teach patient, family, and aide the importance of observing and noting bowel movements between scheduled nursing visits

Obtain patient history related to norms for bowel movements to date (e.g., "All my life I go only every other day")

Bowel management program of stool softeners, laxative of choice, Fleet's enemas prn, and other methods per patient wishes and physician orders

Other interventions, based on patient/family needs

f. *Hydration/Nutrition*

Assess nutrition and hydration statuses

Diet counseling for patient with anorexia

Clinician to teach family about patient's need for small, high-calorie meals of his or her choice

Nutrition/hydration supported by offering patient's choice of favorite or desired foods or liquids

Nutrition/hydration maintained by offering patient high-protein diet and foods of choice as tolerated

Other interventions, based on patient/family needs

g. *Therapeutic/Medication regimens*

Teach new pain or symptom control medication regimen

Teach new medication regimens and side effects

Assess for electrolyte imbalance

Teach and observe regarding side effects of chemotherapy, including constipation, anemia, and fatigue

Medication review, education, and management

Assess the patient's response to therapeutic treatments and interventions, and report any changes or unfavorable responses to the physician

Ongoing observation, assessment, and intervention related to side effects of therapy, including fever, dry skin, mouth pain/sores/ulcers, extreme tiredness, and depression due to symptoms and poor energy level

Teach patient and caregiver use of PCA pump

Nonpharmacological interventions such as progressive muscle relaxation, imagery, positive visualization, music, massage and touch, and humor therapy of patient's choice

Teaching of patient/family, including medications, management program, strength, type, actions, times, and compliance tips

Encourage family/caregivers to give the patient medications on the schedule and around the clock

Medications changed using equianalgesic conversion tables/physician orders (e.g., from oral morphine to an equianalgesic dose of transdermal fentanyl)

Nonpharmacological or other interventions, including relaxation, hot/cold therapy, biofeedback, distraction, guided imagery, humor, music therapy, acupuncture, TENS technology, hypnosis, and massage

Other interventions, based on patient/family needs

h. *Other considerations*

Assess progression of disease process

RN to assess the patient's response to treatments and interventions and to report to the physician changes, unfavorable responses, or reactions

Other interventions, based on patient/family needs

• *Home health aide or certified nursing assistant*

Effective and safe personal care

Safe ADL assistance and support

Respite care and active listening skills

Observation and reporting

Meal preparation

Homemaker services

Comfort care

Other duties

• *Social worker*

Psychosocial assessment of patient and family/caregiver, including adjustment to illness and its implications

Identification of optimal coping strategies

Financial assessment and counseling regarding food acquisition, ability to prepare, and costs of needed medications

Intervention/support related to terminal illness and loss

Emotional/spiritual support

Depression/fear assessed

Facilitate communication among patient, family, and hospice team

Referral/linkage to community services and resources as indicated

Grief counseling and intervention/support related to illness/loss

Patient/caregiver counseling and support

Identification of caregiver role strain necessitating respite/relief measures/support

For patients who live alone with no support system (e.g., able, available, willing caregiver[s]), obtain resources to enable patient to remain in home

Identification of illness-related psychiatric condition necessitating care

Funeral and burial planning assistance

- *Volunteer(s)*

Support, friendship, companionship, and presence

Comfort and dignity maintained/provided for patient and family

Advocacy and respite

Errands and transportation

Other services, based on interdisciplinary team recommendations and patient/caregiver needs

- *Spiritual counselor*

Spiritual assessment and care

Counseling, intervention, and support related to that dimension of life related to life's meaning (consistent with patient's beliefs)

Pray with or for the patient/family, using prayers familiar to patient's religious background (per their wishes)

Support, listening, and presence

Participation in sacred or spiritual rituals or practices

Other supportive care, based on patient/family needs and belief systems

- *Dietitian/Nutritional counseling*

Supportive counseling with patient/family indicating that patient will have a decreased appetite and possible inability to eat/drink

Assessment and recommendations for swallowing difficulties

Teaching and support of family members and caregivers

Evaluation/management of nutritional deficits and needs

Food and dietary recommendations incorporate patient choice and wishes

- *Occupational therapist*

Evaluation of ADLs and functional mobility

Assess for need for adaptive equipment and assistive devices

Safety assessment of patient's environment and ADLs

Assessment for energy conservation training

Teach compensatory techniques

- *Physical therapist*
  Evaluation
  Safety assessment of patient's environment
  Safe transfer training or bed mobility exercises
  Pain assessment/reduction factors
  Strengthening exercises/program
  Assessment of gait safety and home safety measures
  Instruct/supervise caregiver and volunteers on home exercise program
  for conditioning and strength
  Assistive, adaptive devices and evaluation of equipment and teaching

- *Speech-language pathologist*
  Evaluation for speech/swallowing problems
  Food texture recommendations
  Alternative functional communication

- *Bereavement counselor*
  Assessment of the needs of the bereaved family and friends
  Support and intervention, based on assessment and ongoing findings
  Presence and counseling
  Supportive visits, follow-up, and other interventions (e.g., mailings,
  calls)
  Other services related to bereavement work and support

- *Pharmacist*
  Evaluation of hospice patient with constipation on cathartics, stool
  softeners, and other medications for possible food/drug and
  drug/drug interactions
  Medication monitoring regarding therapeutic levels and dosages
  Pain consult and input into interdisciplinary POC related to pain
  control, palliation, and symptom management
  Assessment of medication regimen and plan for safety and compliance

- *Music, massage, art, or other therapies or services*
  Evaluation and intervention based on patient's and caregiver's unique
  wishes and needs that support care, comfort, and death in the setting
  of the patient's choice
  Assessment plan to engage patient and support comfort, quality,
  enjoyment, and dignity
  Pet therapy (including patient's pet, if available) and therapeutic
  intervention

6. **Outcomes for care**

- *Hospice nursing*
  Patient and caregiver verbalize satisfaction with care
  Patient will decide on care and pain intervention and evaluation
  Patient will experience increased comfort and pain control through
  self-report (specify parameters)
  Patient will have palliative care and comfort maintained through death

Patent and infection-free catheter

Patient and caregiver knowledgeable about side effects (e.g., constipation) and interventions needed

Control of pain and other symptoms that affect daily function, quality of life, and ability to interact with friends/family

Teaching related to safety, medications, catheter, and self-care successful as demonstrated by patient's verbalization (specify measurable parameters)

Effective pain control and symptom relief by _____ (specify date)

Patient and caregiver knowledgeable about pain regimen, relief measures, and care for optimal relief/control

Early detection and intervention of problems related to patients with immobility/bedbound status

Patient is protected from injury, has stable respiratory status, and is compliant with medication, safety, and care regimens

Comfort and individualized intervention of patient with immobility/bedbound status (e.g., skin, urinary, musculature, vascular)

Spiritual and psychosocial needs met (specify) as defined by patient and caregiver throughout course of care

Educational tools/plans incorporated in daily care, and patient/caregiver verbalizes understanding of safe, needed care

Patient will decide on care, interventions, and evaluation of care processes

Caregiver is effective in care management, verbalizes changes, and knows whom to call for questions/concerns

Patient will express satisfaction with hospice support received and will experience increased comfort

Patient will be made comfortable at home through death in accordance with the patient's wishes

Effective pain control and symptom control verbalized by patient

Patient verbalizes understanding of and adheres to care and medication regimens

Patient and caregiver supported through patient's death

Comfort maintained through course of care

The patient and family receive hospice support and care, and family members and friends are able to spend quality time with the patient

Caregiver able and verbalizes comfort with role and understands when to call hospice team members

Patient supported through and receives the maximum benefit from palliative chemotherapy and radiation with minimal complications

Patient and caregiver list adverse reactions, potential complications, signs/symptoms of infection (e.g., sputum change, chest congestion)

Comfort maintained through death with dignity

Pain effectively managed, and patient verbalizes comfort

Comfort through death with support and care of hospice team

Mental distress, depression, and fear of dying addressed throughout care by hospice team

Family able to care for and support patient

Patient and caregiver can verbalize symptoms, changes, or accelerations that necessitate call to physician

Patient and family demonstrate compliance with medication regimen and other therapeutic interventions

Patient demonstrates stabilization and increased or enhanced coping skills related to functioning and depression

Pain and symptoms managed/controlled in setting of patient/family choice (e.g., patient/family report ability to eat, sleep, speak with pacing)

Planned and effective bowel program, as evidenced by regular bowel movements and patient/family report of comfort

Death with dignity, and pain/symptoms controlled in setting of patient/family choice

Optimal comfort, support, and dignity provided throughout illness

Death with maximum comfort through effective symptom control with specialized hospice support

Patient and caregiver able to list adverse drug reactions/problems with medication regimen and whom to call for follow-up and resolution

Patient's/family's privacy, independence, and choices supported with respect and maintained through death

Enhancement and support of quality of life

Effective symptom relief and control (e.g., a peaceful and comfortable death at home, depression controlled, some enjoyment of life)

Maximizing the patient's quality of life (e.g., alert and pain free or as patient wishes)

Pharmacological and nonpharmacological interventions, such as localized heat application, biofeedback, massage, positioning, relaxation methods, and music

Patient and caregiver demonstrate appropriate back-up or "rescue" therapies for breakthrough pain or other symptoms (e.g., dyspnea)

Patient cared for and family supported through death with physical, psychosocial, spiritual, and other concerns/needs acknowledged/addressed

Patient- and family-centered hospice care provided based on the patient's/family's unique situation and needs

Infection control and palliation through death in setting of patient's choice

Grief/bereavement expression and support provided

Patient is pain free by next _____ visit

Caregiver demonstrates ability to manage pain, where applicable

Patient maintains comfort and dignity throughout illness

Other outcomes/goals, based on the patient condition with input from the hospice team and patient and family

- ***Home health aide or certified nursing assistant***
  Effective hygiene, personal care, and comfort maintained
  ADL assistance
  Safe environment maintained

- *Social worker*
  Problem identified and addressed, with patient/caregiver linked with
      appropriate support services and plan of care successfully
      implemented
  Patient and caregiver cope adaptively with illness and death
  Adaptive adjustment to changed body and body image
  Psychosocial support and counseling offered to patient/caregivers
      experiencing loss and grief
  Caregiver system assessed, and development of stable caregiver plan
      facilitated
  Funeral and burial planning assistance

- *Volunteer(s)*
  Comfort, companionship, and friendship extended to patient/family
  Support and respite provided as defined by the needs of the
      patient/caregiver
  Patient and family supported by team with care, comfort, and
      companionship

- *Spiritual counselor*
  Spiritual support offered and provided as defined by needs of
      patient/caregiver
  Provision of spiritual support and care as based on the assessed and
      ongoing needs of the patient and family
  Spiritual support offered, and patient and family needs met
  Participation in sacred or spiritual rituals or practices
  Patient and family express relief of symptoms of spiritual suffering
  Support, listening, and presence

- *Dietitian/Nutritional counseling*
  Family and caregiver integrate recommendations into daily meal
      planning (when appropriate)
  Patient and caregiver know whom to call for nutrition- and
      hydration-related questions/concerns
  Nutrition/hydration per patient choices
  Caregiver integrates recommendations into daily meal planning
  Patient and family verbalize comprehension of changing nutritional needs

- *Occupational therapist*
  Patient and caregiver demonstrate maximum independence with ADLs,
      adaptive techniques, and assistive devices
  Patient and caregiver demonstrate maximum safety in ADLs and
      functional mobility
  Patient and caregiver demonstrate effective use of energy conservation
      techniques
  Verbalization/demonstration of improved functional activity level and
      enhanced quality of life
  Patient and caregiver demonstrate effective use of diaphragmatic
      breathing to reduce shortness of breath and relaxation techniques to
      help in pain/symptom management

- *Physical therapist*
  Prevention of complications
  Home exercise and upper-extremity program taught to caregiver
  Optimal strength, mobility, and function maintained/achieved
  Compliance with home exercise program by _____ (date)
  Comfort measures of backrub or hand or other therapeutic massage

- *Speech-language pathologist*
  Communication method implemented, and patient able to be
      understand as self-reported or reported by family/caregivers
  Safe swallowing and functional communication
  Recommended lists of food/textures for safety and patient choice

- *Bereavement counselor*
  Grief support services provided to patient and family
  Well-being and resolution process of grief initiated and followed
      through bereavement services

- *Pharmacist*
  Regimen for bowel regimen successful as self-reported by patient and
      in update at team meeting
  Multiple drug regimen reviewed for food/drug and drug/drug
      interactions in patient on multiple medications
  Stability and safety in complex medication regimen, with maximum
      benefit to patient
  Effective pain and symptom control and management as reported by
      patient/caregiver

- *Music, massage, art, or other therapies or services*
  Therapeutic massage/touch effective for patient as self-reported or
      observed by caregivers/family
  Improved muscle tone, relaxation, and/or sleep
  Patient comfortable and relaxed (e.g., sleeping) after massage
  Music therapy intervention based on assessment to decrease pain
      perception and provide emotional expression and support
  Maintenance of comfort and physical, psychosocial, and spiritual health
  Holistic health maintained and comfort achieved through
      _____ (specify modality)
  Patient has pet's presence as desired—in all care sites, when possible

4

7. **Patient, family, and caregiver educational needs**
   Educational needs are the care regimens that contribute to safe and
   effective care at home between the hospice team's visits. These include
   the following:
       The basic tenets of hospice and the availability of support 24 hours a
           day, 7 days a week
       Home safety assessment and counseling
       The patient's medication regimen
       Safe and proper body mechanics to promote patient comfort and
           prevent caregiver safety problems

Support groups available to patient's family, such as the hospice
program's "Caregiver Support Group" meetings for family
members and friends of the patient

Anticipated disease progression

The availability of adequate pain relief measures

The need for keeping records related to and assessing for constipation

The safe use of oxygen therapy at home

The therapeutic and palliative value of nonpharmacological comfort
measures, such as positioning, massage, progressive muscle
relaxation, and other interventions of patient choice

The patient's medications and their relationship to each other

The importance of around-the-clock analgesia

Teach patient management of hair loss

The importance of medical follow-up

Care of the catheter, changing bags, and signs of catheter problems

The availability of support and hospice programs, if appropriate

Teach about the prevention of infection and the signs and symptoms
of infection

Other teaching specific to the patient's and caregiver's needs

8. Specific tips for quality and reimbursement

Document any variances to executed outcomes. There are many models
of hospice programs.

The Medicare hospice benefit does not require that the patient be
homebound or have identified skilled needs. For further information on
this benefit, please refer to CMS Hospice Manual 21.

Should the patient's status deteriorate and increased personal care
be needed, obtain a telephone order for the increased service, noting
frequency and estimating the duration.

Obtain a telephone order for all medication and treatment changes of
the medical regimen, and document these in the clinical record.

Document changes to the plan of care such as medications, services,
frequency, communication, and concurrence of other team members

Document coordination of services or consultation of the other
members of the IDT

Unless the patient is in a hospice insurance program, some insurers
will not pay for a skilled clinician visit that is made at death if the patient
is dead when the clinician arrives at the home. From a Medicare home care
perspective, the visit at the time of death may be covered when the orders
and clinical record document assessment of the patient's status or signs of
death/life or state law allows pronouncement of death by an RN.

Document patient deterioration

Document dehydration, dehydrating

Document patient change or instability

Document pain, other symptoms not controlled

Document status after acute episode of _____ (specify)

Document positive urine, sputum, etc. culture; patient started
on _____ (specify ordered antibiotic therapy)

Document patient impacted; impaction removed manually per physician's orders

Document RN in frequent communication with physician regarding _____ (specify)

Document febrile at _____, pulse change at _____, irr., irr.

Document change noted in _____

Document bony prominences red, opening

Document RN contacted physician regarding _____ (specify)

Document marked SOB

Document alteration in mental status

Document medications being adjusted, regulated, or monitored and the patient response

Document unable to perform own ADLs, personal care

Document all interdisciplinary team meetings and communications in the POC and in the progress notes of the clinical record

All hospice team members should have input into the POC and document their interventions and goals

Document all patient changes in the clinical record

Document an exacerbation of symptoms

Document unstable, not stable

Document urine culture obtained and the results

Document RN in communication with physician regarding _____ (specify)

Document any POC change in the documentation and obtain orders for all changes

Document the coordination of care and communications among/between disciplines

Document communications and care coordination with other care providers, such as skilled nursing facility or health care home staff, inpatient team members, and hired caregivers

Document the clear progression of symptoms and interventions that demonstrate the overall management of the patient with pain in the clinical notes

Document when/if the patient has respiratory changes, shortness of breath, exacerbation of conditions, dysphagia, changes in pain, and other symptoms and that they are identified and resolved

Remember that the clinical documentation is key to measuring compliance for quality and reimbursement purposes. Care coordination, timely verbal and initial physician orders, and assessment and addressing of spiritual and psychosocial needs should be ongoing and documented in the patient's clinical record

Document that all hospice care supports comfort and dignity while meeting patient/family needs

The documentation should include ongoing assessment and management of pain and other symptoms and the anticipation and prevention of secondary symptoms such as constipation

It is important to note that all team members, including clinicians and social workers, should assess, identify, and "hear" spiritual needs that the patient/family want to be addressed. These spiritual issues are key to the provision of quality hospice care and cannot be addressed effectively and promptly by the spiritual counselor only

Document clearly symptoms, clinical changes, and assessment findings related to pain and patient care

Document weight loss, increased shortness of breath, dyspnea, infection, sepsis, new or changed medications, etc.

Document any skin changes (e.g., inflamed, painful, weeping skin site[s])

Remember that the "litmus test" of care coordination rests on the quality of the clinical documentation by all team members. Review one of your patient's clinical records and ask yourself the following: "If I was unable to give a verbal report/update on this patient's/ family's course of care, would a peer be able to pick up and provide the same level of care and know (from the documentation) the current orders, medications, and other details that contribute to effective hospice care?"

This patient population usually has many clinical changes that should be documented. These include weight loss and multiple and changed medication regimens with varying routes. Side effects to the drug regimen should be observed, noted, documented, and reported

Your assessments, observations, and clinical findings assist in painting a picture to support coverage and documentation requirements for hospice care

Document any hospitalizations and changed clinical findings

Document patient changes, symptoms, and psychosocial issues affecting the patient and the family and POC

Document patient changes, symptoms, and clinical information identified from visits and team conferences that constitute evidence of the need for hospice care and a limited life expectancy

Clearly support in the documentation the rationale that supports/explains the progression of the illness from the chronic to terminal stages

Document mentation, behavioral, and/or cognitive changes

Document dysphagia, weight loss, increased shortness of breath, dyspnea, infection, sepsis, new or changed medications, etc.

Document when the patient is actively dying, deteriorating, or progressing toward death

9. **Queries for quality**

   - *Is patient's pain managed adequately?*
   - *Is patient's anxiety managed adequately?*
   - *What are the patient's symptoms?*
   - *Does patient/family have access to appropriate community resources, and are they documented in the record?*
   - *Have you documented to the interdisciplinary POC?*

10. **Resources for hospice care and practice**

    The National Institutes of Health's National Cancer Institute offers *What You Need to Know About Prostate Cancer, Caring for the Patient with Cancer at Home,* and other information. Call the Cancer Information Service at 1-800-4-CANCER or visit online at www.nci.nih.gov. The American Foundation for Urologic Disease can be reached at (410)468-1800 or 1-800-828-7866. The foundation maintains a network of prostate cancer survivor organizations and services and initiates prostate cancer advocacy programs visit online at www.afud.org

The American Cancer Society has support groups such as "I Can Cope" and other programs. To locate the chapter nearest your patient, call 1-800-ACS-2345.

Facts on Prostate Cancer can be obtained from the American Cancer Society by calling 1-800-ACS-2345 or visit online at www.cancer.org

4

RENAL DISEASE CARE (END STAGE)

1. General conditions

Patients with renal disease, or ESRD, may have a long history of multiple surgeries and treatment interventions related to access sites such as shunts and sometimes transplants and infections, with the devastating cycle of rejection. Other care problems may include DM, CVA, hypertension, and skin care problems. Some patients choose to discontinue dialysis because of illness, whereas others may be referred to hospice because of more acute kidney or other health problems. Please refer to "Bedbound Care," " Cardiac Care (End Stage)," or "Pain Care" should these sections also pertain to your patient.

2. Needs for visit

Physician order for hospice care, specific to the hospice program's
    admission criteria policies
Standard precautions supplies
Vital signs equipment for baseline assessment
Other supplies or equipment, based on physician orders

3. Safety considerations

Infection control/standard precautions
Night-light
Protective skin measures
Identification and report of any skin problems
Tub rail, grab bars for bathroom safety
Supportive and nonskid shoes
Cardiac/diabetes/bleeding precautions based on medication regimen(s)
Fall precautions/protocol
The phone number and name of person to call with a care problem
Safety for home medical equipment (e.g., wheelchair, walker)
Smoke detector and fire evacuation plan
Others, based on the patient's unique condition and environment

4. Potential diagnoses and codes

Acute myocardial infarction	410.90
Acute pyelonephritis	590.10
Acute renal failure	584.9
Anemia	285.9
Angina pectoris	413.9
Ascites	789.5
Benign prostatic hypertrophy	600.0
Bronchitis, acute	466.0
CAPD (continuous ambulatory peritoneal dialysis) (surgical)	54.98
Chronic ischemic heart disease	414.9

Chronic renal failure	585.0
Cirrhosis of the liver	571.5
Congestive heart failure	428.0
Constipation	564.00
Convulsions	780.39
COPD	496
Coronary artery disease (CAD)	414.00
CVA	436
Debility	799.3
Decubitus ulcer (pressure ulcer)	707.0
Dehydration	276.5
Diabetes mellitus, with complications, adult	250.90
Diabetes mellitus, with complications, juv.	250.91
Diabetic nephropathy	250.41 and 583.81
Emphysema	492.8
Failure to thrive, adult	783.7
Gastritis	535.50
Glomerulonephritis	583.9
Heart disease, chronic ischemic	414.9
Heart failure	428.9
Heart failure, left	428.1
Hemiplegia	342.90
Hepatitis	573.3
Hepatitis B	070.30
Hepatitis (viral)	070.9
Hypercalcemia	275.42
Hyperosmolality	276.0
Hypertension	401.9
Hypoglycemia	251.2
Hypopotassemia	276.8
Kidney, cancer of the (renal)	189.0
Kidney transplant (S/P)	V42.0
Kidney transplant (surgical)	55.69
Liver disease	573.9
Lung disease	518.89
Malaise and fatigue	780.79
Malnutrition	263.9
Myocardial infarction	410.90
Nephrosclerosis	403.90
Nephrotic syndrome	581.9
Neuropathy	355.9
Obesity	278.00
Peptic ulcer	533.90
Pericardial effusion	423.9
Pericarditis	423.9
Peripheral neuropathy	356.9
Peripheral vascular disease	443.9
Peritonitis	567.9

4

Pneumonia	486
Postoperative infection	998.59
Postoperative wound disruption	998.32
Pressure ulcer	707.0
Protein-caloric malnutrition	263.9
Psychosis	298.9
Pyelonephritis	590.80
Renal cell cancer, metastatic	198.0
Renal failure, chronic	585
Renal polycystic disease	753.12
Renal transplant (surgical)	55.69
Retention of urine	788.20
Septicemia	038.9
Shunt, arteriovenous (renal dialysis status)	V45.1
Shunt, infected	996.62
Shunt, peritoneovascular (surgical)	54.94
Shunt revision (surgical)	39.42
Skin eruptions, nonspecific	782.1
Stomach ulcer	531.90
Systemic lupus erythematosus	710.0
Tubular necrosis (acute)	584.5
Urinary retention	788.20
Wound debridement, nonexcisional (surgical)	86.28
Wound dehiscence	998.32

5. Skills and services identified

- ### *Hospice nursing*

a. *Comfort and symptom control*

Comprehensive assessment of cardiovascular and all other systems in patient with impaired renal function admitted to hospice for _____ (specify)

Observation and assessment of the patient with RF problem necessitating care

Presentation of hospice philosophy and services

Explain patient rights and responsibilities

Assess patient, family, and caregiver wishes and expectations regarding care

Assess patient, family, and caregiver resources available for care

Assess pain and other symptoms, including site, duration, characteristics, and relief measures

Provision of volunteer support to patient and family

Teach family or caregiver physical care of patient

RN to provide and teach effective oral care and comfort measures

Teach signs and symptoms of bleeding and precautions

RN to teach patient and caregiver self-observational and care skills (e.g., TPR, I and O, BP, weight, and record keeping)

Report changes, including signs and symptoms, to physician

Monitor for signs and symptoms of infection

Teach about effective oral hygiene measures

Monitor blood pressure and other vital signs

Oxygen on at _____ liters per _____ (specify physician orders)

Assess progression of disease process

Identify and monitor pain, symptoms, and relief measures

Teach caregiver or family care of weak, terminally ill patient

RN to instruct in pain-control measures and medications

Teach patient/family use of standardized form/tool to use between hospice team members' visits (and for care coordination between team members)

Teach patient/family principles of effective pain management

Observation and assessment, communication with physician related to signs and symptoms of continuing decompensation and increased symptoms, pain, discomfort, and shortness of breath, and measures to alleviate and control

Effective management of pain and prevention of secondary symptoms

Interventions of symptoms directed toward comfort and palliation

Pain assessment and management q visit, including source of pain (e.g., cancer pain, infection, pathological fracture, other medical problems, such as cardiac or arthritis pain)

RN to assess patient's pain or other symptoms q visit to identify need for change, addition, or other plan or dose adjustment

Teach caregiver/patient use of pain assessment tool/scale and reporting mechanism(s)

Observation, assessment, and comfort measures of neuropathy, encephalopathy, and edema

Teach patient and family about realistic expectations of disease process

Teach care of dying and signs/symptoms of impending death

Presence and support

Other interventions, based on patient/family needs

b. *Safety and mobility considerations*

Provide caregiver with home safety information and instruction related to _____ and documented in the clinical record

Teach family about safety of patient in home

Teach family about energy conservation techniques

Other interventions, based on patient/family needs

c. *Emotional/Spiritual considerations*

Psychosocial assessment of patient and family regarding disease and prognosis

RN to provide emotional support to patient and family

Assess mental status and sleep disturbance changes

Observation and assessment of mental status changes/complaints of depression

Observation of patient for neuropsychiatric complications of illness, including confusion, depression, and anxiety

Clinician to provide support and intervention for depression

Teach patient/family about depression and signs/symptoms of exacerbation that necessitate more intervention

Psychosocial aspects of pain control (e.g., depression) assessed and acknowledged with team support/intervention

Assess for and manage plans for psychosocial and/or spiritual pain (e.g., all pain, anxiety, interpersonal and other distress)

Ongoing acknowledgment of spirituality and related concerns of patient/family

Other interventions, based on patient/family needs

d. *Skin care*

Teach caregiver wound care regimen

Assesment of dressing and teaching to patient and caregiver about access site

Teach application of topical lotion to pruritic areas

Assessment of infection shunt, graft, or fistula sites

Teach caregiver patient's skin care needs, including the need for frequent position changes, appropriate pressure pads and mattresses, and the prevention of breakdown

Pressure ulcer care as indicated

Assess skin integrity

Observation and evaluation of wound and surrounding skin

Evaluate patient's need for equipment, including supplies to decrease pressure, alternating pressure mattress, gel foam seat cushion, and heel and elbow protectors

Teach family to perform dressing changes between RN visits, specifically _____

Teach patient, family, or caregiver about proper body alignment and positioning in bed to prevent skin tears from shearing skin

Observe and apply skilled assessment of areas for possible breakdown, including heels, hips, elbows, ankles, and other pressure-prone areas

Other interventions, based on patient/family needs

e. *Elimination considerations*

Assess bowel regimen, and implement program as needed

Monitor bowel patterns and need for stool softeners, laxatives, and dietary adjustments, and develop bowel management plan

Catheterize patient for residual urine

Assess amount and frequency of urinary output

Teach catheter care to caregiver

RN to teach caregiver daily care of catheter

Teaching and ongoing assessment for the prevention and early identification of constipation and its correction/resolution

Implement bowel assessment and management program

Teach patient, family, and aide the importance of observing and noting bowel movements between scheduled nursing visits

Obtain patient history related to norms for bowel movements to date (e.g., "All my life I go only every other day")

Consider stool softeners, and offer laxative of choice, Fleet's enemas prn, and other methods per patient wishes and physician orders

Other Interventions, based on patient/family needs

f. *Hydration/Nutrition*

Monitoring/reporting of fluid changes in patient (e.g., weight increase, edema, shortness of breath)

Clinician to teach patient and caregiver nutrition and hydration regimen

Instruct about diet (e.g., low protein with fluid or other specified dietary orders and restrictions as specified by physician)

Nutrition/hydration supported by offering patient's choice of favorite or desired foods or liquids

Other interventions, based on patient/family needs

g. *Therapeutic/Medication regimens*

Administer epoetin (EPO) subcutaneously _____ (specify dose and frequency)

Venipuncture to monitor patient's hematocrit related to anemia and EPO therapy

RN to assess for complications of new medication therapy

Obtain venipuncture as ordered q _____ (specify frequency)

Teach new medications and effects

Assess for electrolyte imbalance

Teach patient and caregiver use of PCA pump

Nonpharmacological interventions such as progressive muscle relaxation, imagery, positive visualization, music, massage and touch, and humor therapy of patient's choice

RN to assess the patient's response to therapeutic treatments and interventions, and to report any changes or unfavorable responses to the physician

Teaching of patient/family, including medications, the management program, strength, type, actions, times, and compliance tips

Encourage family/caregivers to give the patient medications on the schedule and around-the-clock

Medications changed using equianalgesic conversion tables/physician orders (e.g., from oral morphine to an equianalgesic dose of transdermal fentanyl)

Other interventions, based on patient/family needs

h. *Other considerations*

Assess progression of disease process

RN to assess the patient's response to treatments and to report to the physician changes, unfavorable responses, or reactions

Other interventions, based on patient/family needs

4

- *Home health aide or certified nursing assistant*
  Effective and safe personal care
  Safe ADL assistance and support
  Respite care and active listening skills
  Observation and reporting
  Meal preparation
  Homemaker services
  Comfort care
  Other duties

- *Social worker*
  Psychosocial assessment of patient and family/caregiver, including
     adjustment to long-term illness and its implications
  Identification of optimal coping strategies
  Financial assessment and counseling regarding food acquisition, ability
     to prepare, and costs of needed medications
  Intervention/support related to terminal illness and loss
  Emotional/spiritual support
  Depression/fear assessed
  Facilitate communication among patient, family, and hospice team
  Referral/linkage to community services and resources as indicated
  Grief counseling and intervention/support related to illness/loss
  Patient/caregiver counseling and support
  For patients who live alone with no support system (e.g., able,
     available, willing caregiver[s]), obtain resources to enable patient
     to remain in the home
  Identification of illness-related psychiatric condition necessitating care
  Funeral and burial planning assistance

- *Volunteer(s)*
  Support, friendship, companionship, and presence
  Advocacy and respite comfort and dignity maintained/provided for
     patient and family
  Errands and transportation
  Other services, based on IDT recommendations and patient/caregiver needs

- *Spiritual counselor*
  Spiritual assessment and care
  Counseling, intervention, and support related to that dimension of life
     related to life's meaning (consistent with patient's beliefs)
  Pray with or for the patient/family, using prayers familiar to patient's
     religious background (per their wishes)
  Support, listening, and presence
  Participation in sacred or spiritual rituals or practices
  Other supportive care based on patient/family needs and belief systems

- *Dietitian/Nutritional counseling*
  Assessment of patient with decreased intake, weight loss, anorexia, and
     increased shortness of breath (e.g., "I don't feel like eating")
  Supportive counseling with patient/family indicating that patient will
     have a decreased appetite and possible inability to eat/drink

Assessment and recommendations for swallowing difficulties
Assessment related to specialized medical nutritional supplements
Teaching and support of family members and caregivers
Support and care with food and nourishment as desired by patient
Evaluation/management of nutritional deficits and needs
Encourage nutritional supplements and snacks to increase protein and caloric intake
Food and dietary recommendations incorporate patient choice and wishes

- *Occupational therapist*
  Evaluation of ADLs and functional mobility
  Assess need for adaptive equipment and assistive devices
  Safety assessment of patient's environment and ADLs
  Assessment for energy conservation training
  Assessment of upper-extremity function, retraining motor skills

- *Physical therapist*
  Evaluation
  Safety assessment of patient's environment
  Safe transfer training or bed mobility exercises
  Pain assessment/reduction factors
  Strengthening exercises/program
  Assessment of gait safety and home safety measures
  Instruct/supervise caregiver and volunteers on home exercise program for conditioning and strength
  Assistive, adaptive devices and evaluation of equipment and teaching

- *Speech-language pathologist*
  Evaluation for speech/swallowing problems
  Food texture recommendations
  Alternate functional communication

- *Bereavement counselor*
  Assessment of the needs of the bereaved family and friends
  Support and intervention, based on assessment and ongoing findings
  Presence and counseling
  Supportive visits, follow-up, and other interventions (e.g., mailings, calls)
  Other services related to bereavement work and support

- *Pharmacist*
  Evaluation of hospice patient with constipation on cathartics, stool softeners, and other medications for possible food/drug and drug/drug interactions
  Medication monitoring regarding therapeutic levels and dosages
  Pain consult and input into interdisciplinary POC related to pain control, palliation, and symptom management
  Assessment of medication regimen and plan for safety and compliance

4

- *Music, massage, art, or other therapies or services*

  Evaluation and intervention based on patient's and caregiver's unique wishes and needs that support care, comfort, and death in the setting of the patient's choice

  Assessment plan to patient and support comfort, quality, enjoyment, and dignity

  Pet therapy (including patient's pet, if available) and therapeutic intervention

6. Outcomes for care

- *Hospice nursing*

  Symptoms controlled in setting of patient/family choice

  Effective pain relief and control (e.g., a peaceful and comfortable death)

  Mental distress, depression, and fear of dying addressed throughout care by hospice team

  Patient and family able to care for and support patient

  Patient and caregiver can verbalize symptoms, changes, or accelerations that necessitate call to physician

  Patient and family demonstrate compliance with medication regimen and other therapeutic interventions

  Patient demonstrates stabilization and increased or enhanced coping skills related to functioning and depression

  Pain and symptoms managed/controlled in setting of patient/family choice (e.g., patient/family report ability to eat, sleep, speak with pacing)

  Planned and effective bowel program, as evidenced by regular bowel movements and patient/family report of comfort

  Death with dignity, and pain/symptoms controlled in setting of patient/family choice

  Optimal comfort, support, and dignity provided throughout illness

  Death with maximum comfort through effective symptom control with specialized hospice support

  Patient and caregiver able to list adverse drug reactions/problems with medication regimen and whom to call for follow-up and resolution

  Patient's/family's privacy, independence, and choices supported with respect and maintained through death

  Enhancement and support of quality of life

  Effective symptom relief and control (e.g., a peaceful and comfortable death at home, depression controlled, some enjoyment of life)

  Maximizing the patient's quality of life (e.g., alert and pain free or as patient wishes)

  Pharmacological and nonpharmacological interventions, such as localized heat application, biofeedback, massage, positioning, relaxation methods, and music

  Patient cared for and family supported through death with physical, psychosocial, spiritual, and other concerns/needs acknowledged/addressed

Patient- and family-centered hospice care provided based on the patient's/family's unique situation and needs

Patient/caregiver verbalizes satisfaction with care

Patient will decide on care, interventions, and evaluation

Patient will experience increased comfort and pain control through self-report (specify parameters)

Patient will have palliative care and comfort maintained through death

Patent and infection-free catheter and other care sites

Skin integrity maintained or improved

Patient and caregiver knowledgeable about side effects (e.g., constipation) and interventions needed

Control of pain and other symptoms that affect daily function, quality of life, and ability to interact with friends/family

Patient and caregiver knowledgeable about and compliant with renal care regimen, relief measures, and care for optimal control

Early detection and intervention regarding problems of patients with immobility/bedbound status (e.g., skin, urinary, musculature, vascular)

Educational tools/plans incorporated in daily care, and patient/caregiver verbalizes understanding of safe, needed care

Patient will decide on care, interventions, and evaluation

Caregiver effective in care management and knows whom to call for questions/concerns

Patient will express satisfaction with hospice support received and will experience increased comfort

Patient will be made comfortable at home through death in accordance with the patient's wishes

Effective pain control and symptom control verbalized by patient

Patient verbalizes understanding of and adheres to care and medication regimens

Patient and caregiver supported through patient's death

Comfort maintained through course of care

The patient and family receive hospice support and care, and family members and friends are able to spend quality time with the patient

Caregiver able and verbalizes comfort with role and understands when to call hospice team members

Patient supported through and receives the maximum benefit from palliative chemotherapy and radiation with minimal complications

Patient/caregiver lists adverse reactions, potential complications, signs/symptoms of infection (e.g., sputum change, chest congestion)

Comfort maintained through death with dignity

Pain effectively managed, and patient verbalizes comfort

Patient states pain is _____ on 0–10 scale by next visit

Patient/caregiver demonstrates appropriate back-up or "rescue" therapies for breakthrough pain or other symptoms (e.g., dyspnea)

Infection control and palliation

Grief/bereavement expression and support provided

4

Patient is pain free by next _____ visit
Caregiver demonstrates ability to manage pain, where applicable
Patient maintains comfort and dignity throughout illness

- ***Home health aide or certified nursing assistant***
  Effective hygiene, personal care, and comfort
  ADL assistance
  Safe environment maintained

- ***Social worker***
  Problem identified and addressed, with patient/caregiver linked with
    appropriate support services and plan of care successfully implemented
  Patient and caregiver cope adaptively with illness and death
  Adaptive adjustment to changed body and body image
  Psychosocial support and counseling offered to patient/caregivers
    experiencing loss and grief
  Resources identified, community linkage as appropriate for patient/family
  Caregiver system assessed, and development of stable caregiver plan
    facilitated
  Funeral and burial planning assistance

- ***Volunteer(s)***
  Comfort, respite, companionship, and friendship extended to
    patient/family
  Support provided as defined by the needs of the patient/caregiver
  Patient and family supported by team with care, comfort, and
    companionship

- ***Spiritual counselor***
  Spiritual support offered and provided as defined by needs of
    patient/caregiver
  Provision of spiritual support and care based on the assessed and
    ongoing needs of the patient and family
  Spiritual support offered, and patient and family needs met
  Patient and family express relief of symptoms of spiritual suffering
  Support, listening, and presence
  Participation in sacred or spiritual rituals or practices
  Pray with or for the patient/family, using prayers familiar to the
    patient's religious background (per their wishes)

- ***Dietitian/Nutritional counseling***
  Family and caregiver integrate recommendations into nutrition teaching
    (where appropriate)
  Patient and caregiver know whom to call for nutrition- and
    hydration-related questions/concerns
  Nutrition/hydration per patient choices
  Caregiver integrates recommendations into daily meal planning
  Patient and family verbalize comprehension of changing nutritional needs

- ***Occupational therapist***
  Patient and caregiver demonstrate maximum independence with ADLs,
    adaptive techniques, and assistive devices

Patient and caregiver demonstrate maximum safety in ADLs and functional mobility

Patient and caregiver demonstrate effective use of energy conservation techniques

Verbalization/demonstration of improved functional activity level and enhanced quality of life

Patient and caregiver demonstrate effective use of diaphragmatic breathing to reduce shortness of breath and relaxation techniques to help in pain/symptom management

Patient and caregiver demonstrate correct use of exercise

- *Physical therapist*
  Prevention of complications
  Home exercise and upper-extremity program taught to caregiver
  Optimal strength, mobility, and function maintained/achieved
  Compliance with home exercise program

- *Speech-language pathologist*
  Communication method implemented, and patient able to be understood as self-reported or reported by family/caregivers
  Safe swallowing and functional communication
  Recommended list of food textures for safety and patient choice

- *Bereavement counselor*
  Support services related to grief provided to patient and family
  Well-being and resolution process of grief initiated and followed through bereavement services

- *Pharmacist*
  Bowel regimen successful as self reported by patient/family and in update at team meeting
  Multiple drug regimen reviewed for food/drug and drug/drug interactions in patient on multiple medications
  Stability and safety in complex medication regimen, with maximum benefit to patient
  Effective pain and symptom control and management as reported by patient/caregiver

- *Music, massage, art, or other therapies or services*
  Therapeutic massage/touch effective for patient as self-reported or observed by caregivers/family
  Improved muscle tone, relaxation, and/or sleep
  Patient comfortable and relaxed (e.g., sleeping) after massage
  Music therapy intervention based on assessment to decrease pain perception and provide emotional expression and support
  Maintenance of comfort and physical, psychosocial, and spiritual health
  Holistic health maintained and comfort achieved through
  _____ (specify modality)
  Patient has pet's presence as desired—in all care sites, when possible

4

7. Patient, family, and caregiver educational needs

Educational needs are the care regimens that contribute to safe and effective care at home between the hospice team's visits. These include the following:

> The basic tenets of hospice and the availability of support 24 hours a day, 7 days a week
>
> Home safety assessment and counseling
>
> The patient's medication regimen
>
> Anticipated disease progression
>
> Safe and proper body mechanics to promote patient comfort and prevent caregiver safety problems
>
> Support groups available to patient's family, such as the hospice program's "Caregiver Support Group" meetings for family members and friends of the patient
>
> Other teaching specific to the patient's and family's unique needs

8. Specific tips for quality and reimbursement

Document any variances to expected outcomes. There are many models of hospice programs.

The Medicare hospice benefit does not require that the patient be homebound or have identified skilled needs. For further information on this benefit, please refer to CMS Hospice Manual 21.

Should the patient's status deteriorate and increased personal care be needed, obtain a telephone order for the increased service, noting frequency and estimating the duration.

Obtain a telephone order for all medication and treatment changes of the medical regimen, and document these in the clinical record.

Document the coordination occurring among team members based on the POC. Have the multidisciplinary conference notes reflected in the clinical record.

> Document coordination of services or consultation with the other members of the IDT
>
> Document communications and care coordination with other care providers, such as skilled health care facility or nursing home staff, inpatient team members, and hired caregivers
>
> Document in the clinical notes the clear progression of symptoms and interventions that demonstrate the overall management of ESRD and attendant needs for hospice support
>
> Document when/if the patient has respiratory changes, shortness of breath, exacerbation of conditions, pain, increased somnolence, and other symptoms and that they are identified and resolved
>
> Remember that the clinical documentation is key to measuring compliance for quality reimbursement purposes. Care coordination, timely verbal and initial physician orders, and assessment and addressing of spiritual and psychosocial needs should be ongoing and documented in the patient's clinical record
>
> Document that all hospice care supports comfort and dignity while meeting patient/family needs

4

The documentation should include ongoing assessment and
management of pain and other symptoms and the anticipation and
prevention of secondary symptoms such as constipation

It is important to note that all team members, including clinicians
and social workers, should assess, identify, and "hear" spiritual
needs that the patient/family want to be addressed. These
spiritual issues are key to the provision of quality hospice care
and cannot be addressed effectively and promptly by the spiritual
counselor only

Document clearly symptoms, clinical changes, and assessment findings
related to pain and patient care

Document patient changes, symptoms, and clinical information
identified from visits and team conferences that constitute evidence
of the need for hospice care and a limited life expectancy

Clearly document the rationale that supports/explains the progression of
the illness from the chronic to terminal stages

Document mentation, behavioral, and/or cognitive changes

Document changes in edema, increased shortness of breath, dyspnea,
infection, sepsis, new or changed medications, etc.

Document any skin changes (e.g., inflamed, painful, weeping skin
site[s])

Document when the patient is actively dying, deteriorating, and
progressing toward death

Remember that the "litmus test" of care coordination rests on the
quality of the clinical documentation by all team members.
Review one of your patient's clinical records and ask yourself the
following: "If I was unable to give a verbal report/update on this
patient, would a peer be able to pick up and provide the same
level of care and know (from the documentation) the current
orders, medications, and other details that contribute to effective
hospice care?"

Your assessments, observations, and clinical findings support coverage
and documentation requirements for hospice care

Document any hospitalizations and changed clinical findings

Document patient changes, symptoms, psychosocial issues impacting
the care, and information gathered at the patient/family visits

Document changes to the POC such as medications, services,
frequency, communication, and concurrence of other team members

The documentation should reflect ongoing effects of the terminal
condition, the patient's/family's difficulty with care or coping, and
the continued desire for hospice care

Unless the patient is in a hospice insurance program, some insurers
will not pay for a skilled clinician visit that is made at death if the patient
is dead when the clinician arrives at the home. From a Medicare home
care perspective, the visit at the time of death may be covered when the
orders and clinical record document assessment of the patient's status or
signs of death/life or state law allows pronouncement of death by
an RN.

Document patient deterioration

Document dehydration, dehydrating

Document patient change or instability

Document pain, other symptoms not controlled

Document status after acute episode of _____ (specify)

Document positive urine, sputum, etc. culture; patient started on _____ (specify ordered antibiotic therapy)

Document any impaction; impaction removed manually

Document RN in frequent communication with physician regarding _____ (specify)

Document febrile at _____, pulse change at _____, irr., irr.

Document change noted in _____

Document bony prominences red, opening

Document RN contacted physician regarding _____ (specify)

Document marked SOB

Document alteration in mental status

Document medications being adjusted, regulated, or monitored and the patient response

Document unable to perform own ADLs, personal care

Document all IDT meetings and communications in the POC and in the progress notes of the clinical record

All hospice team members should have input into the POC and document their interventions and goals

9. Queries for quality

Renal disease care (end stage)
- *Is patient's pain managed adequately?*
- *Is patient's anxiety managed adequately?*
- *What are the patient's symptoms?*
- *Is patient's functional ability/status clearly documented?*
- *Have you documented to the interdisciplinary POC?*

Dialysis therapy
- *Is patient's pain managed adequately?*
- *Is patient's anxiety managed adequately?*
- *What are the patient's symptoms?*
- *What is the status of the patient's shunt/vascular access device?*
- *Is patient's functional ability/status clearly documented?*

10. Resources for hospice care and practice

For more information, contact the National Kidney Foundation at 1-800-622-9010 to order a General Public Materials Catalog, with information on kidney disease, related conditions, and organ donation (www.kidney.org).

Various booklets are available, and *When Stopping Dialysis Treatment Is Your Choice* and *If You Choose Not To Start Dialysis Treatment* are patient education materials. There is also a text entitled *Initiation or Withdrawal of Dialysis in End Stage Renal Disease: Guidelines for the*

Health Care Team that is a comprehensive review of policy considerations related to values, ethics, decision-making, and the dying process. These resources can be obtained by calling 1-800-622-9010.

Another helpful resource is the NHPCO's latest edition of *Medical Guidelines for Determining Prognoses in Selected Non-Cancer Diseases.* Call the NHPCO at (703)243-5900 for more information.

4

SUPPORTIVE CARE: CATHETER, FEEDING TUBE, AND OSTOMY CARE

1. General considerations

Patients with these major alterations in "normal body functions" for eating and elimination, together with their families, will have significant feelings of loss and control. Body image adjustments and grief need to be acknowledged and incorporated into skillful hospice care. Care for a **colostomy, gastrostomy,** and **nasogastric tube feeding** is addressed in this section.

2. Needs for visit

Physician order for hospice care, specific to the hospice program's admission criteria and policies

Standard precautions supplies

Vital signs equipment for baseline assessment

For catheter care: catheter and insertion supplies

For feeding tube or enteral feeding care: related skin care supplies and nutritional supplements

For ostomy care: ostomy bag, belts, and skin care supplies

Other equipment, based on physician orders

3. Safety considerations

Infection control/standard precautions

Night-light

Extra caution on slippery surfaces

Removal of scatter rugs

Tub rail, grab bars for bathroom safety

Supportive and nonskid shoes

Handrail on stairs

Fall precautions/protocol

Protective skin measures

Identification and report of any skin problems

Smoke detector and fire evacuation plan

Assistance with ambulation

Disposal of used catheters and related supplies

Supervised medication administration

Safety for home medical equipment (e.g., use, safe storage)

Safe care of stoma/skin site

The phone number and name of the person to call with a care problem

Others, based on the patient's unique condition and environment

4. Potential diagnoses and codes

Catheter care

Attention to other artificial opening of urinary tract	V55.4
Bladder atony	596.4
Bladder repair (surgical)	57.89
Constipation	564.00
CVA	436
Cystoscopy (surgical)	57.32
Decubitus ulcer	707.0
Fitting and adjustment of urinary devices	V53.6
Hematuria	599.7
Hypertension	401.9
Impaction, bowel	560.30
Incontinence of urine	788.30
Foley catheter insertion	57.94
Neurogenic bladder	596.54
Pressure wound	707.0
Prostate, cancer of the	185
Suprapubic cystostomy (surgical)	57.18
Urinary incontinence	788.30
Urinary tract infection	599.0
Urinary retention	788.20
Vaginitis	616.10

Feeding tube care

Attention to gastrostomy	V55.1
CVA	436
Decubitus ulcer (pressure ulcer)	707.0
Dysphagia	787.2
Foley catheter insertion (surgical)	57.94
Gastrostomy (other) (surgical)	43.19
Gastrostomy, percutaneous (surgical)	43.11
Hemiparesis	342.90
Nasogastric tube feeding	96.6
Nasogastric tube insertion	96.07
Paralysis agitans (Parkinson's)	332.0
Pneumonia	486
Pneumonia, aspiration	507.0
Pressure ulcer	707.0
Urinary incontinence	788.30

4

Ostomy care

Attention to colostomy	V55.3
Attention to cystostomy	V55.5
Attention to ileostomy	V55.2
Attention to other artificial opening of digestive tract	V55.4
Attention to other artificial opening of urinary tract	V55.6

Bladder cancer	188.9
Bowel obstruction	560.9
Bowel perforation	569.83
Bowel resection (surgical)	45.79
Cancer of the colon	153.9
Cancer of the rectosigmoid	154.0
Cancer of the rectum	154.1
Colectomy, sigmoid (surgical)	45.76
Colitis	558.9
Colitis, ulcerative	556.9
Colostomy (surgical)	46.10
Colostomy, attention to	V55.3
Cystostomy, attention to	V55.5
Diverticulitis	562.11
Enteritis, radiation	558.1
Hemicolectomy with colostomy (surgical)	45.75 and 46.10
Ileostomy or other intestinal appliance, fitting and adjustment	V53.5
Ileostomy, attention to	V55.2
Metastases, general	199.1
Proctectomy (surgical)	48.69
Radiation enteritis	558.1
Rectum, cancer of the	154.1
Skin eruptions	782.1
Skin, excoriation of	919.8
Ulcerative colitis	556.9
Urinary devices, fitting and adjustment	V53.6
Wound evisceration, postoperative	998.32

5. Skills and services identified

- *Hospice health care*
  Catheter care

a. *Comfort and symptom control*
   Comprehensive assessment of patient admitted to hospice
       with _____ catheter, due to _____
   Observation and complete systems assessment of the patient with an
       indwelling catheter
   Document catheter (type, size, balloon size) inserted
       on _____ (specify date)
   Presentation of hospice philosophy and services
   Explain patient rights and responsibilities
   Assess patient, family, and caregiver wishes and expectations
       regarding care
   Assess patient, family, and caregiver resources available
       for care
   Provision of volunteer support to patient and family
   Teach family or caregiver physical care of patient

RN to provide and teach effective oral care and comfort measures

Assess pain and other symptoms, including site, duration, characteristics, and relief measures

RN to assess patient's pain q visit to identify need for change, addition, or other plan or dose adjustment

Change catheter number _____ French _____ cc q month

Evaluate the patient for catheter complaints, and contact physician if necessary

Obtain UA/C&S if symptoms of infection are present

Maintain hydration fluid volumes as indicated

Irrigate catheter with 30 cc NSS prn per physician orders

Teach family indwelling catheter are, irrigation of catheter, S/S UTI, adequate hydration, skin care, change of drainage bag, and when to call clinician

Teach family removal of catheter with syringe, how to change bag, and care and positioning of bag

Assess amount, frequency of urinary drainage, intake, and output

Pain assessment and management q visit

Teach family reason for catheter (e.g., bladder atony, retention)

RN to change catheter every 4 weeks and may make 3 prn visits for catheter problems, including patient complaints, signs and symptoms of infection, and other factors necessitating evaluation and possible catheter change

Assess pain, and evaluate pain management's effectiveness

Teach care of bedridden patient

Measure vital signs, including pain, q visit

Assess cardiovascular, pulmonary, and respiratory status

Teach caregivers symptom control and relief measures

Identify and monitor pain, symptoms, and relief measures

Teach caregiver care of weak, terminally ill patient

Comfort measures of backrub and hand/other therapeutic massage

Observation and assessment related to signs/symptoms of urinary infection

Teaching and training about symptoms/changes that necessitate notification of nurse

Observation, assessment, and supportive care to patient and family

Teach patient/family use of standardized form/tool to use between hospice team members' visits (and for care coordination among team members)

Teach patient/family principles of effective pain management

Observation and assessment, communication with physician related to signs and symptoms of continuing decompensation, increased symptoms, pain, discomfort, shortness of breath, and measures to alleviate and control

Effective management of pain and prevention of secondary symptoms

Teach family and caregiver signs and changes to report to clinician and physician

Interventions of symptoms directed toward comfort and palliation

Teach patient and family about realistic expectations of disease process

4

Teach care of dying and signs/symptoms of impending death
Presence and support
Other interventions, based on patient/family needs

b. *Safety and mobility considerations*
Provide caregiver/family with home safety information and instruction
related to _____ and documented in the clinical record
Teach family regarding safety of patient in home
Other interventions, based on patient/family needs

c. *Emotional/Spiritual considerations*
Psychosocial assessment of patient and family regarding disease and
prognosis
RN to provide emotional support to patient and family
Assess mental status and sleep disturbance changes
Observation and assessment of mental status changes/complaints of
depression in new hospice patient with catheter
Observation of patient for neuropsychiatric complications of illness,
including confusion, depression, and anxiety
RN to provide support and intervention/referral for depression
Teach patient/family about depression and signs/symptoms of
exacerbation that require more intervention
Assess for and manage plans for psychosocial and/or spiritual pain
(e.g., all pain, anxiety, interpersonal and other distress)
Psychosocial aspects of pain control (e.g., depression, other) assessed
and acknowledged with team support/intervention
Ongoing acknowledgment of spirituality and related concerns of
patient/family
Other interventions, based on patient/family needs

d. *Skin care*
Maintain skin integrity, and teach care of the immobilized patient,
if indicated
Pressure ulcer care as indicated
Observation and evaluation of wound and surrounding skin
Evaluate patient's need for equipment, including supplies to decrease
pressure, alternating pressure mattress, gel foam seat cushion, and
heel and elbow protectors
RN to teach patient about care of irradiated skin sites
Maintain skin integrity, and teach care of the immobilized patient as
indicated
Teach patient, family, or caregiver about proper body alignment and
positioning in bed to prevent skin tears from shearing skin
Observe and apply skilled assessment of areas for possible breakdown,
including heels, hips, elbows, ankles, and other pressure-prone areas
Teach caregiver regarding skin care needs, including the need for
frequent position changes, appropriate pressure pads and mattresses,
and the prevention of breakdown
Teach family to perform dressing changes between RN visits
Other interventions, based on patient/family needs

e. *Elimination considerations*

Assess bowel regimen, and implement program as needed

Assess amount and frequency of urinary output

RN to evaluate the patient's bowel patterns and need for stool softeners, laxatives, and dietary adjustments, and to develop bowel management plan

Check for and remove impaction as needed

Condom catheter or indwelling catheter as indicated

Teaching and ongoing assessment for the prevention and early identification of constipation and its correction/resolution

Implement bowel assessment management program

Teach patient, family, and aide the importance of observing and noting bowel movements between scheduled health care visits

Obtain patient history related to norms for bowel movements to date (e.g., "All my life I go only every other day")

Bowel management program of stool softeners, laxative of choice, Fleet's enemas prn, and other methods per patient wishes and physician orders

Teach catheter care to caregiver

RN to teach caregiver daily care of catheter

RN to change catheter (specify type, size) q _____ (specify ordered frequency)

RN to change catheter every 4 weeks and may make 3 prn visits for catheter problems, including patient complaints, signs and symptoms of infection, and other factors necessitating evaluation and possible catheter change

Observation and complete systems assessment of patient with an indwelling catheter

Other interventions, based on patient/family needs

f. *Hydration/Nutrition*

Assess nutrition/hydration status

Teach feeding-tube care to family

Nutrition/hydration supported by offering patient's choice of favorite or desired foods or liquids

Nutrition/hydration maintained by offering patient high-protein diet and foods of choice as tolerated

Teach patient and family to expect decreased nutritional and fluid intake as disease progresses

Other interventions, based on patient/family needs

g. *Therapeutic/Medication regimens*

Medication management related to antibiotics and food/drug and drug/drug interactions

RN to assess the patient's response to therapeutic treatments and interventions and report any changes or unfavorable responses to the physician

Medication assessment and management q visit

Teach new medication regimens and side effects

Assess for electrolyte imbalance

Teach patient and caregiver use of PCA pump

Nonpharmacological interventions such as progressive muscle relaxation imagery, positive visualization, music, massage and touch, and humor therapy of patient's choice implemented

Teach and observe regarding side effects of palliative chemotherapy, including constipation, anemia, and fatigue

Teaching of patient/family, including medications, management program, strength, type, actions, times, and compliance tips

Encourage family/caregivers to give the patient medications on the schedule and around the clock

RN to instruct in pain control measures and medications

Medications changed using equianalgesic conversion tables/physician orders (e.g., from oral morphine to an equianalgesic dose of transdermal fentanyl)

Nonpharmacological or other interventions of relaxation, hot/cold therapy, biofeedback, distraction, guided imagery, humor, music therapy, acupuncture, TENS technology, hypnosis, massage, or others as patient and family wish

Other interventions, based on patient/family needs

h. *Other considerations*

Assess disease process progression

RN to assess the patient's response to treatments and interventions and to report to the physician any changes, unfavorable responses, or reactions

Other interventions, based on patient/family needs

- *Feeding tube care*

a. *Comfort and symptom control*

Skilled observation and systems assessment of patient with feeding tube _____ (specify type, site) due to _____ (specify)

Comprehensive assessment of patient with feeding tube

Observation, assessment, and supportive care to patient with feeding tube _____ (specify type) and family

Presentation of hospice philosophy and services

Explain patient rights and responsibilities

Assess patient, family, and caregiver wishes and expectations regarding care

Assess patient, family, and caregiver resources available for care

Provision of volunteer support to patient and family

Teach family or caregiver physical care of patient

RN to provide and teach effective oral care and comfort measures

Assess pain and other symptoms, including site, duration, characteristics, and relief measures

RN to assess patient's pain q visit to identify need for change, addition, or other plan or dose adjustment

Measure vital signs

Teach family or caregiver about enteral feeding

Teach about equipment for feeding, preparation, and storage of feeding supplies/solution product

Teach patient and caregiver protocols of changing feeding bags and administration tubing per physician orders

RN to observe q visit for leaking, movement, discomfort, or other change

Instruct patient and family in jejunostomy or other tube feedings

RN/wound ostomy care nurse/WOCN to evaluate patient and peristomal skin to identify health care needs

Teach the importance of verifying the tube's placement before every feeding

Teach family mouth and oral hygiene care

Teach caregiver regarding irrigation with water or per protocol

Teach family observational skills, including record keeping of intake and output, nutritional solution or supplement, and rate, frequency, amount, and time of ordered feedings

Pain assessment and management q visit

Monitor for complications, including diarrhea

Teach care of feeding tube

Teach family or caregiver gastrostomy feeding

Teach family or caregiver equipment care and preparation

Teach Dobhoff tube care, including _____ (specify)

Weigh daily or weekly per physician order(s)

Monitor amount and sites of edema

Assess gastric tube for proper placement and patency, and teach patient or family regarding care

Cleanse gastric tube site q _____ with hydrogen peroxide and water

Teach family or caregiver care of gastric tube

Assess respiratory and cardiovascular statuses

Gastric tube feedings of _____ in 24 hours at _____ cc/hr

Change and reinsert tube prn per physician orders

Teach patient/family use of standardized form/tool to use between hospice team members' visits (and for care coordination between team members)

Teach patient/family principles of effective pain management

Observation and assessment, communication with physicians related to signs and symptoms of continuing decompensation, increased symptoms, pain, discomfort, shortness of breath, and measures to alleviate and control

Effective management of pain and prevention of secondary symptoms

Pain assessment and management q visit, including source of pain (e.g., neuropathy, phantom pain, claudification, infection, and other problems such as cardiac or arthritis pain)

Oxygen on at _____ liters per _____ (specify physician orders)

Identify and monitor pain, symptoms, and relief measures

Teach caregiver care of weak, terminally ill patient

Comfort measures of backrub and hand or other therapeutic massage

Assess pain, and evaluate pain management's effectiveness

Teach care of bedridden patient

4

Measure vital signs, including pain, q visit
Assess cardiovascular, pulmonary, and respiratory status
Teach caregivers symptom control and relief measures
Interventions of symptoms directed toward comfort and palliation
Teach patient and family about realistic expectations of disease process
Teach care of dying and signs/symptoms of impending death
Presence and support
Other interventions, based on patient/family needs

b. *Safety and mobility considerations*
Provide caregiver/family with home safety information and instruction
   related to _____ and documented in the clinical record
Teach regarding elevated position of head in bed for safety
Teach family regarding safety of patient in home
Other interventions, based on patient/family needs

c. *Emotional/Spiritual considerations*
Psychosocial assessment of patient and family regarding disease and
   prognosis
Clinician to provide emotional support to patient and family
Assess mental status and sleep disturbance changes
Observation and assessment of mental status and changes/complaints of
   depression in new hospice patient
Observation of patient for neuropsychiatric complications of illness,
   including confusion, depression, and anxiety
RN to provide support and intervention/referral for depression
Teach patient/family about depression and signs/symptoms of
   exacerbation that require more intervention
Assess for and manage plans for psychosocial and/or spiritual pain
   (e.g., all pain, anxiety, interpersonal and other distress)
Psychosocial aspects of pain control (e.g., depression, other) assessed
   and acknowledged with team support/intervention
Ongoing acknowledgment of spirituality and related concerns of
   patient/family
Other interventions, based on patient/family needs

d. *Skin care*
Wound care to abdominal site
Pressure ulcer care as indicated
Assess skin integrity
Observation and evaluation of wound and surrounding skin
Evaluate patient's need for equipment, including supplies to decrease
   pressure, alternating pressure mattress, gel foam seat cushion, and
   heel and elbow protectors
RN to teach patient about care of irradiated skin sites
Teach patient, family, or caregiver about proper body alignment
   and positioning in bed to prevent skin tears from
   shearing skin
Teach family to perform dressing changes between RN visits

Observe areas for possible breakdown, including heels, hips, elbows, ankles, and other pressure-prone areas

Teach caregiver about skin care needs, including the need for frequent position changes, appropriate pressure pads and mattresses, and the prevention of breakdown

Other interventions, based on patient/family needs

e. *Elimination considerations*

Assess bowel regimen, and implement program as needed

Observation and assessment of patient's bowel patterns

Teaching and ongoing assessment for the prevention and early identification of constipation and its correction/resolution

Initiate bowel management program per physician

Implement bowel assessment management program

Teach patient, family, and aide the importance of observing and noting bowel movements between scheduled health care visits

Obtain patient history related to norms for bowel movements to date (e.g., "All my life I go only every other day")

Bowel management program of stool softeners, offer laxative of choice, Fleet's enemas prn, and other methods per patient wishes and physician orders

Assess amount and frequency of urinary output

RN to evaluate the patient's bowel patterns and need for stool softeners, laxatives, and dietary adjustments and to develop bowel management plan

RN to teach daily catheter care

Assess bowel regimen, and implement program as needed

Check for and remove impaction as needed

Condom catheter or indwelling catheter as indicated

Other interventions, based on patient/family needs

4

f. *Hydration/Nutrition*

Teach and monitor for signs of dehydration and diarrhea

Assess nutrition/hydration status

Diet counseling for patient with anorexia

Nutrition/hydration supported by offering patient's choice of favorite or desired foods or liquids

Nutrition/hydration maintained by offering patient high-protein diet and foods of choice as tolerated

Teach patient and family to expect decreased nutritional and fluid intake as disease progresses

Teach feeding-tube care to family

Other interventions, based on patient/family needs

g. *Therapeutic/Medication regimens*

RN to assess the patient's response to therapeutic treatments and interventions and to report to the physician any changes or unfavorable responses

Teaching of patient/family, including medications and the management program (e.g., strength, type, actions, times, compliance tips)

Encourage family/caregivers to give the patient medications on the schedule and around the clock

Medications changed using equianalgesic conversion tables/physician orders (e.g., from oral morphine to an equianalgesic dose of transdermal fentanyl)

Nonpharmacological or other interventions of relaxation, hot/cold therapy, biofeedback, distraction, guided imagery, humor, music therapy, acupuncture, TENS technology, hypnosis, massage, or others as patient and family wish

Teach about and observe side effects of palliative chemotherapy, including constipation, anemia, and fatigue

Teach new medication regimens and side effects

RN to instruct in pain control measures and medications

Assess for electrolyte imbalance

Teach patient and caregiver use of PCA pump

Nonpharmacological interventions such as progressive muscle relaxation imagery, positive visualization, music, massage and touch, and humor therapy of patient's choice implemented

Teach new pain and symptom control medication regimen

Medication assessment and management

Other interventions, based on patient/family needs

h. *Other considerations*

Assess disease process progression

RN to assess the patient's response to treatments and interventions and to report to the physician any changes, unfavorable responses, or reactions

Other interventions, based on patient/family needs

• ***Ostomy care***

a. *Comfort and symptom control*

Skilled observation and systems assessment of patient with a
_____ (specify) ostomy due to _____ (specify)

Comprehensive assessment of patient with ostomy

Presentation of hospice philosophy and services

Explain patient rights and responsibilities

Assess patient, family, and caregiver wishes and expectations regarding care

Assess patient, family, and caregiver resources available for care

Provision of volunteer support to patient and family

Teach family or caregiver physical care of patient

RN to provide and teach effective oral care and comfort measures

Assess pain and other symptoms, including site, duration, characteristics, and relief measures

RN to assess patient's pain q visit to identify need for change, addition, or other plan or dose adjustment

Teach ostomy care

Adjust size of karaya seal

Teach patient modification of appliance to preserve skin integrity

Closely assess stoma and wound progress

Help patient find best ostomy equipment and supplies, based on patient needs and price

Teach regarding irrigation procedure(s)

Consult with WOCN for review of care and care planning

Assess for allergy to sealant or appliances

Teach patient to be prepared for "accidents" and have cosmetic bag with supplies, one of each appliance used, and small plastic bag for disposal of soiled materials

WOCN contacted for care and care plan review

Comfort measures of backrub and hand or other therapeutic massage

Assess pain, and evaluate pain management's effectiveness

Teach care of bedridden patient

Measure vital signs, including pain, q visit

Assess cardiovascular, pulmonary, and respiratory status

Teach caregivers symptom control and relief measures

Oxygen on at _____ liters per _____ (specify physician orders)

Identify and monitor pain, symptoms, and relief measures

Teach caregiver care of weak, terminally ill patient

Teach patient/family use of standardized form/tool to use between hospice team members' visits (and for care coordination among team members)

Observation, assessment, and supportive care to patient and family

Teach patient/family principles of effective pain management

Effective management of pain and prevention of secondary symptoms

Observation and assessment, communication with physician related to signs and symptoms of continuing decompensation, increased symptoms, pain, discomfort, shortness of breath, and measures to alleviate and control

Teach caregiver/patient use of pain assessment tool/scale and reporting mechanism(s)

Interventions directed toward comfort and palliation of symptoms

Teach patient and family about realistic expectations of disease process

Teach care of dying and signs/symptoms of impending death

Presence and support

Other interventions, based on patient/family needs

b. *Safety and mobility considerations*

Provide caregiver and family with home safety information and instruction related to _____ and documented in the clinical record

Teach family regarding safety of patient in home

Teach patient and family regarding energy conservation techniques

Other interventions, based on patient/family needs

4

c. *Emotional/Spiritual considerations*

Psychosocial assessment of patient and family regarding disease and prognosis

Document emotional or physical barriers to learning or coping (e.g., severe arthritis of hands)

RN to provide emotional support to patient and family

Assess mental status and sleep disturbance changes

Observation and assessment of mental status and changes/complaints of depression in new hospice patient with ostomy

Observation of patient for neuropsychiatric complications of illness, including confusion, depression, and anxiety

Clinician to provide support and intervention/referral for depression

Teach patient/family about depression and signs/symptoms of exacerbation that require more intervention

Assess for and manage plans for psychosocial and/or spiritual pain (e.g., all pain, anxiety, interpersonal and other distress)

Psychosocial aspects of pain control (e.g., depression) assessed and acknowledged with team support/intervention

Assessment and care/support related to depression, changed body image concerns, fever, mouth sores/ulcers, complaints of extreme tiredness, and dry/cracking skin in patient receiving palliative chemotherapy

Ongoing acknowledgment of spirituality and related concerns of patient/family

Other interventions, based on patient/family needs

d. *Skin care*

Instruct patient regarding skin care and air-dry procedures

Teach about skin care to protect from irritation and infection

Pressure ulcer care as indicated

Assess skin integrity

Teach family to perform dressing changes between RN visits

Observation and evaluation of wound and surrounding skin

Evaluate patient's need for equipment, including supplies to decrease pressure, alternating pressure mattress, gel foam seat cushion, and heel and elbow protectors

RN to teach patient about care of irradiated skin sites

Teach patient, family, or caregiver about proper body alignment and positioning in bed to prevent skin tears from shearing skin

Observe and apply skilled assessment of areas for possible breakdown, including heels, hips, elbows, ankles, and other pressure-prone areas

Teach caregiver about skin care needs, including the need for frequent position changes, appropriate pressure pads and mattresses, and the prevention of breakdown

Other interventions, based on patient/family needs

e. *Elimination considerations*

Assess bowel regimen, and implement program as needed

Check for and remove impaction as needed

Condom catheter or indwelling catheter as indicated

Assess amount and frequency of urinary output

RN to evaluate the patient's bowel patterns and need for stool softeners, laxatives, and dietary adjustments and to develop bowel management plan

RN to teach daily catheter care

Teach patient, family, and aide the importance of observing and noting bowel movements between scheduled health care visits

Obtain patient history related to norms for bowel movements to date (e.g., "All my life I go only every other day")

Teaching and ongoing assessment for the prevention and early identification of constipation and its correction/resolution

Implement bowel assessment management program

Bowel management program of stool softeners, laxative of choice, Fleet's enemas prn, and other methods per patient wishes and physician orders

Observation and complete systems assessment of the patient with an indwelling catheter

RN to change catheter every 4 weeks and to make 3 prn visits for catheter problems, including patient complaints, signs and symptoms of infection, and other factors necessitating evaluation and possible catheter change

Other interventions, based on patient/family needs

f. *Hydration/Nutrition*

Teach patient about avoidance of gas-producing foods such as cauliflower, cabbage, beans, cucumbers, and onions

Teach about appropriate diet

Assess nutrition/hydration status

Diet counseling for patient with anorexia

Nutrition/hydration supported by offering patient's choice of favorite or desired foods or liquids

Nutrition/hydration maintained by offering patient high-protein diet and foods of choice as tolerated

Teach patient and family to expect decreased nutritional and fluid intake as disease progresses

Teach feeding tube care to family

Assessment and plan related to anorexia/cachexia, tube feedings, difficulty swallowing, and/or transitional feedings (e.g., TPN to oral)

Assessment and interventions/plan related to patient/family complaints of dry mouth, with painful chewing, difficulty speaking, and denture fit concerns after radiation and surgery

Other interventions, based on patient/family needs

g. *Therapeutic/Medication regimens*

RN to assess the patient's response to therapeutic treatments and interventions, and to report any changes or unfavorable responses to the physician

4

Teach and observe regarding side effects of palliative chemotherapy, including constipation, anemia, and fatigue

Teach new pain and symptom control medication regimen

Medication assessment and management

Venipuncture q _____ (specify ordered frequency) for monitoring platelet count

Obtain venipuncture as ordered q _____ (specify ordered frequency)

Teach about new medication and effects

RN to instruct in pain control measures and medications

Assess for electrolyte imbalance

Teach patient and caregiver use of PCA pump

Teaching of patient/family, including medications and the management program (e.g., strength, type, actions, times, and compliance tips)

Encourage family/caregivers to give the patient medications on the schedule and around the clock

Medications changed using equianalgesic conversion tables/physician orders (e.g., from oral morphine to an equianalgesic dose of transdermal fentanyl)

Nonpharmacological or other interventions of relaxation, hot/cold therapy, biofeedback, distraction, guided imagery, humor, music therapy, acupuncture, TENS technology, hypnosis, massage, or others as patient and family wish

Other interventions, based on patient/family needs

h. *Other considerations*

Assess disease process progression

RN to assess the patient's response to treatments and interventions and to report to the physician any changes, unfavorable responses, or reactions

Other interventions, based on patient/family needs

4

- **Home health aide or certified nursing assistant**

Effective and safe personal care

Safe ADL assistance and support

Observation and reporting

Respite care and active listening skills

Meal preparation

Homemaker services

Comfort care

Other duties

- **Social worker**

Psychosocial assessment of patient and family/caregiver, including adjustment to illness and its implications

Identification of optimal coping strategies

Financial assessment and counseling regarding food acquisition, ability to prepare, and costs of needed medications

Intervention/support related to terminal illness and loss

Emotional/spiritual support

Depression/fear assessed

Facilitate communication among patient, family, and hospice team

Referral/linkage to community services and resources as indicated

Grief counseling and intervention/support related to illness/loss

Patient/caregiver counseling and support

For patients who live alone with no support system (e.g., able, available, willing caregiver[s]), identify/review possible resources to enable patient to remain in home

Identification of illness-related psychiatric condition necessitating care

Caregiver system assessed, and development of stable caregiver plan facilitated

Identification of caregiver role strain necessitating respite/relief measures/support

Funeral and burial planning assistance

- *Volunteer(s)*

  Support, friendship, companionship, and presence

  Comfort and dignity maintained/provided for patient and family

  Errands and transportation

  Advocacy and respite

  Other services, based on IDT recommendations and patient/caregiver needs

- *Spiritual counselor*

  Spiritual assessment and care

  Counseling, intervention, and support related to that dimension of life related to life's meaning (consistent with patient's beliefs)

  Support, listening, and presence

  Participation in sacred or spiritual rituals or practices

  Pray with or for the patient/family, using prayers familiar to patient's religious background (per their wishes)

  Other supportive care, based on patient's/family's needs and belief systems

  Patient and family express relief of symptoms of spiritual suffering

- *Dietitian/Nutritional counseling*

  Assessment of patient with decreased intake, weight loss, anorexia, and increased shortness of breath (e.g., "I don't feel like eating")

  Supportive counseling with patient/family indicating that patient may have a decreased appetite and usually at some point may not eat/drink

  Assessment and recommendations for swallowing difficulties

  Teaching and support of family members and caregivers

  Support and care, with food and nourishment as desired by patient

  Evaluation/management of nutritional deficits and needs

  Encourage nutritional supplements and snacks to increase protein and caloric intake

  Food and dietary recommendations incorporate patient choice and wishes

  Patient and family verbalize comprehension of changing nutritional needs

- *Occupational therapist*

  Evaluation of ADLs and functional mobility

  Assess for need for adaptive equipment and assistive devices

4

Safety assessment of patient's environment and ADLs
Assessment for energy conservation training
Assessment of upper-extremity function, retraining motor skills

- *Physical therapist*
Evaluation
Assessment of patient's environment for safety
Safe transfer training or bed mobility exercises
Pain assessment/reduction factors
Strengthening exercises/program
Assessment of gait safety and home safety measures
Instruct/supervise caregiver and volunteers on home exercise program
   for conditioning and strength
Assistive, adaptive devices and evaluation of equipment and teaching

- *Speech-language pathologist*
Evaluation for speech/swallowing problems
Food texture recommendations
Alternate functional communication

- *Bereavement counselor*
Assessment of the needs of the bereaved family and friends
Support and intervention, based on assessment and ongoing findings
Presence and counseling
Supportive visits, follow-up, and other interventions (e.g., mailings, calls)
Other services related to bereavement work and support

- *Pharmacist*
Evaluation of hospice patient with constipation on cathartics, stool
   softeners, and other medications for possible food/drug, drug/drug
   interactions
Medication monitoring regarding therapeutic levels and dosages
Pain consult and input into interdisciplinary POC related to pain
   control, palliation, and symptom management
Assessment of medication regimen and plan for safety and compliance

- *Music, massage, art, or other therapies or services*
Evaluation and intervention based on patient's and caregiver's unique
   wishes and needs that support care, comfort, and death in the setting
   of the patient's choice
Assessment plan to engage patient and support comfort, quality,
   enjoyment, and dignity
Pet therapy (including patient's pet, if available) and therapeutic
   intervention

6. Outcomes for care

- *Hospice Nursing*

Catheter care
Patient and caregiver verbalize comfort with and understand of care
Infection-free, patent urinary catheter

No skin breakdown, and family able to provide care as taught

Support and care from hospice team facilitate patient's death per wishes (setting, symptoms controlled, etc.)

Mental distress, depression, and fear of dying addressed throughout care by hospice team

Patient and family able to care for and support patient

Patient and caregiver can verbalize symptoms, changes, or accelerations that necessitate call to physician

Patient and family demonstrate compliance with medication regimen and other therapeutic interventions

Patient demonstrates stabilization and increased or enhanced coping skills related to functioning and depression

Pain and symptoms managed/controlled in setting of patient/family choice (e.g., patient/family report ability to eat, sleep, speak with pacing)

Planted and effective bowel program, as evidenced by regular bowel movements and patient/family report of comfort

Death with dignity, and pain/symptoms controlled in setting of patient/family choice

Optimal comfort, support, and dignity provided throughout illness

Death with maximum comfort through effective symptom control with specialized hospice support

Patient and caregiver able to list adverse drug reactions/problems with medication regimen and whom to call for follow-up and resolution

Patient's/family's privacy, independence, and choices supported with respect and maintained through death

Enhancement and support of quality of life

Effective symptom relief and control (e.g., a peaceful and comfortable death at home, depression controlled, some enjoyment of life)

Maximizing the patient's quality of life (e.g., alert and pain free or as patient wishes)

Pharmacological and nonpharmacological interventions such as localized heat application, biofeedback, massage, positioning, relaxation methods, and music

Patient cared for and family supported through death, with physical, psychosocial, spiritual and others concerns/needs acknowledged/addressed

Patient- and family-centered hospice care provided based on the patient's/family's unique situation and needs

Infection control and palliation

Grief/bereavement expression and support provided

Patient is pain free by next _____ visit

Caregiver demonstrates ability to manage pain, where applicable

Patient maintains comfort and dignity throughout illness

Educational tools/plans incorporated in daily care, and patient/caregiver verbalizes understanding of safe, needed care

Patient will decide on care, interventions, and evaluation

Caregiver effective in care management and knows whom to call for questions/concerns

4

Patient will express satisfaction with hospice support received and will experience increased comfort

Patient will be made comfortable at home through death in accordance with the patient's wishes

Effective pain control and symptom control verbalized by patient

Patient verbalizes understanding of and adheres to care and medication regimens

Patient and caregiver supported through patient's death

Comfort maintained through course of care

The patient and family receive hospice support and care, and family members and friends are able to spend quality time with the patient

Caregiver able and verbalizes comfort with role and lists when to call hospice team members

Patient supported through and receives the maximum benefit from palliative chemotherapy and radiation with minimal complications

Patient and caregiver list adverse reactions, potential complications, signs/symptoms of infection (e.g., sputum change, chest congestion)

Comfort maintained through death with dignity

Pain effectively managed, and patient verbalizes comfort

Patient has stable respiratory status with patent airway

Patient is protected from injury, has stable respiratory status, and is compliant with medication, safety, and care regimens

Comfort and individualized intervention of patient with immobility/bed-bound status (e.g., skin, urinary, musculature, vascular)

Spiritual and psychosocial needs met (specify) as defined by patient and caregiver throughout course of care

Other outcomes/goals, based on the patient condition with input from the hospice team and patient and family

4

- *Feeding tube care*

Patent tube with correct placement, and skin site infection free

Adherence to POC as demonstrated and verbalized by caregiver and demonstrated by patient findings by _____ (specify date)

Caregiver effective in care management and knows whom to call for questions/concerns

Patient verbalizes understanding of and adheres to medication regimens

Patient and caregiver verbalize satisfaction with care

Educational tools/plans incorporated in daily care, and patient/caregiver verbalizes understanding of safe, needed care

Patient and caregiver compliant with medications and tube-feeding schedules as demonstrated to visiting team members

Support and care from hospice through symptom-controlled death

Mental distress, depression, and fear of dying addressed throughout care by hospice team

Patient and family able to care for and support patient

Patient and caregiver can verbalize symptoms, changes, or accelerations that necessitate call to physician

Patient and family demonstrate compliance with medication regimen and other therapeutic interventions

Patient demonstrates stabilization and increased or enhanced coping skills related to functioning and depression

Pain and symptoms managed/controlled in setting of patient/family choice (e.g., patient/family report ability to eat, sleep, speak with pacing)

Planned and effective bowel program, as evidenced by regular bowel movements and patient/family report of comfort

Death with dignity, and pain/symptoms controlled in setting of patient/family choice

Optimal comfort, support, and dignity provided throughout illness

Death with maximum comfort through effective symptom control with specialized hospice support

Patient and caregiver able to list adverse drug reactions/problems with medication regimen and whom to call for follow-up and resolution

Patient's/family's privacy, independence, and choices supported with respect and maintained through death

Enhancement and support of quality of life

Effective symptom relief and control (e.g., a peaceful and comfortable death at home, depression controlled, some enjoyment of life)

Maximizing the patient's quality of life (e.g., alert and pain free or as patient wishes)

Pharmacological and nonpharmacological interventions such as localized heat application, biofeedback, massage, positioning, relaxation methods, and music

Patient cared for and family supported through death, with physical, psychosocial, spiritual, and other concerns/needs acknowledged/addressed

Patient- and family-centered hospice care provided based on the patient's/family's unique situation and needs

Infection control and palliation

Grief/bereavement expression and support provided

Patient is pain free by next _____ visit

Caregiver demonstrates ability to manage pain, where applicable

Patient maintains comfort and dignity throughout illness

Patient and caregiver verbalize satisfaction with care

Educational tools/plans incorporated in daily care, and patient and caregiver verbalize understanding of safe, needed care

Patient will decide on care, interventions, and evaluation

Caregiver effective in care management and knows whom to call for questions/concerns

Patient will express satisfaction with hospice support received and will experience increased comfort

Patient will be made comfortable at home through death in accordance with the patient's wishes

Effective pain control and symptom control verbalized by patient

Patient verbalizes understanding of and adheres to care and medication regimens

Patient and caregiver supported through patient's death

Comfort maintained through course of care

Patient and family receive hospice support and care, and family members and friends are able to spend quality time with the patient

Caregiver able and verbalizes comfort with role and lists when to call hospice team members

Patient supported through and receives the maximum benefit from palliative chemotherapy and radiation with minimal complications

Patient and caregiver list adverse reactions, potential complications, signs/symptoms of infection (e.g., sputum change, chest congestion)

Comfort maintained through death with dignity

Patient is protected from injury, has stable respiratory status, and is compliant with medication, safety, and care regimens

Comfort and individualized intervention of patient with immobility/bedbound status (e.g., skin, urinary, musculature, vascular)

Spiritual and psychosocial needs met (specify) as defined by patient and caregiver throughout course of care

Other outcomes/goals, based on the patient condition with input from the hospice team and patient and family

- **Ostomy care**

  Patient and caregiver verbalize satisfaction with care

  Educational tools/plans incorporated in daily care, and patient/caregiver verbalize understanding of safe, needed care

  Stoma site and incision free of signs/symptoms of infection

  Patient and caregiver effective in providing skin care

  Patient able to care for ostomy through self-report and demonstration

  Patient and caregiver effective in care management and know whom to call for questions/concerns

  Patient verbalizes understanding of and adheres to pain and other medication regimens

  Patient and caregiver demonstrate understanding of care and associated regimens

  Support and care from hospice through symptom-controlled death

  Mental distress, depression, and fear of dying addressed throughout care by hospice team

  Patient and family able to care for and support patient

  Patient and caregiver can verbalize symptoms, changes, or accelerations that necessitate call to physician

  Patient and family demonstrate compliance with medication regimen and other therapeutic interventions

  Patient demonstrates stabilization and increased or enhanced coping skills related to functioning and depression

  Pain and symptoms managed/controlled in setting of patient/family choice (e.g., patient and family report ability to eat, sleep, speak with pacing)

Planned and effective bowel program, as evidenced by regular bowel movements and patient/family report of comfort

Death with dignity, and pain/symptoms controlled in setting of patient/family choice

Optimal comfort, support, and dignity provided throughout illness

Death with maximum comfort through effective symptom control with specialized hospice support

Patient and caregiver able to list adverse drug reactions/problems with medication regimen and whom to call for follow-up and resolution

Patient's/family's privacy, independence, and choices supported with respect and maintained through death

Enhancement and support of quality of life

Effective symptom relief and control (e.g., a peaceful and comfortable death at home, depression controlled, some enjoyment of life)

Maximizing the patient's quality of life (e.g., alert and pain free or as patient wishes)

Pharmacological and nonpharmacological interventions such as localized heat application, biofeedback, massage, positioning, elaxation methods, and music

Patient cared for and family supported through death, with physical, psychosocial, spiritual, and other concerns/needs acknowledged/addressed

Patient- and family-centered hospice care provided based on the patient's family's unique situation and needs

Infection control and palliation

Grief/bereavement expression and support provided

Patient is pain free by next _____ visit

Caregiver demonstrates ability to manage pain, where applicable

Patient maintains comfort and dignity throughout illness

Patient and caregiver verbalize satisfaction with care

Educational tools/plans incorporated in daily care, and patient and caregiver verbalize understanding of safe, needed care

Patient will decide on care, interventions, and evaluation

Caregiver effective in care management and knows whom to call for questions/concerns

Patient will express satisfaction with hospice support received and will experience increased comfort

Patient will be made comfortable at home through death in accordance with the patient's wishes

Effective pain control and symptom control verbalized by patient

Patient verbalizes understanding of and adheres to care and medication regimens

Patient and caregiver supported through patient's death

Comfort maintained through course of care

Patient and family receive hospice support and care, and family members and friends are able to spend quality time with the patient

Caregiver able and verbalizes comfort with role and lists when to call hospice team members

4

Patient supported through and receives the maximum benefit from palliative chemotherapy and radiation with minimal complications

Patient and caregiver list adverse reactions, potential complications, signs/symptoms of infection (e.g., sputum change, chest congestion)

Comfort maintained through death with dignity

Pain effectively managed, and patient verbalizes comfort

Patient has stable respiratory status with patent airway

Patient and caregiver demonstrate appropriate back-up or "rescue" therapies for breakthrough pain or other symptoms (e.g., dyspnea)

Patient is protected from injury, has stable respiratory status, and is compliant with medication, safety, and care regimens

Comfort and individualized intervention of patient with immobility/ bedbound status (e.g., skin, urinary, musculature, vascular)

Spiritual and psychosocial needs met (specify) as defined by patient and caregiver throughout course of care

Other outcomes/goals, based on the patient condition with input from the hospice team and patient and family

- *Home health aide or certified nursing assistant*
  Effective hygiene, personal care, and comfort
  ADL assistance
  Safe environment maintained
  Catheter/feeding tube/ostomy care, as indicated
  Advocacy and respite

- *Social worker*
  Problem identified and addressed, with patient/caregiver linked with appropriate support services and POC successfully implemented
  Patient and caregiver cope adaptively with illness and death
  Adaptive adjustment to changed body and body image
  Psychosocial support and counseling offered to patient/caregivers experiencing loss and grief
  Funeral and burial planning assistance

- *Volunteer(s)*
  Comfort, companionship, and friendship extended to patient/family
  Support provided as defined by the needs of the patient/caregiver
  Patient and family supported by team with care, comfort, and companionship

- *Spiritual counselor*
  Spiritual support offered and provided as defined by needs of patient/caregiver
  Provision of spiritual support and care as based on the assessed and ongoing needs of the patient and family
  Spiritual support offered, and patient and family needs met
  Support, listening, and presence

Pray with or for the patient/family, using prayers familiar to the patient's religious background (per their wishes)

- *Dietitian/Nutritional counseling*
  Family and caregiver integrate recommendations into nutrition teaching (where appropriate)
  Patient and caregiver know whom to call for nutrition- and hydration-related questions/concerns
  Nutrition/hydration per patient's choices
  Caregiver integrates recommendations into daily meal planning

- *Occupational therapist*
  Patient and caregiver demonstrate maximum independence with ADLs, adaptive techniques, and assistive devices
  Patient and caregiver demonstrate maximum safety in ADLs and functional mobility
  Patient and caregiver demonstrate effective use of energy conservation
  Verbalization/demonstration of improved functional activity level and enhanced quality of life
  Patient and caregiver demonstrate effective use of diaphragmatic breathing to reduce shortness of breath and relaxation techniques to help in pain/symptom management
  Patient and caregiver demonstrate correct use of exercise and splints for maximum upper-extremity function and joint position

- *Physical therapist*
  Prevention of complications
  Home exercise and upper-extremity program taught to caregiver
  Optimal strength, mobility, and function maintained/achieved
  Compliance with home exercise program by _____ (specify date)

- *Speech-language pathologist*
  Communication method implemented, and patient able to be understood as self-reported or reported by family/caregivers
  Safe swallowing and functional communication
  Recommended lists of foods/textures for safety and patient choice

- *Bereavement counselor*
  Support services related to grief provided to patient and family
  Well-being and resolution process of grief initiated and followed through bereavement services

- *Pharmacist*
  Regimen for bowel regimen successful as self-reported by patient and in update at team meeting
  Multiple drug regimen reviewed for food/drug and drug/drug interactions in patient on multiple medications
  Stability and safety in complex medication regimen, with maximum benefit to patient
  Effective pain and symptom control and symptom management as reported by patient/caregiver

4

Other outcomes/goals, based on the patient's condition, with input from
the hospice team and patient and family

- *Music, massage, art, or other therapies or services*
Therapeutic massage/touch effective for patient as self-reported or
observed by caregivers/family
Improved muscle tone, relaxation, and/or sleep
Patient comfortable and relaxed (e.g., sleeping) after massage
Music therapy intervention based on assessment to decrease pain
perception and provide emotional expression and support
Maintenance of comfort and physical, psychosocial, and spiritual health
Patient has pet's presence as desired—in all care sites, when possible
Holistic health maintained and comfort achieved through
_____ (specify modality)

7. **Patient, family, and caregiver educational needs**
Educational needs are the care regimens that contribute to safe and
effective care at home between the hospice team's visits. These include
the following:
The basic tenets of hospice and the availability of support 24 hours a
day, 7 days a week
Home safety assessment and counseling
Anticipated disease progression
The patient's medication regimen
Safe and proper body mechanics to promote patient comfort and
avoid caregiver safety problems
Other teaching specific to the patient's and family's unique needs
Support groups available to patient's family, such as the hospice
program's "Caregiver Support Group" meetings for family
members and friends of the patient

- *Catheter care*
The symptoms of a urinary tract or other infection that necessitate
calling the RN or physician
The importance of keeping the bag below the patient's waist or lower
than the catheter insertion site
Skin care and hygiene regimens in the patient with an indwelling catheter
Aspects of infection control, including effective hand washing
and catheter site care and the importance of keeping the bag off
the floor
Safety issues that the caregiver needs to be aware of in safely caring for
the homebound patient
Other specific teaching as needed based on the patient's unique medical
condition and the caregiver's needs

- *Feeding tube care*
Peristomal skin site care routines
Teach caregiver all aspects of the particular tube (e.g., teach care of
percutaneous gastrostomy tube)

Teach about continuous infusion or other ordered method of
administration

All aspects of safe enteral feeding preparation and delivery

Teach effective handwashing and infection control techniques,
including safe storage of feedings and care and changing of supplies

Other information that this patient and family need to know to function
safely and effectively

- ***Ostomy care***

Care of ostomy, including bag changes, skin care, and signs and
symptoms to report

Teach patient/family observational skills regarding skin and other care
regimens

The patient's medications and effect(s) on ostomy function

Symptoms/changes that necessitate calling the hospice clinician

Other instructions as needed, based on the patient's unique medical
condition and other needs

8. Specific tips for quality and reimbursement

Document any variances to expected outcomes. There are many models
of hospice programs.

The Medicare hospice benefit does not require that the patient be
homebound or have identified skilled needs. For further information on
this benefit, please refer to CMS Hospice Manual 21.

Should the patient's status deteriorate and increased personal care
be needed, obtain a telephone order for the increased service, noting
frequency and estimating the duration.

Obtain a telephone order for all medication and treatment changes of
the medical regimen, and document these in the clinical record.

Unless the patient is in a hospice insurance program, some insurers
will not pay for a skilled clinician visit that is made at death if the patient
is dead when the clinician arrives at the home. From a Medicare home care
perspective, the visit at the time of death may be covered when the orders
and clinical record document assessment of the patient's status or signs
of death/life or state law allows pronouncement of death by an RN.

Document patient deterioration

Document dehydration, dehydrating

Document patient change or instability

Document pain, other symptoms not controlled

Document status after acute episode of _____ (specify)

Document positive urine, sputum, etc. culture; patient started on
_____ (specify ordered antibiotic therapy)

Document patient impacted; impaction removed manually per
physician's orders

Document RN in frequent communication with physician
regarding _____ (specify)

Document febrile at _____, pulse change at _____, irr., irr.

Document change noted in _____

4

Document bony prominences red, opening

Document RN contacted physician regarding _____ (specify)

Document marked SOB

Document alteration in mental status

Document medications being adjusted, regulated, or monitored

Document unable to perform own ADLs, personal care

Document all IDT meetings and communications in the POC and in the progress notes of the clinical record

All hospice team members should have input into the POC and document their interventions and goals

Document changes to the POC, such as medications, services, frequency, communication, and concurrence of other team members

Document coordination of services or consultation of the other members of the IDT

Document communications and care coordination with other care providers, such as skilled nursing facility or nursing home staff, inpatient team members, hired caregivers, and others

- **Catheter care**

  Documentation should include the size and type of catheter, the frequency of change, and other physician orders

  Document color, appearance of urine, and urine C&S results in your clinical documentation

  Document the continuing need for personal care services of the home health aide

  Implement new or changed POC, teach or communicate to the patient or family, and document in the clinical record

  Document specific teaching needs, teaching accomplished, and the behavioral outcomes of that teaching

  Document your catheter supplies, including type and size

  Document the following:

  Constipation and resulting pressure on the bladder

  A urinary infection, catheter position change, or the need for a different size or kind of catheter

  Bladder spasms that can occur after catheter change

  Increased sediment, sometimes indicating need for bladder irrigation

  Catheter draining, but leaking apparent also and other catheter problems based on their unique history

- **Feeding tube care**

  Document the gastrostomy site wound, and indicate color, any drainage, amount, and the specific care rendered

  Communicate any POC changes

  Document the reason for the tube feeding and the type of tube chosen

  Document progress in wound healing or deterioration in wound status in the clinical documentation

  Document the supplies needed on the POC, and obtain physician orders for all supplies or equipment

Obtain a telephone order for any additional visits not projected on the
original POC and state why (e.g., RN to visit × 1 to reinsert tube).
Better yet, obtain prn orders for tube dislodgment (e.g., prn × 3),
patient complaint, or other tube problem needing evaluation

Document any learning barriers

Document the specific care and teaching accomplished and the
behavioral and objective outcomes of that teaching

Document patient's level of independence in care

Document that the nutritional solutions are the patient's sole source of
nutrition, when appropriate. Medicare and many other insurers will
pay only if it is the *sole* source of nutrition (e.g., Ensure)

Document any problems with the skin site surrounding the tube and
care provided

Document the specific type and size of tube. Specify the insertion date
and site, the ordered feeding schedule, and teaching needs identified
and accomplished.

Document need for disease-specific nutrition products when standard
formula is unsuccessful

- ***Ostomy care***

Document up with assistance only

Document any changes, including specific care provided

Document physician changed medications to _____ (specify)

Document new onset (any problem)

Document pain not controlled effectively

Document increased gas pain and discomfort

Document the specific type of ostomy, the type and size of the ordered
appliances, and frequency of changes needed

Document the patient's skin condition and the specific skin care
regimen ordered and provided

Document the patient's level of self-care and progress toward
predetermined, patient-centered goals

The patient with a new colostomy or the patient with a new
caregiver must be taught the established care regimens. These include the
following:

Observation and assessment skills

Ostomy care, including healing, complications, and body image

Wound care (hands-on teaching and wound assessment/reassessment)

Teaching the safe care regimens to caregivers

Document in the clinical notes the clear progression of symptoms and
interventions that demonstrate the overall management
of the patient with _____ (specify)

Document when/if the patient has respiratory changes, shortness of
breath, exacerbation of conditions, dysphagia, changes in pain,
and/or other symptoms and that they are identified and resolved

Remember that the clinical documentation is key to measuring
compliance for quality and reimbursement purposes. Care coordination, timely verbal and initial physician orders, and assessment and

4

addressing of spiritual and psychosocial needs should be ongoing and documented in the patient's clinical record

Document that all hospice care supports comfort and dignity while meeting patient/family needs

The documentation should include ongoing assessment and management of pain and other symptoms and the anticipation and prevention of secondary symptoms such as constipation

It is important to note that all team members, including clinicians and social workers, should assess, identify, and "hear" spiritual needs that the patient and family want to be addressed. These spiritual issues are key to the provision of quality hospice care and cannot be addressed effectively and promptly by the spiritual counselor only

Document clearly symptoms, clinical changes, and assessment findings related to pain and patient care

Document patient changes, symptoms, and clinical information identified from visits and team conferences that constitute evidence of the need for hospice care and a limited life expectancy

Clearly support in the documentation the rationale that supports/explains the progression of the illness from the chronic to terminal stages

Document mentation, behavioral, and/or cognitive changes

Document dysphagia, weight loss, increased shortness of breath, dyspnea, infection, sepsis, new or changed medications, etc.

Document any skin changes (e.g., inflamed, painful, weeping skin site[s])

Document when the patient is actively dying, deteriorating, or progressing toward death

Remember that the "litmus test" of care coordination rests on the quality of the clinical documentation by all team members. Review one of your patient's clinical records and ask yourself the following: "If I was unable to give a verbal report/update on this patient, would a peer be able to pick up and provide the same level of care and know (from the documentation) the current orders, medications, and other details that contribute to effective hospice care?"

This patient population usually has many clinical changes that should be documented. These include weight loss and multiple and changed medication regimens with varying routes. Side effects to the drug regimen should be observed, noted, documented, and reported

9. Queries for quality

Supportive care: Catheter, feeding tube, and ostomy care

- Is patient's pain managed adequately?
- Is patient's anxiety managed adequately?
- Is patient's functional ability/status clearly documented?
- Does patient/family have access to appropriate medical supplies, and are the sources documented in the record?
- Have you documented to the interdisciplinary POC?

Catheter care

- Is patient's pain managed adequately?

- *Is patient's anxiety managed adequately?*
- *Is patient's functional ability/status clearly documented?*
- *What is the character, amount, and odor of the patient's urine?*
- *Have you documented to the interdisciplinary POC?*

Feeding tube care
- *Is patient's pain managed adequately?*
- *Is patient's anxiety managed adequately?*
- *Is patient's functional ability/status clearly documented?*
- *Does patient/family have access to appropriate medical supplies, and are the sources documented in the record?*
- *Have you documented to the interdisciplinary POC?*

Ostomy care
- *Is patient's pain managed adequately?*
- *Is patient's anxiety managed adequately?*
- *Is patient's functional ability/status clearly documented?*
- *Does patient/family have access to appropriate medical supplies, and are the sources documented in the record?*
- *Have you documented to the interdisciplinary POC?*

10. Resources for hospice care and practice

- **Catheter care**

    Available free from the Agency for Health Care Policy and Research (AHCPR) are these four resources: *Clinical Practice Guideline: Urinary Incontinence in Adults; Quick Reference Guide for Clinicians: Urinary Incontinence in Adults; Urinary Incontinence in Adults: A Patient's Guide;* and *Caregiver Guide: Helping People with Incontinence.* To receive these publications, call the AHCPR at 1-800-358-9295.

- **Feeding tube care and ostomy care**

    For resources or support for patients, there are two organizations that your patients can contact: The United Ostomy Association at 1-800-826-0826 or 1-800-826-0826 (www.uoa.org) or the Crohn's and Colitis Foundation of America at 1-800-932-2423 or visit www.ccfa.org.

4

WOUND AND PRESSURE ULCER CARE

1. **General considerations**
   Pressure ulcers, malignant cutaneous wounds, and other draining or leaking skin sites are commonly seen in patients in the home setting and are cared for sensitively and skillfully by the hospice team. The enterostomal therapist may be consulted. The enterostomal therapist plays an important role in providing this special patient population with quality care.

2. **Needs for visit**
   Physician order for hospice care, specific to the hospice program's admission criteria and policies
   Standard precautions supplies
   Vital signs equipment for baseline assessment
   Dressing supplies
   Other supplies or equipment, based on physician orders

3. **Safety considerations**
   Infection control/standard precautions
   Night light
   Extra caution on slippery surfaces
   Removal of scatter rugs
   Tub rail, grab bars for bathroom safety
   Supportive and nonskid shoes
   Handrail on stairs
   Fall precautions/protocol
   The phone number of whom to call with a care problem
   The need to report changes in skin integrity
   Protective skin measures
   Smoke detector and fire evacuation plan
   Assistance with ambulation
   Others, based on the patient's unique condition and environment

4. **Potential diagnoses and codes**

Amputation, infected right or left BKA, AKA	997.62
Amputation, transmetatarsal (right or left) (surgical)	84.12
Anal rectal abscess	566
Arterial graft (surgical)	39.58
Arterial insufficiency	447.1
Arterial occlusive disease	444.22
Bullous pemphigoid	694.5
Catheter (Foley, indwelling) insertion (surgical)	57.94
Cellulitis of the arm	682.3
Cellulitis of the trunk	682.2
Cellulitis RLE, LLE	682.6

4

Chronic ischemic heart disease	414.9
Congestive heart failure (CHF)	428.0
Coronary artery disease	414.00
CVA	436
Debridement, excisional (surgical)	86.22
Decubitus ulcer (pressure ulcer)	707.0
Diabetes mellitus, with complications (NIDDM)	250.90
Diabetes mellitus, with complications (IDDM)	250.91
Diabetic neuropathy	250.60 and 357.2
Diabetic retinopathy	250.50 and 362.01
Excoriation of skin	919.8
Femoral-popliteal bypass (right or left) (surgical)	39.29
Foot abscess	682.7
Foot wound, open	707.10
Gangrene, toe	785.4
Heel ulcer, right or left	707.14
Hypertension	401.9
I and D, skin (surgical)	86.04 and 998.59
Infection, postoperative	998.59
Leg injury	959.7
Open wound, ulcer, lower leg (right or left)	707.10
Open wound, ulcer, upper leg (right or left)	707.10
Osteomyelitis, acute	730.00
Osteomyelitis, foot, acute	730.07
Osteomyelitis, lower leg (right or left)	730.06
Peripheral vascular disease	443.9
Peritonitis	567.9
Pressure ulcer	707.0
Protein-caloric malnutrition	263.9
Quadriplegia	344.00
Septicemia	038.9
Skin eruption	782.1
Skin, excoriation of	919.8
Skin graft (surgical)	86.69
Staph infection	041.10
Stasis ulcer	454.2
Stitch abscess and excisional debridement (surgical)	998.59 and 86.22
Surgical wound, open	998.32
Thrombophlebitis	451.9
Ulcer, heel with cellulitis	682.7
Ulcer, right or left heel	707.14
Urinary incontinence	788.30
Varicose leg ulcer	454.9
Vascular insufficiency	459.9
Vascular shunt bypass (surgical)	32.29
Venous insufficiency	459.81
Venous ulcer	454.0

4

Wound evisceration	998.32
Wound, open ulcer, lower leg (right or left)	707.10

5. Skills and services identified

- ### *Hospice nursing*

a. *Comfort and symptom control*

Skilled observation and systems assessment of patient with a _____ (specify site or type) wound

Skilled observation and all systems assessment of patient with a pressure ulcer

Presentation of hospice philosophy and services

Explain patient rights and responsibilities

Assess patient, family, and caregiver wishes and expectations regarding care

Assess patient, family, and caregiver resources available for care

Provision of volunteer support to patient and family

Teach family or caregiver physical care of patient

RN to provide and teach effective oral care and comfort measures

Skilled observation and assessment of wound q visit

Assess pain and other symptoms, including site, duration, characteristics, and relief measures

RN to assess patient's pain q visit to identify need for change, addition, or other plan or dose adjustment

Assessment of healing process and site for sign of infection

Comprehensive risk assessment of patient with a wound

Pack wound with _____, cover with _____ (per physician orders)

Culture wound PRN

Teach patient or caregiver wound packing and irrigation techniques

Soak foot in _____ (per physician orders)

Pain assessment and effectiveness of pain management every visit

Cover wound with _____ (specify orders)

Wrap site

Assess wound on left extremity for signs and symptoms of infection

Measure vital signs q visit

RN to contact enterosotomal therapist for assessment of wound and recommendation of plan

RN to provide aseptic wound care to site (specify supplies, frequency, and specific wound orders)

RN to evaluate patient's pain and to implement pain control/relief program

Teach patient and caregiver regarding wound infection control measures

Observe for signs and symptoms of infection

Assess healing process

Change packing q _____ (specify)

Teach family or caregiver wound procedure and care regimen(s)

Pack wound with _____ (specify)

Apply wet to dry dressing of _____ (specify)

Soak site with _____ (specify)

Assess peripheral circulation

Instruct patient in dressing change

Assess wound drainage and amount

Cover with sterile 4×4

Remove dressing using normal saline solution

Repack wound with _____ (specify)

Pain assessment and management q visit

Assess wound for symptoms of infection, decreased circulation, or other problems

Elevate leg whenever sitting

TEDs or Ace wrap whenever up

Wash site gently with _____ (specify)

RN to consult with enterostomal therapist clinician for evaluation and POC and to report findings and recommendations to physician

Measure the site(s) for baseline and progress, including length, width, and depth

RN to teach infection control measures of wound care

Observation and skilled assessment of other areas for possible breakdown, including heels, hips, elbows, ankles, and other pressure-prone areas

RN to monitor for infection, necrosis, and increased exudate or other problems and to report to physician

Comfort measures of backrub and hand or other therapeutic massage

Assess pain, and evaluate the pain management's effectiveness

Teach care of bedridden patient

Measure vital signs, including pain, q visit

Assess cardiovascular, pulmonary, and respiratory statuses

Teach caregivers symptom control and relief measures

Oxygen on at _____ liters per _____ (specify physician orders)

Identify and monitor pain, symptoms, and relief measures

Teach caregiver care of weak, terminally ill patient

Observation, assessment, and supportive care to patient and family

Teach patient/family use of standardized form/tool to use between hospice team members' visits (and for care coordination among team members)

Supportive care and scopolamine patches per physician orders

Observation, assessment, and supportive care to patient and family

Teach patient/family principles of effective pain management

Effective management of pain and prevention of secondary symptoms

Observation and assessment, communication with physician related to signs and symptoms of continuing decompensation, increased symptoms, pain, discomfort, shortness of breath, and measures to alleviate and control

Pain assessment and management q visit, including source of pain (e.g., neuropathy, phantom pain, claudication, infection, other problems such as cardiac or arthritis pain)

Interventions of symptoms directed toward comfort and palliation

Teach patient and family about realistic expectations of disease process

4

Teach care of dying and signs/symptoms of impending death
Presence and support
Other interventions, based on patient/family needs

b. *Safety and mobility considerations*
Provide caregiver/family with home safety information and
instruction related to _____ and documented in the clinical
record
Teach family about safety of patient in home
Teach patient and family about energy conservation techniques
Other interventions, based on patient/family needs

c. *Emotional/Spiritual considerations*
Psychosocial assessment of patient and family regarding disease and
prognosis
RN to provide emotional support to patient and family
Assess mental status and sleep disturbance changes
Observation and assessment of mental status changes/complaints of
depression in new hospice patient with large draining wound
Observation of patient for neuropsychiatric complications of illness,
including confusion, depression, and anxiety
Clinician to provide support and intervention/referral for depression
Teach patient/family about depression and signs/symptoms of
exacerbation that require more intervention
Assess for and manage plans for psychosocial and/or spiritual pain
(e.g., all pain, anxiety, interpersonal or other distress)
Psychosocial aspects of pain control (e.g., depression) assessed and
acknowledged with team support/intervention
Ongoing acknowledgment of spirituality and related concerns of
patient/family
Other interventions, based on patient/family needs

d. *Skin care*
Pressure ulcer care as indicated
Assess skin integrity
Observation and evaluation of wound and surrounding skin
Evaluate patient's need for equipment, including supplies to decrease
pressure, alternating pressure mattress, gel foam seat cushion, and
heel and elbow protectors
Teach family to perform dressing changes between RN visits
RN to teach patient regarding care of irradiated skin sites
Teach patient, family, or caregiver about proper body alignment and
positioning in bed to prevent skin tears from shearing skin
Observe and apply skilled assessment of areas for possible breakdown,
including heels, hips, elbows, ankles, and other pressure-prone areas
Teach caregiver about skin care needs, including the need for frequent
position changes, appropriate pressure pads and mattresses, and the
prevention of breakdown
Other interventions, based on patient/family needs

e. *Elimination considerations*

Assess bowel regimen, and implement program as needed

Check for impaction and remove in bedbound patient per physician orders

Condom catheter or indwelling catheter as indicated

Assess amount and frequency of urinary output

RN to evaluate the patient's bowel patterns and need for stool softeners, laxatives, and dietary adjustments and to develop bowel management plan

RN to teach daily catheter care

Teaching and ongoing assessment for the prevention and early identification of constipation and its correction/resolution

Initiate bowel management program per hospice physician

Teach patient, family, and aide the importance of observing and noting bowel movements between scheduled nursing visits

Obtain patient history related to norms for bowel movements to date (e.g., "All my life I go only every other day")

Implement bowel assessment management program

Bowel management program of stool softeners, laxative of choice, Fleet's enemas prn, and other methods per patient wishes and physician orders

Other interventions, based on patient/family needs

f. *Hydration/Nutrition*

Teach patient/family role of adequate nutrition in wound healing; promote intake of high biological value proteins

Assess nutrition/hydration status

Diet counseling for patient with anorexia

Nutrition/hydration supported by offering patient's choice of favorite or desired foods or liquids

Nutrition/hydration maintained by offering patient high-protein diet and foods of choice as tolerated

Teach patient and family to expect decreased nutritional and fluid intake as disease progresses

Teach feeding-tube care to family

Other interventions, based on patient/family needs

g. *Therapeutic/Medication regimens*

Assess the patient's response to therapeutic treatments and interventions, and report to the physician any changes or unfavorable responses

Teach about new antibiotic regimen

Teach about medication and medication management

RN to instruct in pain control measures and medications

Teach and observe regarding side effects of palliative chemotherapy, including constipation, anemia, and fatigue

Venipuncture q _____ (specify ordered frequency) for monitoring platelet count

Medication assessment and management

Teach new medication and effects

Assess for electrolyte imbalance

Teach patient and caregiver use of PCA pump

RN to instruct in pain control measures and medications

Nonpharmacological interventions of progressive muscle relaxation imagery, positive visualization, music, massage and touch, and humor therapy of patient's choice implemented

Teaching of patient/family, including medications and the management program, including strength, type, actions, times, and compliance tips

Encourage family/caregivers to give the patient medications on the schedule and around the clock

Medications changed using equianalgesic conversion tables/physician orders (e.g., from oral morphine to an equianalgesic dose of transdermal fentanyl)

Nonpharmacological or other interventions of relaxation, hot/cold therapy, biofeedback, distraction, guided imagery, humor, music therapy, acupuncture, TENS technology, hypnosis, massage, or others as patient/family wishes

Other interventions, based on patient/family needs

h. *Other considerations*

Assess disease process progression

Other interventions, based on patient/family needs

RN to assess the patient's response to treatments and interventions and to report to physician any changes, unfavorable responses, or reactions

- *Home health aide or certified nursing assistant*

Effective and safe personal care

Safe ADL assistance and support

Respite care and active listening skills

Observation and reporting

Meal preparation

Homemaker services

Comfort care

Other duties

- *Social worker*

Psychosocial assessment of patient and family/caregiver, including adjustment to illness and its implications

Identification of optimal coping strategies

Financial assessment and counseling regarding food acquisition, ability to prepare, and costs of needed medications or wound care supplies

Intervention/support related to terminal illness and loss

Emotional/spiritual support

Depression/fear assessed

Facilitate communication among patient, family, and hospice team

Identification of caregiver role strain necessitating respite/relief measures/support

Referral/linkage to community services and resources as indicated

Grief counseling and intervention/support related to illness/loss

Patient/caregiver counseling and support

For patients who live alone with no support system (e.g., able, available, willing caregiver[s]), obtain resources to enable patient to remain in home

Identification of illness-related psychiatric condition necessitating care

Funeral and burial planning assistance

- *Volunteer(s)*
  Support, friendship, companionship, and presence
  Comfort and dignity maintained/provided for patient and family
  Errands and transportation
  Advocacy and respite
  Other services, based on interdisciplinary team recommendations and patient/caregiver needs

- *Spiritual counselor*
  Spiritual assessment and care
  Counseling, intervention, and support related to that dimension of life related to life's meaning (consistent with patient's beliefs)
  Support, listening, and presence
  Pray with or for the patient/family, using prayers familiar to patient's religious background (per their wishes)
  Participation in sacred or spiritual rituals or practices
  Other supportive care, based on patient's/family's needs and belief systems

- *Dietitian/Nutritional counseling*
  Supportive counseling with patient/family indicating that patient will have a decreased appetite and usually at some point may not eat/drink
  Assessment and recommendations for swallowing difficulties
  Teaching and support of family members and caregivers
  Support and care with food and nourishment as desired by patient
  Encourage oral nutritional supplements for increased caloric and protein intake
  Encourage adequate fluids
  Evaluation/management of nutritional deficits and needs
  Food, dietary recommendations incorporate patient choice and wishes

- *Occupational therapist*
  Evaluation of ADLs and functional mobility
  Assess for need for adaptive equipment and assistive devices
  Safety assessment of patient's environment and ADLs
  Assessment for energy conservation training
  Assessment of upper-extremity function, retraining motor skills, and/or splinting for contracture(s)

4

- *Physical therapist*
  Evaluation
  Assessment of patient's environment for safety
  Instruct in transfer training or bed mobility exercises and positioning to facilitate healing
  Pain assessment/reduction factors
  Strengthening exercises/program
  Assessment of gait safety and home safety measures
  Instruct/supervise caregiver and volunteers on home exercise program for conditioning and strength
  Assistive, adaptive devices and evaluation of equipment and teaching
  Progressive mobility
  Assist with selection of pressure-relieving devices

- *Speech-language pathologist*
  Evaluation for speech/swallowing problems
  Food texture recommendations
  Alternate functional communication

- *Bereavement counselor*
  Assessment of the needs of the bereaved family and friends
  Support and intervention, based on assessment and ongoing findings
  Presence and counseling
  Supportive visits, follow-up, and other interventions (e.g., mailings, calls)
  Other services related to bereavement work and support

- *Pharmacist*
  Evaluation of hospice patient with constipation on cathartics, stool softeners, and other medications for possible food/drug and drug/drug interactions
  Medication monitoring regarding therapeutic levels and dosages
  Pain consult and input into interdisciplinary plan of care related to pain control, palliation, and symptom management
  Assessment of medication regimen and plan for safety and compliance

- *Music, massage, art, or other therapies or services*
  Evaluation and intervention based on patient's and caregiver's unique wishes and needs that support care, comfort, and death in the setting of the patient's choice
  Pet therapy (including patient's pet, if available) and therapeutic intervention
  Assessment plan to engage patient and support comfort, quality, enjoyment, and dignity

6. **Outcomes for care**

- *Hospice nursing*
  Patient and caregiver verbalize satisfaction with care
  Educational tools/plans incorporated in daily care, and patient and caregiver verbalize understanding of safe, needed care

Patient will decide on care, interventions, and evaluation

Caregiver effective in care management and knows whom to call for questions/concerns

Patient will express satisfaction with hospice support received and will experience increased comfort

Patient will be made comfortable at home through death in accordance with the patient's wishes

Effective pain control and symptom control verbalized by patient

Patient verbalizes understanding of and adheres to care and medication regimens

Patient and caregiver supported through patient's death

Comfort maintained through course of care

Patient and family receive hospice support and care, and family members and friends are able to spend quality time with the patient

Caregiver able and verbalizes comfort with role and lists when to call hospice team members

Patient supported through and receives the maximum benefit from palliative chemotherapy and radiation with minimal complications

Patient and caregiver list adverse reactions, potential complications, and signs/symptoms of infection (e.g., sputum change, chest congestion)

Comfort maintained through death with dignity

Pain effectively managed, and patient verbalizes comfort

Patient is protected from injury, has stable respiratory status, and is compliant with medication, safety, and care regimens

Comfort and individualized intervention of patient with immobility/bedbound status (e.g., skin, urinary, musculature, vascular)

Spiritual and psychosocial needs met (specify) as defined by patient and caregiver throughout course of care

Patient and caregiver will demonstrate _____ % behavioral compliance with instructions related to medications, diet, and skin care

Infection-free wound healing by _____ (specify date)

Patient states pain is _____ on 0–10 scale by next visit

Patient and caregiver demonstrate appropriate back-up or "rescue" therapies for breakthrough pain or other symptoms (e.g., dyspnea)

Patient and caregiver correctly demonstrate/provide incisional or other wound care

Optimal circulation and nutrition for patient to support healing

Adherence to POC by patient and caregivers and ability to demonstrate safe and supportive care

Behavioral compliance with home care regimen

Patient and caregiver compliant with comprehensive wound care program, including pressure reduction, pain management, nutritional support, and positioning regimen

Wound site healing and infection free by _____ (specify date)

Wound closure occurring in patient with burns as demonstrated by measurements that show a decrease in wound size (specify)

Patient and caregiver will demonstrate _____ % behavioral compliance with instructions related to medications, diet, and wound/skin care

4

Optimal nutrition/hydration needs maintained/addressed as evidenced
by patient's weight maintained/decreased by/increased by _____ lbs

Patient will be maintained in home stating/demonstrating adherence
to POC

Adherence to multiple medication regimen

Laboratory values (specify) will be improved/WNL for patient

Caregiver and patient able to self-manage care, ADLs, diet, safety,
medications, and exercise regimens

Medications regulated as demonstrated by stable blood levels

Caregiver and patient verbalize symptoms that necessitate calling the
physician and intervention/follow-up

Supportive and skillful care to patient with draining wound

Comfort through death with support and care of hospice team

Mental distress, depression, and fear of dying addressed throughout
care by hospice team

Patient and family able to care for and support patient

Patient and caregiver can verbalize symptoms, changes, or accelerations
that necessitate call to physician

Patient and family demonstrate compliance to medication and other
therapeutic interventions

Patient demonstrates stabilization and increased or enhanced coping
skills related to functioning and depression

Pain and symptoms managed/controlled in setting of patient/family
choice (e.g., patient/family report ability to eat, sleep, speak with
pacing)

Planned and effective bowel program, as evidenced by regular bowel
movements and patient/family report of comfort

Death with dignity and pain/symptoms controlled in setting of
patient/family choice

Optimal comfort, support, and dignity provided throughout illness

Death with maximum comfort through effective symptom control with
specialized hospice support

Patient and caregiver able to list adverse drug reactions/problems
with medication regimen and whom to call for follow-up and
resolution

Patient's/family's privacy, independence, and choices supported with
respect and maintained through death

Enhancement and support of quality of life

Effective symptom relief and control (e.g., a peaceful and comfortable
death at home, depression controlled, some enjoyment of life)

Maximizing the patient's quality of life (e.g., alert and pain free or as
patient wishes)

Pharmacological and nonpharmacological interventions such as
localized heat application, biofeedback, massage, positioning,
relaxation methods, and music

Patient cared for and family supported through death with physical,
psychosocial, spiritual, and other concerns/needs
acknowledged/addressed

4

Patient- and family-centered hospice care provided based on the
   patient's/family's unique situation and needs

Infection control and palliation through death in setting of patient's choice

Grief/bereavement expression and support provided

Patient is pain free by next _____ visit

Caregiver demonstrates ability to manage pain, where applicable

Patient maintains comfort and dignity throughout illness

Other outcomes/goals, based on the patient condition with input from
   the hospice team and patient and family

- *Home health aide or certified nursing assistant*
   Effective hygiene, personal care, and comfort
   ADL assistance
   Safe environment maintained
   Respite and advocacy
   Reinforce wound dressings, as indicated

- *Social worker*
   Problem identified and addressed, with patient/caregiver linked with
      appropriate support services and plan of care successfully implemented
   Patient and caregiver cope adaptively with illness and death
   Adaptive adjustment to changed body and body image
   Psychosocial support and counseling offered to patient/caregivers
      experiencing loss and grief
   Caregiver system assessed, and development of stable caregiver plan
      facilitated
   Funeral and burial planning assistance

- *Volunteer(s)*
   Comfort, companionship, and friendship extended to patient/family
   Support provided as defined by the needs of the patient/caregiver
   Patient and family supported by team with care, comfort, and
      companionship

- *Spiritual counselor*
   Spiritual support offered and provided as defined by needs of
      patient/caregiver
   Provision of spiritual support and care based on the assessed and
      ongoing needs of the patient and family
   Spiritual support offered, and patient and family needs met
   Patient and family express relief of symptoms of spiritual suffering
   Support, listening, and presence
   Participation in sacred or spiritual rituals or practice
   Pray with or for the patient/family, using prayers familiar to patient's
      religious background (per their wishes)

- *Dietitian/Nutritional counseling*
   Patient and family verbalize comprehension of changing nutritional needs
   Family and caregiver integrate dietary recommendations into nutrition
      teaching (where appropriate)

4

Patient and caregiver know whom to call for nutrition- and
hydration-related questions/concerns
Nutrition/hydration per patient's choices
Caregiver integrates recommendations into daily meal planning

* *Occupational therapist*
Patient and caregiver demonstrate maximum independence with ADLs,
adaptive techniques, and assistive devices
Patient and caregiver demonstrate maximum safety in ADLs and
functional mobility
Patient and caregiver demonstrate effective use of energy conservation
Verbalization/demonstration of improved functional activity level and
enhanced quality of life
Patient and caregiver demonstrate effective use of diaphragmatic
breathing to reduce shortness of breath and relaxation techniques to
help in pain/symptom management
Patient and caregiver demonstrate correct use of exercise and splints for
maximum upper-extremity function and joint position

* *Physical therapist*
Prevention of complications
Home exercise and upper-extremity program taught to caregiver
Optimal strength, mobility, and function maintained/achieved
Compliance with home exercise program by _____ (specify date)

* *Speech-language pathologist*
Communication method implemented, and patient able to be
understood as self-reported or reported by family/caregivers
Safe swallowing and functional communication
Recommended lists of food/textures for safety and patient choice

* *Bereavement counselor*
Support services related to grief provided to patient and family
Well-being and resolution process of grief initiated and followed
through bereavement services

* *Pharmacist*
Regimen for bowel regimen successful as self-reported by patient and
in update at team meeting
Multiple drug regimen reviewed for food/drug and drug/drug
interactions in patient on multiple medications
Stability and safety in complex medication regimen with maximum
benefit to patient
Effective pain and symptom control and symptom management as
reported by patient/caregiver

* *Music, massage, art, or other therapies or services*
Therapeutic massage/touch effective for patient as self-reported or
observed by caregivers/family
Improved muscle tone, relaxation, and/or sleep
Patient comfortable and relaxed (e.g., sleeping) after massage

Music therapy intervention based on assessment to decrease pain
  perception and provide emotional expression and support
Maintenance of comfort and physical, psychosocial, and spiritual health
Patient has pet's presence as desired—in all care sites, when possible
Holistic health maintained and comfort achieved through
        _____ (specify modality)

7. **Patient, family, and caregiver educational needs**
   Educational needs are the care regimens that contribute to safe and effec-
   tive care at home between the hospice team's visits. These include the
   following:
   The basic tenets of hospice and the availability of support 24 hours a
     day, 7 days a week
   Home safety assessment and counseling
   The patient's medication regimen
   Anticipated disease progression
   Safe and proper body mechanics to promote patient comfort and
     prevent caregiver safety problems
   Other teaching specific to the patient's and family's unique needs
   Support groups available to patient's family, such as the hospice
     program's "Caregiver Support Group" meetings for family
     members and friends of the patient
   All aspects of the specific care related to wound care, including
     effective handwashing techniques, safe disposal of soiled dress-
     ings, and other infection control measures
   The importance of optimal nutrition and, when possible, exercise to
     speed the healing process
   Medication instruction, including schedule, route, functions, and
     possible side effects
   Other aspects of care, based on patient's unique medical condition
     and needs

8. **Specific tips for quality and reimbursement**
   Document any variances to expected outcomes. There are many models
   of hospice programs.
   The Medicare hospice benefit does not require that the patient be
   homebound or have identified skilled needs. For further information on
   this benefit, please refer to CMS Hospice Manual 21.
   Should the patient's status deteriorate and increased personal care
   be needed, obtain a telephone order for the increased service, noting
   frequency and estimating the duration.
   Obtain a telephone order for all medication and treatment changes of
   the medical regimen, and document these in the clinical record.
   Unless the patient is in a hospice insurance program, some insurers
   will not pay for a skilled clinician visit that is made at death if the patient
   is dead when the clinician arrives at the home. From a Medicare home
   care perspective, the visit at the time of death may be covered when the
   orders and clinical record document assessment of the patient's status or

signs of death/life or state law allows pronouncement of death by an RN.

Document patient deterioration

Document dehydration, dehydrating

Document patient change or instability

Document pain, other symptoms not controlled

Document status after acute episode of _____ (specify)

Document positive urine, sputum, etc. culture; patient started on _____ (specify ordered antibiotic therapy)

Document any impaction; impaction removed manually

Document RN in frequent communication with physician regarding _____ (specify)

Document febrile at _____, pulse change at _____, irr., irr.

Document change noted in ——

Document bony prominences red, opening

Document RN contacted physician regarding _____ (specify)

Document marked SOB

Document alteration in mental status

Document medications being adjusted, regulated, or monitored

Document unable to manage ADLs, personal care

Document all interdisciplinary team meetings and communication in the POC and in the progress notes of the clinical record

All hospice team members involved should have input into the POC and document their interventions and goals

Document all teaching accomplished with family or caregiver

Document progress toward goals, when identified

Document description of pressure ulcer

Document infected area

Document any discharge and odor and amount

Document draining wound

Document up only with assistance

Document can only transfer safely

Document length, width, depth of wound, drainage, odor, surrounding tissue

Document any changes, including specific care provided

Document medication(s) changed or medication(s) being regulated

Document RN contacted physician regarding _____ (specify)

Document any change in the patient's status or POC

Take photograph of wound(s) to substantiate findings, document at onset of care have patient sign release, photograph for the clinical record

Specify any learning barriers, such as arthritic hands, poor eyesight, and language barriers

Document the specific teaching accomplished and the behavioral outcomes of that teaching

Document clearly the status of the pressure ulcer and the clinical progress toward healing and patient-centered goal achievement

It is the professional nurse's responsibility to remember that it is not just the dressing change that occurs. When a nurse makes a home visit, an assessment of the wound healing or deterioration and teaching occur. There should also be observation and assessment of the wound and the surrounding skin. These skills usually require the skills of a clinician. All these components contribute to safe, effective wound care.

Document progress toward wound healing

Document patient or wound deterioration

Document any change that affects the provision of safe care

Document wound draining, amount, and site

Document any medication change(s)

Document progress or deterioration in wound healing, and take measurements at least once a week

The way to help third-party payors understand these components is to clearly record the care you provided on each skilled visit. The specifics related to the wound size, drainage, odor, involvement of tissues/structures, and your skilled assessment of the healing or potential for healing will be helpful to those having to make a payment decision about the services provided.

Wound dressing or care orders should always include the specific orders such as aseptic or clean technique, wound location, frequency of change, and any special supplies needed to safely and effectively follow the POC.

Document coordination of services or consultation of the other members of the IDT

Document communications and care coordination with other care providers, such as skilled health care facility or nursing home staff, inpatient team members, and hired caregivers

Document in the clinical notes the clear progression of symptoms and interventions that demonstrate the overall management of _____ (specify)

Document when/if the patient has respiratory changes, shortness of breath, exacerbation of conditions, dysphagia, changes in pain, and/or other symptoms and that they are identified and resolved

Remember that the clinical documentation is key to measuring compliance for quality and reimbursement purposes. Care coordination, timely verbal and initial physician orders, and assessment and addressing of spiritual and psychosocial needs should be ongoing and documented in the patient's clinical record

The documentation should support that all hospice care supports comfort and dignity while meeting patient/family needs

The documentation should include ongoing assessment and management of pain and other symptoms and the anticipation and prevention of secondary symptoms such as constipation

It is important to note that all team members, including clinician and social workers, should assess, identify, and "hear" spiritual needs that the patient/family want to be addressed. These spiritual issues are key to the provision of quality hospice care and cannot be addressed effectively and promptly by the spiritual counselor only

4

Document clearly symptoms, clinical changes, and assessment findings related to pain and patient care

Document patient changes, symptoms, and clinical information identified from visits and team conferences that support hospice care and a limited life expectancy

Clearly support in the documentation the rationale that supports/explains the progression of the illness from the chronic to terminal stages

Document mentation, behavioral, and/or cognitive changes

Document dysphagia, weight loss, increased shortness of breath, dyspnea, infection, sepsis, new or changed medications, etc.

Document changes to the POC such as medications, services, frequency, communication, and concurrence of other team members

Your assessments, observations, and clinical findings are information that assists in painting a picture to support coverage and documentation requirements for hospice care

Document any hospitalizations and changed clinical findings

Document patient changes, symptoms, psychosocial issues impacting the care, and information gathered at the patient/family visits and during team meetings

The documentation should reflect ongoing effects of the terminal condition, the patient's/family's difficulty with care or coping, and the continued desire for hospice care

Document any skin changes (e.g., inflamed, painful, weeping skin site[s])

Document when the patient is actively dying, deteriorating, or progressing toward death

Remember that the "litmus test" of care coordination rests on the quality of the clinical documentation by all team members. Review one of your patient's clinical records and ask yourself the following: "If I was unable to give a verbal report/update on this patient, would a peer be able to pick up and provide the same level of care and know (from the documentation) the current orders, medications, and other details that contribute to effective hospice care?"

This patient population usually has many clinical changes that should be documented. These include weight loss and multiple and changed medication regimens with varying routes. Side effects to the drug regimen should be observed, noted, documented, and reported

9. Queries for quality

Wound and pressure ulcer care
- *Is patient's pain managed adequately?*
- *Is patient's anxiety managed adequately?*
- *Is patient's functional ability/status clearly documented?*
- *What is the status of the patient's pressure ulcer, treatment regimen, and support surfaces?*
- *Have you documented to the interdisciplinary POC?*

Pressure ulcer care
- *Is patient's pain managed adequately?*
- *Is patient's anxiety managed adequately?*
- *Is patient's functional ability/status clearly documented?*
- *What is the status of the patient's pressure ulcer, treatment regimen and support surfaces?*
- *Have you documented to the interdisciplinary POC?*

10. **Resources for hospice care and practice**
    The Agency for Health Care Policy and Research has *Pressure Ulcers: Prediction and Prevention, Pressure Ulcers: Treatment, Treating Pressure Sores: Consumer Guide,* and *Preventing Pressure Ulcers: Patient Guide,* which can be ordered by calling 1-800-358-9295. The Wound Care Institute, Inc. offers *Wound Care Information,* a newsletter on computer disk. For more information, or to order, send a fax request to (305)944-6260 or order via their web site at woundcare.org

PART FIVE

HOSPICE CARE OF CHILDREN
Special Patients and Families

OUTLINE FOR CARE GUIDELINES

1. **General Considerations**

2. **Needs for Visit**

3. **Safety Considerations**

4. **Potential Diagnoses and Codes**

5. **Skills and Services Identified**
   * Hospice Nursing
     a. Comfort and Symptom Control
     b. Safety and Mobility Considerations
     c. Emotional/Spiritual Considerations
     d. Skin Care
     e. Elimination Considerations
     f. Hydration/Nutrition
     g. Therapeutic/Medication Regimens
     h. Other Considerations
   * Home Health Aide or Certified Nursing Assistant
   * Social Worker
   * Volunteer(s)
   * Spiritual Counselor
   * Dietitian/Nutritional Counseling
   * Occupational Therapist
   * Physical Therapist
   * Speech-Language Pathologist
   * Bereavement Counselor
   * Pharmacist (for some diagnoses)
   * Music, Massage, Art, or Other Therapies or Services

6. **Outcomes for Care**

7. **Patient, Family, and Caregiver Educational Needs**

8. **Specific Tips for Quality and Reimbursement**

9. **Queries for Quality**

10. **Resources for Hospice Care and Practice**

5

ACQUIRED IMMUNE DEFICIENCY SYNDROME (AIDS) (CARE OF THE CHILD WITH)

1. **General considerations**

   Children with HIV and AIDS are susceptible to numerous infections, including encephalopathy with associated developmental delays, cardiomyopathy, diarrhea, and thrush. The hospice team and the child and family work together to meet these children's myriad needs for care, love, infection control, and symptom relief.

   Please refer to "Care of the Medically Fragile Child," "Care of the Child with Cancer," or "Infusion Care" should these sections also pertain to your patient.

2. **Needs for visit**

   Physician order for hospice care, specific to the hospice program's admission criteria and policies

   Standard precautions supplies

   Vital signs equipment for baseline assessment

   Other supplies or equipment, based on physician orders

3. **Safety considerations**

   Infection control/standard precautions

   Night-light

   Medication safety and storage

   Infant/Child safety considerations (e.g., car seat, electrical outlet protection, sleeping position)

   Municipal water source/safety

   Pet care (e.g., infection control)

   Symptoms that necessitate immediate reporting/assistance

   Safety related to home medical equipment

   Smoke detector and fire evacuation plan

   Others, based on patient's unique condition and environment

4. **Potential diagnoses and codes**

AIDS (general)	042
Anemia	042 and 285.9
Bacterial infections, recurrent with AIDS	042
Candidiasis and AIDS	042 and 112.9
Candidiasis, esophageal and AIDS	042 and 112.84
Candidiasis, oral and AIDS	042 and 112.0
Candidiasis, vaginal and AIDS	042 and 112.1
Cardiomyopathy and AIDS	042 and 425.4
Cervical cancer and AIDS	042 and 180.9
Chorioretinitis and AIDS	042 and 363.20
Cytomegalovirus and AIDS	042 and 078.5, and 363.20
Cytomegalovirus retinitis and AIDS	042, 078.5, and 363.20
Developmental delays, neurological	042
Diarrhea and AIDS	042 and 787.91

Encephalitis and AIDS	042 and 323.0
Encephalopathy and AIDS	042 and 348.30
Endocarditis and AIDS	042 and 424.90
Esophagitis and AIDS	042 and 530.10
Failure to thrive and AIDS	042 and 783.7
Herpes simplex and AIDS	042 and 054.9
Herpes zoster and AIDS	042 and 053.9
Histoplasmosis and AIDS	042 and 115.90
HTLV III and AIDS	042
Kaposi's sarcoma and AIDS	042 and 176.9
Lymphocytic interstitial pneumonia and AIDS	042 and 516.8
Meningitis and AIDS	042 and 321.2
Mycobacterium avium intracellulare and AIDS	042 and 031.0
Neurological development delays and AIDS	042 and 315.9
Neuropathy, peripheral and AIDS	042 and 357.4
Neutropenia and AIDS	042 and 288.0
Peripheral neuropathy and AIDS	042 and 357.4
Pneumocystis carinii pneumonia and AIDS	042 and 136.3
Pneumonia (bacterial) and AIDS	042 and 482.9
Pneumonia (NOS) and AIDS	042 and 486
Pneumonia (viral) and AIDS	042 and 480.9
Polymyositis and AIDS	042 and 710.4
Polyradiculopathy and AIDS	042 and 357.4
Protein-caloric malnutrition and AIDS	042 and 263.9
Quadriplegia and AIDS	042 and 344.00
Retinal detachment and AIDS	042 and 361.9
Retinal hemorrhage and AIDS	042 and 362.81
Seizures and AIDS	042 and 780.39
Sepsis and AIDS	042 and 038.9
Shigella and AIDS	042 and 004.9
Shigella, dysentery, and AIDS	042 and 004.9
Thrombocytopenia and AIDS	042 and 287.5
Toxoplasmosis and AIDS	042 and 130.9
Tuberculosis (pulmonary) and AIDS	042 and 011.90
Wasting syndrome and AIDS	042 and 799.4

5. **Skills and services identified**

- *Hospice nursing*

    a. *Comfort and symptom control*
       Complete initial assessment of the child with an impaired
          immune response and multiple system infections
       Presentation of hospice philosophy and services
       Explain patient rights and responsibilities to parents
       Assess child, family, and caregiver wishes and expectations
          regarding care
       Assess child, family, and caregiver resources available for care
       Teach family or caregiver physical care of child

5

Provision of volunteer support to child and family

Assess pain and other symptoms, including site, duration, characteristics, and relief measures

RN to provide and teach effective oral care and comfort measures

RN assessment of pulmonary status, including dyspnea, changed or abnormal breath sounds, retractions, respiratory rate, flaring, and other symptoms of respiratory compromise

RN to observe and assess all systems and symptoms every visit

RN to report changes or new symptoms to physician

RN to assess and monitor child's use of and response to aerosol therapy medication

RN to assess child for candidal diaper rash or oral thrush

RN to evaluate caregiving ability, particularly if parents or other caregivers are HIV+

RN to monitor child's blood pressure and other vital signs

Instruct child, parents, and caregivers in all aspects of effective handwashing techniques and proper care of bodily fluids and excretions

RN to instruct parents and caregivers to call physician for symptoms of fever, increased irritability, vomiting, diarrhea, suspected ear or other infection, decreased appetite, new cough, or any new symptom or complaint

RN to instruct parents regarding the need to isolate HIV+ child from anyone with known infections, such as other children at school who have chicken pox, measles, or other communicable infections that are life threatening for the child with AIDS

RN to instruct parents or caregivers regarding signs and symptoms that necessitate calling RN or physician

RN to provide support to child with new tumor necessitating surgery, chemotherapy, or radiation

RN to address sexuality concerns of young adolescent with AIDS and the importance of safe sexual expression, including the use of condoms, abstinence, or other techniques

Teach child/family about realistic expectations of disease process

Teach care of dying and signs/symptoms of impeding death

Presence and support

Other interventions, based on child/family needs

b. *Safety and mobility considerations*

Provide child with home safety information and instruction related to _____ and documented in the clinical record

Instruct on pet care and avoidance of cross-contamination, and check with physician about certain types of pets

RN to teach child and parents safe use of oxygen therapy

RN to instruct child and family about safety and standard precautions in the home

RN to teach parents and caregiver about all aspects of child's needed care for safe and effective management at home

Other interventions, based on child/family needs

c. *Emotional/Spiritual considerations*

Psychosocial assessment of child and family regarding disease and prognosis

Clinician to provide emotional support to child and caregivers with chronic/terminal illness and associated implications, especially if parent is HIV+

Assess grief, denial, and guilt of parents and caregivers

Other interventions, based on child/family needs

d. *Skin care*

RN to teach parents and caregivers all aspects of wound care, including safe disposal of dressing supplies

Other interventions, based on child/family needs

e. *Elimination considerations*

Assess bowel regimen, and implement program as needed

RN to closely monitor parenteral feeding catheter side for infection and other problems

Other interventions, based on child/family needs

f. *Hydration/Nutrition*

Weigh child q visit and review intake diary

Instruct parents or caregivers regarding prescribed diet

Monitor for adverse effects of medication, particularly steroids

Teach parents and caregivers about the importance of optimal hydration and nutrition

Other interventions, based on child/family needs

g. *Therapeutic/Medication regimens*

RN to teach parents and caregivers about new medications

RN to instruct parents or caregivers on all aspects of medications, including schedule, functions, and side effects

RN to assess the child's unique response to treatments and interventions and to report to the physician changes, unfavorable responses, or reactions

Other interventions, based on child/family needs

h. *Other considerations*

Assess disease process progression

Other interventions, based on child/family needs

- **Home health aide or certified nursing assistant**

Effective and safe personal care

Safe ADL assistance and support

Respite care

Active listening skills

Meal preparation

Observation and reporting

Homemaker services

Assist with diversional therapy (e.g., playing games)

Comfort care

Other duties

5

- *Social worker*
  Psychosocial assessment (age appropriate) of patient and family/care-
      giver, including adjustment to long-term illness and its implications
  Identification of optimal coping strategies
  Financial assessment and counseling regarding food acquisition,
      ability to prepare, and costs of needed medications
  Intervention/support related to terminal illness and loss
  Emotional/Spiritual support
  Depression/fear assessed and addressed
  Facilitate communication among patient, family and hospice team
  Referral/Linkage to community services and resources as indicated
  Grief counseling and intervention/support related to illness/loss
  Patient/Caregiver counseling and support
  Identification of illness-related psychiatric condition necessitating care
  Funeral and burial planning assistance

- *Volunteer(s)*
  Support, friendship, companionship, and presence
  Comfort and dignity maintained/provided for patient and family
  Errands and transportation
  Other services, based on interdisciplinary team recommendations and
      patient/caregiver needs

- *Spiritual counselor*
  Spiritual assessment and care
  Counseling, intervention, and support related to that dimension of life
      related to life's meaning (consistent with child's beliefs)
  Support, listening, and presence
  Pray with or for the patient/family, using prayers familiar to the
      patient's religious background (per their wishes)
  Participation in sacred or spiritual rituals or practices
  Other supportive care, based on patient's/family's needs and belief
      systems
  Pray with or for the patient/family, using prayers familiar to patient's
      religious background (per their wishes)

- *Dietitian/Nutritional counseling*
  Supportive counseling with patient/family indicating that patient
      will have a decreased appetite and usually at some point may
      not eat/drink
  Assessment and recommendations for swallowing difficulties
  Teaching and support of family members and caregivers
  Support and care with food and nourishment as desired by patient
  Evaluation/Management of nutritional deficits and needs
  Food and dietary recommendations incorporate child's choices
      and wishes

- *Occupational therapist*
  Evaluation of activities of daily living (ADLs) and functional mobility
  Assess for need for adaptive equipment and assistive devices
  Safety assessment of patient's environment and ADLs

5

Assessment for energy conservation training
Assessment of upper-extremity function, retraining motor skills

- *Physical therapist*
Evaluation
Assessment of patient's environment for safety
Safe transfer training or bed mobility exercises
Pain assessment/reduction factors
Strengthening exercises/program
Assessment of gait safety and home safety measures
Instruct/Supervise caregiver and volunteers on home exercise pro-
gram for conditioning and strength
Assistive, adaptive devices and evaluation of equipment and teaching

- *Speech-language pathologist*
Evaluation for speech/swallowing problems
Food texture recommendations
Alternate functional communication

- *Bereavement counselor*
Assessment of the needs of the bereaved family and friends
Support and intervention, based on assessment and ongoing findings
Presence and counseling
Supportive visits, follow-up, and other interventions
(e.g., mailings, calls)
Other services related to bereavement work and support

- *Pharmacist*
Evaluation of hospice patient with constipation on cathartics, stool
softeners, and other medications for possible food/drug and
drug/drug interactions
Medication monitoring regarding therapeutic levels and dosages
Pain consult and input into interdisciplinary plan of care (POC)
related to pain control, palliation, and symptom management
Assessment of medication regimen and plan for safety and compliance

- *Music, massage, art, or other therapies or services*
Evaluation and intervention based on patient's and caregiver's unique
wishes and needs that support care, comfort, and death in the setting of the patient's choice
Assessment plan to engage patient and support comfort, quality,
enjoyment, and dignity
Promote expressions of grief and grieving through therapeutic activities **5**

6. **Outcomes for care**
- *Hospice nursing*
Comfort through death for child and family with support and care of
hospice team
Parent/Caregiver able to care for and support child with hospice
assistance
Parent/Caregiver can verbalize symptoms, changes, or questions that
necessitate call to hospice

Parent/Caregiver demonstrates compliance to medication and other care and therapeutic interventions

Pain and symptoms managed/controlled in setting of family choice

Death with dignity and pain/symptoms controlled in setting of family choice

Optimal comfort, support, and dignity provided to child throughout illness

Death with maximum comfort through effective symptom control with specialized hospice support

Parent/Caregiver able to list adverse drug reactions/problems with medication regimen and whom to call for follow-up and resolution

Enhancement and support of child's/family's quality of life

Effective symptom relief and control (e.g., a peaceful and comfortable death at home, pain and other symptoms controlled, and some enjoyment of life and play)

Pharmacological and nonpharmacological interventions used effectively for comfort and supportive care through illness

Child/Family cared for and family supported through death with physical, psychosocial, developmental, spiritual, and other concerns/needs acknowledged/addressed

Infection control and palliation through illness in setting of child/family choice

Grief/Bereavement expression and support provided to family

Patient is pain free by next _____ visit

Parent and caregiver demonstrate ability to manage pain and other symptoms, where applicable

Parent and caregiver demonstrate appropriate backup or "rescue" therapies for breakthrough pain or other symptoms (e.g., dyspnea)

Parent/Caregiver and child verbalize satisfaction with care

Support growth and developmental tasks of childhood

Successful pain and symptom management as verbalized by patient/caregiver

Patient will demonstrate adequate breathing patterns as evidenced by a lack of respiratory distress symptoms

Patient will be comfortable through illness

Patient and caregiver will demonstrate _____ % compliance with instructions related to care

Patient and caregiver demonstrate and practice effective hand washing and other infection-control measures (specify, e.g., disposal of waste, cleaning linens, other aspects of care at home)

Adherence to POC by patient and caregivers and able to demonstrate safe and supportive care of child

Nutritional needs maintained/addressed as evidenced by patient's weight maintained/increased by _____ lbs.

Patient's pulmonary status will be maintained/improved

Child and parent integrate information and care regarding implications of disease and terminal nature

Lab values (specify) will be improved/WNL for child

Catheter will remain patent and infection free

Caregiver adheres to/demonstrates compliance with multiple medication regimens (e.g., times, storage, refrigeration)

Child's educational play, and support needs met as verbalized by caregiver and adherence to plan

Palliative and symptomatic interventions to ensure optimal level of functioning in child

- ***Home health aide or certified nursing assistant***
  Effective hygiene, personal care, and comfort
  ADL assistance
  Safe environment maintained
  Comfort and life enjoyment, including play and activities of choices

- ***Social worker***
  Problem identification and addressed with child/caregiver and linked with appropriate support services and plan of care successfully implemented
  Patient/Caregiver copes adaptively with illness and death
  Adaptive adjustment to changed body and body image
  Psychosocial support and counseling offered/initiated to patient/caregivers experiencing loss and grief

- ***Volunteer(s)***
  Comfort, companionship, and friendship extended to patient/family
  Support provided as defined by the needs of the patient/caregiver
  Patient and family supported by team with care, comfort, and companionship

- ***Spiritual counselor***
  Spiritual support offered and provided as defined by needs of patient/caregiver
  Provision of spiritual support and care based on the assessed and ongoing needs of the patient and family
  Spiritual support offered, and patient and family needs met
  Patient and family express relief of symptoms of spiritual suffering

- ***Dietitian/Nutritional counseling***
  Family and caregiver integrate recommendations into nutrition teaching (where appropriate)
  Patient and parent know whom to call for nutrition- and hydration-related questions/concerns
  Nutrition/Hydration per patient's choices
  Caregiver integrating recommendations into daily meal planning (age dependent)
  Parent and caregiver verbalize comprehensive of changing nutritional needs

- ***Occupational therapist***
  Patient and caregiver demonstrate maximum independence with ADLs, adaptive techniques, and assistive devices

5

Patient and caregiver demonstrate maximum safety in ADLs and
functional mobility

Patient and caregiver demonstrate effective use of energy conservation

Verbalization/demonstration of improved functional activity level and
enhanced quality of life

Patient and caregiver demonstrate effective use of diaphragmatic
breathing to reduce shortness of breath and relaxation techniques
to help in pain/symptom management

- *Physical therapist*
  Prevention of complications
  Home exercise and upper-extremity program taught to parent/caregiver
  Optimal strength, mobility, and function maintained/achieved
  Compliance with home exercise program by _____ (specify date)

- *Speech-language pathologist*
  Communication method implemented, and patient able to be
  understood as self-reported or reported by family/caregivers
  Safe swallowing and functional communication
  Recommended lists of foods/textures for safety and choice

- *Bereavement counselor*
  Support services related to grief provided to patient and family
  Well-being and resolution process of grief initiated and followed
  through bereavement services

- *Pharmacist*
  Regimen for bowel regimen successful as self-reported by patient and
  in update at team meeting
  Multiple drug regimen reviewed for food/drug and drug/drug
  interactions in patient on multiple medications
  Stability and safety in complex medication regimen, with maximum
  benefit to patient
  Effective pain and symptom control and symptom management as
  reported by patient/caregiver

- *Music, massage, art, or other therapies or services*
  Therapeutic massage/touch effective for child as self-reported or
  observed by caregiver/family
  Improved muscle tone, relaxation, and/or sleep
  Patient comfortable and relaxed (e.g., sleeping) after massage
  Music therapy intervention based on assessment to decrease pain
  perception, provide emotional expression and support
  Maintenance of comfort, physical, psychosocial, and spiritual health
  Holistic health maintained and comfort achieved through
  _____ (specify modality)
  Patient/Family participate in grief work through art theraphy

7. **Patient, family, and caregiver educational needs**
   Educational needs are the care regimens that contribute to safe and effective
   care at home between the hospice team's visits. These include the following:

The basic tenets of hospice and the availability of support 24 hours a
day, 7 days a week

Home safety assessment and counseling

Anticipated disease progression

The patient's medication regimen

Safe and proper body mechanics to promote comfort and avoid caregiver safety problems

Other teaching specific to the child's and family's unique needs

Symptom management

Importance of adequate hydration and nutrition

Standard precaution protocols

Home safety concerns, issues, and teaching

The avoidance and prevention of infection, when possible

The importance of medical follow-up

Support groups and resources in the community available to the parent
and child

Other identified information needed, based on the child's and family's
unique medical and other needs

8. **Specific tips for quality and reimbursement**

Document any variances to expected outcomes. The care provided
is directed toward symptom and infection control and treatment.
These children and adolescents are usually so ill that there are many
skills the professional nurse and other team members must provide.
Document the coordination occurring among team members based
on the POC. The interdisciplinary conference notes should be reflected
in the clinical record. Refer to these meetings or communications
on any form used by third-party payors (e.g., your program's
update form). *In addition:*

Write the specific care and teaching instructions provided

Document your progress toward goals

Document any exacerbation of symptoms that necessitated another
visit, and be sure there is a physician order for care

Document all POC changes

Document all interactions/communications with the physician

Document the skills used in the provision of professional practice when
caring for the child (e.g., teaching, training, observation, assessment,
catheters, IV site care)

Many times these children are closely case managed to identify
problem early on; communicate information about the child's and
family's statuses and course of care necessitating intervention

Discuss other measurable changes and information that communicate
the status of the child and the need for skilled home care services

Document changes to the POC, such as medications, services,
frequency, communication, and concurrence of other team members

Document coordination of services or consultation of the other
members of the IDT

5

Document communications and care coordination with other care providers, such as inpatient team members and hired caregivers

Document in the clinical notes the clear progression of symptoms and interventions that demonstrate the overall management of symptoms_____ (specify)

Document when/if the patient has respiratory changes, shortness of breath, exacerbation of conditions, changes in pain, and/or other symptoms and that they are identified and resolved

Remember that the clinical documentation is key to measuring compliance for quality and reimbursement purposes. Care coordination, timely verbal and initial physician orders, and assessment and addressing of spiritual and psychosocial needs should be ongoing and documented in the patient's clinical record

Document that all hospice care supports comfort and dignity while meeting child/family needs

The documentation should include ongoing assessment and management of pain and other symptoms and the anticipation and prevention of secondary symptoms such as constipation

It is important to note that all team members, should assess, identify, and "hear" spiritual needs that the patient/family want to be addressed. These spiritual issues are key to the provision of high-quality hospice care and cannot be addressed effectively and promptly by the spiritual counselor only

Document clearly symptoms, clinical changes, and assessment findings related to pain and patient care

Document weight loss, increased shortness of breath, dyspnea, infection, sepsis, new or changed medications, etc.

Document any skin changes (e.g., inflamed, painful, weeping skin site[s])

Remember that the "litmus test" of care coordination rests on the quality of the clinical documentation by all team members. Review one of your patient's clinical records and ask yourself the following: "If I was unable to give a verbal report/update on this child/family's course of care, would a peer be able to pick up and provide the same level of care and know (from the documentation) the current orders, medications, and other details that contribute to effective hospice care?"

This patient population usually has many clinical changes that should be documented. These include weight loss and multiple and changed medication regimens with varying routes. Side effects to the drug regimen should be observed, noted, documented, and reported

Your assessments, observations, and clinical findings are information that assists in painting a picture to support coverage and documentation requirements for hospice care

Document any hospitalizations and changed clinical findings

Document patient changes, symptoms, psychosocial issues impacting the care, and information gathered at the child/family visits and during team meetings

Document all care provided and outcomes of that care

5

Document the child's/parent's responses to care, changes, and
   communications with the physician and other hospice team members
Document the course of care, including why the infant/child was
   admitted for care, the plan, and support provided

9. **Queries for quality**

   - *Is the child's pain managed adequately?*

   - *Is the child's anxiety managed adequately?*

   - *What infection control measures are implemented?*

   - *What are the child's symptoms?*

   - *Have you documented to the interdisciplinary POC?*

10. **Resources for hospice care and practice**
    The Centers for Disease Control and Prevention (CDC)
    National AIDS Hotline: 1-800-342-2437 or 1-800-342-AIDS
    The National AIDS Information Clearinghouse: 1-800-458-5231
    The AIDS Pediatric Clinical Trials Information Service:
       1-800-TRIALS-A (1-800-874-2572)
    The National Hemophiliac Foundation: 1-212-431-8541
    The CDC National AIDS Clearinghouse offers *Adolescents and HIV
       Disease* and *HIV and Your Child: Consumer Guide.* For more
       information, call 1-800-458-5231.
    *Guidelines for the Use of Antiretroviral Agents in Pediatric HIV
       Infection* is available free from the Department of Health
       and Human Services (HHS) by calling 1-800-458-5231 or
       1-800-448-0440.
    The Candlelighters Childhood Cancer Foundation offers many services
       for parents and children, including resources, services, advocacy,
       and support. Call 1-301-657-8401 or 1-800-366-2223 (CCCF) for
       information: or visit online at *www.candlelighters.org*
    Children's Hospice International: 703-684-0330 or
    web site: *www.chionline.org*
    Ann Armstrong–Davey and Sarah Zarbock (eds) (2001): *Hospice Care
       for children*, Oxford University Press.
    Institute of Medicine (2003). *When Children Die: Improving Palliative
       and End-of-life Care for Children and Their Families.* Washington,
       DC, National Academies Press. For full report and summary go to
       web site: *www.nap.edu.*

5

CANCER (CARE OF THE CHILD WITH)

1. **General considerations**

   The news that a child's prognosis is terminal is devastating. Brain tumors, leukemias, and solid tumors, such as Wilms', are some of the cancers seen in pediatric hospice. It is said that cancer is the leading cause of death from disease in children who are 3 to 15 years old and the second cause of death from all causes, surpassed only by death from injuries.

   Cancer care in children utilizes all facets of nursing and other skills. Death at any age is sad, but the suffering and death of children magnify the emotional turmoil. Parents know their child best, and in this role they are the teachers for care providers. Parental control should be maintained as much as possible. The child, the siblings, and the parents become the unit of care for comfort, support, and intervention.

   Please refer to "AIDS (Care of the Child With)," "Care of the Medically Fragile Child," and "Infusion Care" should these sections also pertain to your patients.

2. **Needs for visit**

   Physician order for hospice care, specific to the hospice program's admission criteria and policies

   Standard precautions supplies

   Vital signs equipment for baseline assessment

   Other supplies or equipment, based on physician orders

3. **Safety considerations**

   Infection control/standard precautions

   Night-light

   Medication safety and storage

   Child safety considerations (e.g., car seat, electrical outlet protection, sleeping position)

   Symptoms that necessitate immediate reporting/assistance

   Safety related to home medical equipment

   Smoke detector and fire evacuation plan

   Others, based on the patient's unique condition and environment

4. **Potential diagnoses and codes**

Acute lymphocytic leukemia	204.00
Acute myelogenous leukemia	205.00
Aplastic anemia	284.9
Astrocytoma	191.9
Bone marrow transplant (surgical)	41.00
Chronic leukemia	208.10
Chronic myelogenous leukemia	205.10
Ewing's tumor	170.9
Glioblastoma	191.9
Leukopenia	288.00

5

Metastases, general	199.1
Neuroblastoma	194.0
Wilm's tumor	189.0

5. **Skills and services identified**

- *Hospice nursing*

a. *Comfort and system control*

Admission of infant/child to hospice with _____ (specify)

Presentation of hospice philosophy and services

Explain patient rights and responsibilities to parents

Assess parent and caregiver wishes and expectations regarding care

Assess parent, family, and caregiver resources available for care

Teach parent or caregiver physical care of child

Provision of volunteer support to child and family

Assess pain and other symptoms, including site, duration, characteristics, and relief measures

RN to provide and teach effective oral care and comfort measures

Anticipate and encourage child and family input into care regimen(s)

Teach caregivers observational aspects of care, including fever, bleeding, bruising, and other signs unique to the disease or treatment

RN to monitor for seizure activity and perform neurological checks q visit

Teach the importance of effective hand washing and other infection-control measures, including the prevention and avoidance of infection when possible

RN to instruct caregiver to call physician for symptoms of fever, irritability, vomiting, diarrhea, suspected ear or other infection, decreased appetite, cough, or other complaint

Ongoing assessment and observation of cardiovascular, pulmonary, and respiratory statuses

Teach new pain and symptom control measures to parent

Identify and monitor pain, symptoms, and relief measures

Observation, assessment, and supportive care to child and family

Teach child/family use of standardized form/tool for pain to use between hospice team members' visit (and for care coordination between team members and child/family)

Teach parent principles of effective pain management

Effective management of pain and prevention of secondary symptoms

Interventions of symptoms directed toward comfort and palliation

Observation and assessment and communication with physician related to signs, new symptoms, increasing irritability, thrush, others

Pain assessment and management q visit, including source of pain

Teach parent/family about realistic expectations of disease process

Teach care of dying and signs/symptoms of impending death

Presence and support

Other interventions, based on child/family needs

5

b. *Safety and mobility considerations*
   Parent and caregiver provided with home safety information and
      instruction
   Teach parent regarding home safety and infection-control measures
   Other interventions, based on child/family needs

c. *Emotional/Spiritual considerations*
   Psychosocial assessment of child and family regarding disease and
      prognosis
   RN to provide emotional support to child and family
   Assess child's and parent's coping skills
   RN to provide emotional support to child and family with chronic or
      terminal illness and associated implications
   Assess for and manage plans for psychosocial and/or spiritual pain
      (e.g., fear, anxiety, interpersonal and other distress)
   Observation of child for neuropsychiatric complications of illness,
      including pain, irritability, and depression.
   Psychosocial aspects of pain control (e.g., depression) assessed and
      acknowledged with team support/intervention
   Ongoing acknowledgment of spiritually and related concerns of
      child/family and their belief systems
   Other interventions, based on child/family needs

d. *Skin care*
   RN to teach parents and caregivers all aspects of skin care
   Other interventions, based on child/family needs

e. *Elimination considerations*
   Assess bowel regimen, and implement program as needed
   Other interventions, based on child/family needs

f. *Hydration/Nutrition*
   Teach the importance of optimal nutrition and hydration
   Assessment and referral for child with thrush and painful
      swallowing
   Nutrition/hydration supported by offering foods/beverages of child's
      choice, when possible
   Other interventions, based on child/family needs

g. *Therapeutic/Medication regimens*
   Symptom control for side effects of radiation or chemotherapy
   RN to assess the child's unique response to treatments and
      interventions and to report to the physician changes, unfavorable
      responses, or reactions
   Teach new medications and effects
   Teach parent about medications and the management program,
      including strength, type, actions, times, and compliance tips
   Encourage parent to give the child medications on the schedule and
      around the clock
   Nonpharmacological or other interventions of relaxation, guided
      imagery, humor, music therapy, art therapy, bubble blowing, magic

5

presentations and wands, and massage for comfort during painful interventions

Other interventions, based on child/family needs

h. *Other considerations*

Assess disease process progression

Other interventions, based on child/family needs

- **Home health aide or certified nursing assistant**
  Effective and safe personal care
  Safe ADL assistance and support
  Respite care and active listening
  Observation and reporting
  Meal preparation
  Assist with diversional therapy (e.g., playing games)
  Homemaker services
  Comfort care
  Other duties

- **Social worker**
  Psychosocial assessment of patient and parent/caregiver, including adjustment to long-term illness and its implications
  Identification of optimal coping strategies
  Financial assessment and counseling regarding food acquisition, ability to prepare food, and costs of needed medications
  Intervention/support related to terminal illness and loss
  Emotional/spiritual support
  Depression/fear assessed and addressed
  Facilitate communication among patient, family, and hospice team
  Referral/Linkage to community services and resources as indicated
  Grief counseling and intervention/support related to illness/loss
  Patient and caregiver counseling and support
  Illness-related psychiatric condition necessitating care
  Funeral and burial planning assistance

- **Volunteer(s)**
  Support, friendship, companionship, presence, fun, and play (based on child's illness/age)
  Comfort and dignity maintained/provided for patient and family
  Errands and transportation
  Other services, based on interdisciplinary team recommendations and patient/caregiver needs

- **Spiritual counselor**
  Spiritual assessment and care
  Counseling, intervention, and support related to that dimension of life related to life's meaning (consistent with patient's beliefs)
  Support, listening, and presence
  Pray with or for the patient/family, using prayers familiar to patient's religious background (per their wishes)
  Participation in sacred or spiritual rituals or practices

5

Other supportive care, based on patient's/family's needs and belief
systems

- **_Dietitian/Nutritional counseling_**
  Supportive counseling with patient/parent indicating that patient will
  have a decreased appetite and usually at some point may not eat/drink
  Assessment and recommendations for swallowing difficulties
  Teaching and support of family members and caregivers
  Support and care with food and nourishment as desired by patient
  Evaluation/Management of nutritional deficits and needs
  Food and dietary recommendations incorporate patient's choice and
  wishes
  Allow child to eat whatever and whenever desired, with small, frequent
  feedings
  Tube feeding, as necessary
  Teach child to manage own tube feedings, "special care," when possible

- **_Occupational therapist_**
  Evaluation
  Energy conservation techniques
  Adaptive, assistive, and safety supports/devices and training
  ADL training
  Teach compensatory techniques

- **_Physical therapist_**
  Evaluation
  Assessment of patient's environment for safety
  Safe transfer training or bed mobility exercises
  Pain assessment/reduction factors
  Strengthening exercises/program
  Assessment of gait safety and home safety measures
  Instruct/Supervise caregiver and volunteers on home exercise program
  for conditioning and strength
  Assistive, adaptive devices and evaluation of equipment and teaching

- **_Speech-language pathologist_**
  Evaluation for speech/swallowing problems
  Food texture recommendations
  Alternate functional communication

- **_Bereavement counselor_**
  Assessment of the needs of the bereaved family and friends
  Support and intervention, based on assessment and ongoing findings
  Presence and counseling
  Supportive visits, follow-up, and other interventions (e.g., mailings, calls)
  Other services related to bereavement work and support

- **_Pharmacist_**
  Evaluation of hospice patient with constipation on cathartics, stool
  softeners, and other medications for possible food/drug and
  drug/drug interactions

Medication monitoring regarding therapeutic levels and dosages

Pain consult and input into interdisciplinary POC related to pain control, palliation, and symptom management

Assessment of medication regimen and plan for safety and compliance

- *Music, massage, art, or other therapies or services*

    Evaluation and intervention based on patient's and caregiver's unique wishes and needs that support care, comfort, and death in the setting of the patient's choice

    Assessment plan to engage patient and support comfort, quality, enjoyment, and dignity (e.g., play)

6. Outcomes for care

- *Hospice nursing*

    Comfort through death for child and family with support and care of hospice team

    Parent able to care for and support child with hospice support

    Parent can verbalize changes or symptoms that necessitate call to hospice

    Parent demonstrates compliance to medication and other care and therapeutic interventions

    Pain and symptoms managed/controlled in setting of family choice

    Death with dignity and pain/symptoms controlled in setting of family choice

    Optimal comfort, support, and dignity provided throughout illness

    Death with maximum comfort through effective symptom control with specialized hospice support

    Parent able to list adverse drug reactions/problem with medication regimen and whom to call for follow-up and resolution

    Enhancement and support of child's/family's quality of life

    Effective symptom relief and control (e.g., a peaceful and comfortable death at home, pain and other symptoms controlled, some enjoyment of life and play)

    Pharmacological and nonpharmacological interventions used effectively for comfort and supportive care through illness

    Child/Family cared for and family supported through death with physical, psychosocial, developmental, spiritual, and other concerns/needs acknowledged/addressed

    Infection control and palliation through illness in setting of patient's choice

    Grief/Bereavement expression and support provided to family

    Patient is pain free by next _____ visit

    Parent and caregiver demonstrate ability to manage pain and other symptoms, where applicable

    Observation and assessment of child's behavior, including expressions, usual activity level, and changes noted, to assist in pain identification and management

    Patient and parent verbalize satisfaction with care

5

Educational tools/plans incorporated in daily care, and child and
  caregiver verbalize understanding of safe, needed care

Patient and parent decide on care, interventions, and evaluation

Caregiver effective in care management and knows whom to call for
  questions/concerns

Parent and caregiver will express satisfaction with hospice support
  received and will experience increased comfort

Child will be made comfortable at home through death in accordance
  with the family/parent wishes

Effective pain control and symptom control communicated by child

Parent and caregiver verbalize understanding of and adhere to care and
  medication regimens

Child and family supported through patient's death

Comfort maintained through course of care

The patient and family receive support and care, and family members
  and friends are able to spend quality time with the patient

Child and caregivers supported through and receive the maximum
  benefit from surgery, chemotherapy, and/or radiation

Patient and caregiver list adverse reactions, potential complications, and
  signs/symptoms of infection (e.g., sputum change, chest congestion)

Comfort maintained through death with dignity

Patient protected from injury and compliant with medication, safety,
  and care regimens

Comfort and individualized intervention of child with cancer

Spiritual and psychosocial needs met (specify) as defined by
  child/parent/caregiver throughout course of care

Patient states pain is _____ on 0–10 scale by next visit

Patient/Caregiver demonstrates appropriate backup or "rescue" therapies for breakthrough pain or other symptoms (e.g., dyspnea)

Other outcomes/goals, based on the patient condition with input from
  the hospice team and patient and family

- *Home health aide or certified nursing assistant*
  Effective hygiene, personal care, and comfort
  ADL assistance
  Safe environment maintained

- *Social worker*
  Problems identified and addressed, with patient/parent linked with appro-
    priate support services and plan of care successfully implemented
  Patient and parent cope adaptively with illness and death
  Adaptive adjustment to changed body and body image
  Psychosocial support and counseling offered to patient/caregivers
    experiencing loss and grief
  Funeral and burial planning assistance

- *Volunteer(s)*
  Comfort, companionship, respite, and friendship extended to
    child/family
  Support provided as defined by the needs of the patient/caregiver

5

Patient and family supported by team with care, comfort, and companionship

- *Spiritual counseling*
  Spiritual support offered and provided as defined by needs of patient/caregiver
  Provision of spiritual support and care as based on the assessed and ongoing needs of the patient and family
  Spiritual support offered, and patient and family needs met
  Patient and family express relief of symptoms of spiritual suffering
  Pray with or for the patient/family, using prayers familiar to the patient's religious background (per their wishes)

- *Dietitian/Nutritional counseling*
  Family and caregiver integrate recommendations into nutrition teaching (where appropriate)
  Parent and caregiver know whom to call for nutrition- and hydration-related questions/concerns
  Nutrition/Hydration per child's choices
  Parent integrating recommendations into daily meal planning
  Parent and caregiver verbalize comprehension of changing nutritional needs
  Pray with or for the patient/family, using prayers familiar to the patient's religious background (per their wishes)

- *Occupational therapist*
  Maximize independence in ADLs for patient/caregiver
  Optimal function maintained/attained
  Patient and caregiver demonstrate ADL program for maximum safety
  Patient and caregiver demonstrate maximum independence with ADLs, adaptive techniques, and assistive devices
  Patient and caregiver demonstrate maximum safety in ADLs and functional mobility
  Patient and caregiver demonstrate effective use of energy conservation
  Verbalization/demonstration of improved functional activity level and enhanced quality of life
  Patient and caregiver demonstrate effective use of diaphragmatic breathing to reduce shortness of breath and relaxation techniques to help in pain/symptom management

- *Physical therapist*
  Prevention of complications
  Home exercise and upper extremity program taught to parent or other team member (e.g., HHA)
  Optimal strength, mobility, and function maintained/achieved
  Compliance with home exercise program by _____ (specify date)

- *Speech-language pathologist*
  Communication method implemented, and child able to be understood as self-reported or reported by family/caregivers

Safe swallowing and functional communication
Recommended lists of foods/textures for safety and patient choice

- ***Bereavement counselor***
  Support services related to grief provided to patient and family
  Well-being and resolution process of grief initiated and followed
    through bereavement services

- ***Pharmacist***
  Regimen for bowel regimen successful as self-reported by patient
    and in update at team meeting
  Multiple drug regimen reviewed for food/drug and drug/drug
    interactions in patient on multiple medications
  Stability and safety in complex medication regimen, with maximum
    benefit to patient
  Effective pain and symptom control and symptom management as
    reported by patient/caregiver

- ***Music, massage, art, or other therapies or services***
  Therapeutic massage/touch effective for patient as self-reported or
    observed by caregiver/family
  Improved muscle tone, relaxation, and/or sleep
  Patient comfortable and relaxed (e.g., sleeping, playing) after massage
  Music therapy intervention based on assessment to decrease pain
    perception and provide emotional expression and support
  Maintenance of comfort and physical, psychosocial, and
    spiritual health
  Holistic health maintained and comfort achieved through
    _____ (specify modality)
  Patient/Family participate in grief work through art therapy

7. **Patient, family, and caregiver educational needs**
   Educational needs are the care regimens that contribute to safe and
   effective care at home between the hospice team's visits.
   These include the following:
   The basic tenets of hospice and the availability of support 24 hours a
     day, 7 days a week
   Home safety assessment and counseling
   The patient's medication regimen
   Anticipated disease progression
   Safe and proper body mechanics to promote patient comfort and avoid
     caregiver safety problems
   Other teaching specific to the patient's and family's unique needs
   Support groups available to patient's family, such as the hospice
     program's "Caregiver Support Group" meetings for family
     members and friends
   The medication regimen, including schedule, route, functions, and
     side effects
   Signs and symptoms that necessitate calling the physician or RN

The importance of round-the-clock medications for pain control
Pain and other symptom control measures
Information about the disease process
Other support services for the patient, parents, and caregivers

8. **Specific tips for quality and reimbursement**
Document coordination of services or consultation of the other
members of the IDT
Document all care provided and outcomes of that care
Document the child's/parent's responses to care, changes, and
communications with the physician and other hospice team
members
Document the course of care, including why the infant/child was
admitted for care, the plan, and support provided
Document in the clinical notes the clear progression, of symptoms,
interventions, and overall management of
_____ (specify)
Document when/if the patient has respiratory changes, shortness of
breath, exacerbation of conditions, changes in pain, and/or other
symptoms and that they are identified and resolved
Remember that the clinical documentation is key to measuring
compliance for quality and reimbursement purposes. Care
coordination, timely verbal and initial physician orders, and
assessment and addressing of spiritual and psychosocial needs
should be ongoing and documented in the patient's clinical record
Document that all hospice care supports comfort and dignity while
meeting child's/family's needs
The documentation should include ongoing assessment and
management of pain and other symptoms and the anticipation
and prevention of secondary symptoms such as constipation
It is important to note that all team members should assess, identify,
and "hear" spiritual needs that the patient/family want to be
addressed. These spiritual issues are key to the provision of quality
hospice care and cannot be addressed effectively and promptly by
the spiritual counselor only
Document clearly symptoms, clinical changes, and assessment findings
related to pain and patient care
Document weight loss, increased shortness of breath, dyspnea,
infection, sepsis, new or changed medications, etc.
Document any skin changes (e.g., inflamed, painful, weeping skin
site[s])
Remember that the "litmus test" of care coordination rests on the
quality of the clinical documentation by all team members.
Review one of your patient's clinical records and ask yourself the
following: "If I was unable to give a verbal report/update on this
child's/family's course of care, would a peer be able to pick up and
provide the same level of care and know (from the documentation)

5

the current orders, medications, and other details that contribute to effective hospice care?"

This patient population usually has many clinical changes that should be documented. These include weight loss, multiple and changed medication regimens with varying routes. Side effects to the drug regimen should be observed, noted documented, and reported

Your assessments, observations, and clinical findings are information that assists in painting a picture to support coverage and documentation requirements for hospice care

Document any hospitalizations and changed clinical findings

Document patient changes, symptoms, psychosocial issues impacting the care, and information gathered at the child/family visits and during team meetings

Document communications and care coordination with other care providers, such as inpatient team members and hired caregivers

Document changes to the POC, such as medications, services, frequency, communication, and concurrence of other team members

9. **Queries for quality**
   - *Is the child's pain managed adequately?*
   - *Is the child's anxiety managed adequately?*
   - *What are the child's symptoms?*
   - *What support systems are in place for the child/parent(s)/family?*
   - *Have you documented to the interdisciplinary POC?*

10. **Resources for hospice care and practice**
    The American Brain Tumor Association *www.abta.org*, offers helpful resources for children and parents about the varying types of tumors and other information. *When Your Child Is Ready To Return to School* addresses homework and important safety details should the patient/child wish to continue school and learning, depending on the pathology and course of care and illness. Another is *Alex's Journey,* which is the story of a child with a brain tumor. Information and these free resources can be obtained by calling 1-800-886-2282.

    Radiotherapy Days, a 20-page, four-color paperback for children ages 8 to 12, is useful to caregivers who need to explain radiotherapy to children. To order, send $5.00 per copy to Mount Sinai Medical Center, Radiotherapy Days, Department of Pediatric Hematology/Oncology, Box 1208. One Gustave L. Levy Place, New York, NY 10029. Make check payable to MSMC.

5

The Make-A-Wish Foundation fulfills special wishes for children with a life-threatening illness and their families. Call 1-800-722-WISH (9474) or visit online at *www.wish.org*

The Wisconsin Pain Initiative offers *Children's Cancer Pain Can Be Relieved* by calling 1-608-262-0978. *Acute Pain Management in Infants, Children, and Adolescents: Operative and Medical Procedures* is available free through the Agency for Health Care Policy and Research at 1-800-358-9295.

The Candlelighters Childhood Cancer Foundation offers many services for parents and children, including resources, services, advocacy, and support. Call 1-800-366-2223 (CCCF) for information or visit online at *www.candlelighters.org*

5

CARE OF THE MEDICALLY FRAGILE CHILD

1. **General considerations**
   The news that a child's prognosis is terminal is devastating. Congenital anomalies, accidents, or progressive disease include some of the problems or diagnoses when an infant or child is referred and admitted to hospice. The child, the siblings, and the parents become the unit of care for comfort, support, and intervention.

   Please refer to "Care of the Child with AIDS," "Care of the Child with Cancer," and "Infusion Care" should these sections also pertain to your patients.

2. **Needs for visit**
   Physician order for hospice care, specific to the hospice program's
   admission criteria and policies
   Standard precautions supplies
   Vital signs equipment for baseline assessment
   Other supplies or equipment, based on physician orders

3. **Safety considerations**
   Infection control/standard precautions
   Night-light
   Infant/child safety considerations (e.g., car seat, electrical outlet
   protection, sleeping position, immunizations)
   Phone number of whom to call with a problem
   Medication access and storage
   Oxygen safety
   Equipment safety (if there is home medical equipment/technology)
   Symptoms and problems that necessitate emergency call to 911
   If ventilator, TPN, or infusion patient _____ adequate elec-
   tricity, refrigerator, clean storage area, and access to a
   telephone
   Smoke detector and fire evacuation plan
   Others, based on the patient's unique condition and environment

4. **Potential diagnoses and codes**

AIDS	042
Apnea	786.03
Apnea (newborn)	770.81
Asthma	493.90
Bacteriuria	791.9
Biliuria	791.4
Bone marrow transplant (surgical)	41.00
Brain injury, traumatic	854.00
Bronchial pulmonary dysplasia	770.7
Bronchiolitis	466.19
Cardiac dysrhythmia	427.9
Cerebral palsy	343.9

Child maltreatment syndrome	995.50
Cholelithiasis	574.20
Chronic renal failure	585
Cleft lip	749.10
Cleft palate	749.00
Cystic fibrosis	277.00
Dehydration	276.5
Diabetes mellitus, with complic.	250.90
Diarrhea	787.91
Down's syndrome	758.0
Encephalitis	323.9
Failure to thrive	783.41
Fetal/neonatal jaundice	774.6
Immaturity, extreme	765.00
Jaundice	782.4
Liver transplant (surgical)	50.59
Meningitis, bacterial	320.9
Meningitis, viral	047.9
Metabolism disorder	277.9
Muscular dystrophy	359.1
Nasogastric tube (surgical)	96.07
Newborn feeding problems	779.3
Normal delivery	650, Report *only* on mother's record
Normal development, lack of	783.4
Pancreatitis, acute	577.0
Pneumonia	486.
Preterm infant with low birth weight	765.00
Pulmonary insufficiency, newborn	770.89
Reactive airway disease	493.90
Rectal prolapse	569.1
Respiratory problem, postbirth	770.89
Respiratory syncytial virus	079.6
Seizure disorder	780.39
Sickle cell anemia	282.60
Sickle cell crisis	282.62
Sickle cell trait	282.5
Spina bifida	741.90
Spinal cord injury	952.9
Tracheal stenosis, congenital	748.3
Tracheomalacia, congenital	748.3
Tracheostomy, attention to	V55.0
Wasting syndrome	799.4

5

5. **Skills and services identified**

- *Hospice nursing*

a. *Comfort and system control*
   Admission of infant/child to hospice with _____ (specify)

Comprehensive skilled assessment of all systems of infant/child
with _____ (specify) admitted

Presentation of hospice philosophy and services

Explain to parents patient rights and responsibilities

Assess child, family, and caregiver wishes and expectations regarding
care

Assess child, family, and caregiver resources available for care

Teach family or caregiver physical care of child

Provision of volunteer support to child and family

Assess pain and other symptoms, including site, duration,
characteristics, and relief measures

RN to provide and teach effective oral care and comfort measures

Support play, growth and development, and health maintenance through
length of care

Establish an environment of mutual trust and respect to enhance
learning

Communicate only brief amounts of complex information related to
the infant's care at any given time

Assess respiratory rate and depth and lung sounds for improvement or
deterioration

Teach parent management of cardiorespiratory monitor

Teach parent oxygen administration and safety considerations with
infant at risk for hydroxemia and history of bradycardia and apnea

Ongoing assessment and observation of cardiovascular, pulmonary, and
respiratory statuses

Teach new pain and symptom control measures to parents

Identify and monitor pain, symptoms, and relief measures

Observation, assessment, and supportive care to child and family

Teach child/family use of standardized form/tool for pain to use
between hospice team members' visit (and for care coordination
between team members and child/family)

Teach parent principles of effective pain management

Effective management of pain and prevention of secondary symptoms

Interventions of symptoms directed toward comfort and palliation

Observation and assessment and communication with physician related
to signs, new symptoms, increasing irritability, thrush, others

Pain assessment and management q visit, including source of pain
(e.g., neuropathy, infection, muscles, thrush/swallowing,
dental disease, otitis)

Teach parent/family about realistic expectations of disease process

Teach care of dying, signs/symptoms of impending death

Presence and support

Other interventions, based on child/family needs

b. *Safety and mobility considerations*

Child and parent provided with home safety information and
instruction related to _____ and documented in the
clinical record

Teach parent about home safety and infection-control measures

Encourage family members to refrain from smoking or allowing others to smoke in the home

Schedule frequent rest periods with activities to promote optimal oxygenation

Parent provided with home safety information and instruction

Other interventions, based on child/family needs

c. *Emotional/Spiritual considerations*

Psychosocial assessment of patient and family regarding disease and prognosis

RN to provide emotional support to child and family

Observation of child for neuropsychiatric complications of illness, including pain, irritability, and depression

Assess for and manage plans for psychosocial and/or spiritual pain (e.g., fear, anxiety, interpersonal and other distress)

Psychosocial aspects of pain control (e.g., depression) assessed and acknowledged with team support/intervention

Ongoing acknowledgment of spiritually and related concerns of child/family and their belief systems

Other interventions, based on child/family needs

d. *Skin care*

RN to teach parents and caregivers all aspects of skin care

Other interventions, based on child/family needs

e. *Elimination considerations*

Assess bowel regimen, and implement program as needed

Other interventions, based on child/family needs

f. *Hydration/Nutrition*

Monitor length, weight, head circumference, and review of food diary for infant with failure to thrive

Reinforce feeding techniques and intake and output diary

Teach the importance of optimal nutrition and hydration

Assessment and referral for child with thrush and painful swallowing

Nutrition/Hydration supported by offering foods/beverages of child's choice, when possible

Other interventions, based on child/family needs

g. *Therapeutic/Medication regimens*

Administer prescribed medications as ordered, including aerosol treatments, and monitor for adverse effects

Instruct regarding medication administration and side effects

RN to assess the child's unique response to treatments and interventions and to report to the physician changes, unfavorable responses, or reactions

Teach new medications and effects

Teach parent about medications and the management program, including strength, type, actions, times, and compliance tips

5

Encourage parent to give the child medications on the schedule and around the clock

Nonpharmacological interventions of relaxation, guided imagery, humor, music therapy, art therapy, bubble blowing, magic presentations and wands, and massage for comfort during painful interventions

Other interventions, based on child/family needs

h. *Other considerations*

Assess disease process progression

Other interventions, based on child/family needs

- **Home health aide or certified nursing assistant**

  Effective and safe personal care

  Safe ADL assistance and support

  Respite care

  Observation and reporting

  Meal preparation

  Assist with diversional therapy (e.g., playing games)

  Homemaker services

  Comfort care

  Other duties

- **Social worker**

  Psychosocial assessment of patient and family/caregiver, including adjustment to long-term illness and its implications

  Identification of optimal coping strategies

  Financial assessment and counseling regarding food acquisition, ability to prepare food, and costs of needed medications

  Intervention/Support related to terminal illness and loss

  Emotional/Spiritual support

  Depression/Fear assessed and addressed

  Facilitate communication among patient, family, and hospice team

  Referral/Linkage to community services and resources as indicated

  Grief counseling and intervention/support related to illness/loss

  Patient and caregiver counseling and support

  Identification of illness-related psychiatric condition necessitating care

  Funeral and burial planning assistance

- **Volunteer(s)**

  Comfort, dignity, and respite maintained/provided for patient and family

  Errands and transportation

  Other services, based on interdisciplinary team recommendations and patient/caregiver needs

- **Spiritual counselor**

  Spiritual assessment and care

  Counseling, intervention, and support related to that dimension of life related to life's meaning (consistent with patient's beliefs)

  Support, listening, and presence

Pray with or for the patient/family, using prayers familiar to patient's religious background (per their wishes)

Participation and scared or spiritual rituals or practices

Other supportive care, based on patient/family needs and belief systems

- *Dietitian/Nutritional counseling*

  Supportive counseling with parent/family indicating that child will have a decreased appetite and usually at some point may not eat/drink

  Assessment and recommendations for swallowing difficulties

  Teaching and support of family members and caregivers

  Support and care with food and nourishment as desired by patient

  Evaluation/Management of nutritional deficits and needs

  Food and dietary recommendations incorporate patient choice and wishes

- *Occupational therapist*

  Evaluation of ADLs and functional mobility

  Assess for need for adaptive equipment and assistive devices

  Safety assessment of patient's environment and ADLs

  Assessment for energy conservation training

  Assessment of upper-extremity function, retraining motor skills and/or splinting for contracture(s)

- *Physical therapist*

  Evaluation

  Assessment of environment for safety

  Safe transfer training or bed mobility exercises

  Pain assessment/reduction factors

  Strengthening exercises/program

  Assessment of gait safety and home safety measures

  Instruct/Supervise parents and volunteers on home exercise program for conditioning and strength

  Assistive, adaptive devices and evaluation of equipment and teaching

- *Speech-language pathologist*

  Evaluation for speech/swallowing problems

  Food texture recommendations

  Alternate functional communication

- *Bereavement counselor*

  Assessment of the needs of the bereaved family and friends

  Support and intervention, based on assessment and ongoing findings

  Presence and counseling

  Supportive visits and follow-up, and other interventions (e.g., mailings, calls)

  Other services related to bereavement work and support

- *Pharmacist*

  Evaluation of hospice patient with constipation on cathartics, stool softeners, and other medications for possible food/drug, drug/drug interactions

5

Medication monitoring regarding therapeutic levels and dosages

Pain consult and input into interdisciplinary POC related to pain control, palliation, and symptom management

Assessment of medication regimen and plan for safety and compliance

- ***Music, massage, art, or other therapies or services***

  Evaluation and intervention based on child's/parent's unique wishes and needs that support care, comfort, and death in the setting of the patient's choice

  Assessment plan to engage child and support comfort, quality, enjoyment, and dignity and quality of life

6. **Outcomes for care**

- ***Hospice nursing***

  Comfort through death for child and family with support and care of hospice team

  Parent able to care for and support child with hospice support

  Parent can verbalize symptoms, changes, or symptoms that necessitate call to hospice

  Parent demonstrates compliance with medication regimen and other care and therapeutic interventions

  Pain and symptoms managed/controlled in setting of family choice

  Death with dignity and pain/symptoms controlled in setting of family choice

  Optimal comfort, support, and dignity provided throughout illness

  Death with maximum comfort through effective symptom control with specialized hospice support

  Parent able to list adverse drug reactions/problems with medication regimen and whom to call for follow-up and resolution

  Enhancement and support of child's/family's quality of life

  Effective symptom relief and control (e.g., a peaceful and comfortable death at home, pain and other symptoms controlled, some enjoyment of life and play)

  Pharmacological and nonpharmacological interventions used effectively for comfort and supportive care through illness

  Child/Family cared for and family supported through death with physical, psychosocial, developmental, spiritual, and other concerns/needs acknowledged/addressed

  Infection control and palliation through illness in setting of choice

  Grief/Bereavement expression and support provided to family

  Child/Adolescent is pain free by next _____ visit

  Parent and caregiver demonstrate ability to manage pain and other symptoms, where applicable

  Observation and assessment of child's behavior, including expressions, usual activity level, and changes noted, to assist in pain identification and management

  Parent and child verbalize satisfaction with care

5

Educational tools/plans related to care of infant with _____ incorporated into care routines (e.g., rest, fluids)

Safe and infection-free delivery of total parenteral nutrition at home

Child remains at home without or with minimal complications

Infant or child is pain free and comfortable

Child will demonstrate an adequate breathing pattern as evidenced by lack of respirtory distress (e.g., no retractions, not using accessory muscles, appears comfortable)

Child will maintain a patient airway and mobilization of secretions by use of respiratory treatments, oral medications, and effective cough

Child will maintain sufficient fluid intake to prevent dehydration(_____ cc in 24 hours)

Parent and caregiver will identify factors/triggers that seem to cause exacerbations

Prevention of multiple hospital admissions for infusion therapy with case management and phone intervention program by _____ (specify date)

Parent and caregiver will meet the developmental and play needs of child

Parent and caregiver demonstrate the ability to perform taught/learned health-related behaviors

Parent can list medications, their schedule, use, and side effects

Parent experiences decreased worry

Family bonding evidenced by loving relationship with infant

Parent effective in child's health maintenance and knows whom to call for questions/concerns

Patient and caregiver demonstrate appropriate backup or "rescue" therapies for breakthrough pain or other symptoms (e.g., dyspnea)

- *Home health aide or certified nursing assistant*
  Effective hygiene, personal care, and comfort
  ADL assistance
  Safe environment maintained

- *Social worker*
  Problems identified and addressed, with patient/caregiver linked with appropriate support services and POC successfully implemented
  Patient and caregiver cope adaptively with illness and death
  Adaptive adjustment to changed body and body image
  Psychosocial support and counseling offered/initiated to patient/caregivers experiencing loss and grief
  Funeral and burial planning assistance

- *Volunteer(s)*
  Comfort, companionship, and friendship extended to patient/family
  Support provided as defined by the needs of the patient/caregiver
  Patient and family supported by team with care, comfort, and companionship

- *Spiritual counseling*
  Spiritual support offered and provided as defined by needs of
      patient/caregiver
  Provision of spiritual support and care as based on the assessed and
      ongoing needs of the patient and family
  Parent and caregiver verbalize comprehension of changing
      nutritional needs
  Pray with or for the patient/family, using prayers familiar to the
      patient's religious background (per their wishes)

- *Dietitian/Nutritional counseling*
  Family and caregiver integrate recommendations into nutrition teaching
      (where appropriate)
  Parent and caregiver known whom to call for nutrition- and
      hydration-related questions/concerns
  Nutrition/Hydration per patient choices
  Caregiver integrates recommendations into daily meal planning

- *Occupational therapist*
  Patient and caregiver demonstrate maximum independence with ADLs,
      adaptive techniques, and assistive devices
  Patient and caregiver demonstrate maximum safety in ADLs and
      functional mobility
  Patient and caregiver demonstrate effective use of energy
      conservation
  Verbalization/Demonstration of improved functional activity level and
      enhanced quality of life
  Patient and caregiver demonstrate effective use of diaphragmatic
      breathing to reduce shortness of breath and relaxation techniques to
      help in pain/symptom management
  Patient and caregiver demonstrate correct use of exercise and splints for
      maximum upper extremity function and joint position devices to
      increase functioning

- *Physical therapist*
  Prevention of complications
  Home exercise and upper-extremity program taught to parent
  Optimal strength, mobility, and function maintained/achieved
  Compliance with home exercise program by _____ (specify date)

- *Speech-language pathologist*
  Communication method implemented and child able to be understood
      as self-reported or reported by family/caregivers
  Safe swallowing and functional communication
  Recommended lists of foods/textures for safety and
      child choice

- *Bereavement counselor*
  Support services related to grief provided to patient and family
  Well-being and resolution process of grief initiated and followed
      through bereavement services

- *Pharmacist*

    Bowel regimen successful as self-reported by patient and in update
    at team meeting

    Multiple drug regimen reviewed for food/drug and drug/drug interac-
    tions in patient on multiple medications

    Stability and safety in complex medication regimen, with maximum
    benefit to patient

    Effective pain and symptom control and symptom management as
    reported by patient/parent

- *Music, massage, art, or other therapies or services*

    Therapeutic massage/touch effective for patient as self-reported or
    observed by caregivers/family

    Improved muscle tone, relaxation, and/or sleep

    Patient comfortable and relaxed (e.g., sleeping, playing) after massage

    Music therapy intervention based on assessment to decrease pain
    perception and provide emotional expression and support

    Maintenance of comfort and physical, psychosocial, and spiritual health

    Holistic health maintained and comfort achieved through _____
    (specify modality)

    Patient/Family participate in grief work through art therapy

7. **Patient, family, and caregiver educational needs**

    Educational needs are the care regimens that contribute to safe and
    effective care at home between the hospice team's visits. These
    include the following: The basic tenets of hospice and the
    availability of support 24 hours a day, 7 days a week

    Home safety assessment and counselling

    Anticipated disease progression

    The patient's medication regimen

    Safe and proper body mechanics to promote patient comfort and
    prevent caregiver safety problems

    Other teaching specific to the patient's and family's unique needs

    Support groups available to patient's family, such as the hospice
    program's "Caregiver Support Group" meetings for family
    members and friends of the patient

    Health maintenance and growth and development information

    The importance of immunizations

    Signs and symptoms that necessitate calling the physician

    Potential complications of new technologies (e.g., TPN)

    Home medical equipment vendor's name and number should be
    readily accessible in the home care clinical record should there
    be a problem

    Other information, based on the child's unique condition

8. **Specific tips for quality and reimbursement**

    Document all care provided and outcomes of that care

    Document the child's/parent's responses to care, changes, and
    communications with the physician and other hospice team members

Document the course of care including why the infant/child was admitted for care, the plan, and support provided

Document in the clinical notes the clear progression of symptoms, interventions, and overall management of _____ (specify)

Document when/if the patient has respiratory changes, shortness of breath, exacerbation of conditions, changes in pain, and/or other symptoms and that they are identified and resolved

Remember that the clinical documentation is key to measuring compliance for quality and reimbursement purposes. Care coordination, timely verbal and initial physician orders, and assessment and addressing of spiritual and psychosocial needs should be ongoing and documented in the patient's clinical record

Document changes to the POC such as medications, services, frequency, communication, and concurrence of other team members

Document coordination of services or consultation of the other members of the IDT

Document communications and care coordination with other care providers such as inpatient team members and hired caregivers

Document that all hospice care supports comfort and dignity while meeting child/family needs

The documentation should include ongoing assessment and management of pain and other symptoms and the anticipation and prevention of secondary symptoms such as constipation

It is important to note that all team members should assess, identify, and "hear" spiritual needs that the patient/family want to be addressed. These spiritual issues are key to the provision of quality hospice care and cannot be addressed effectively and promptly by the spiritual counselor only

Document clearly symptoms, clinical changes, and assessment findings related to pain and patient care

Document weight loss, increased shortness of breath, dyspnea, infection, sepsis, new or changed medications, etc.

Document any skin changes (e.g., inflamed, painful, weeping skin site[s])

Remember that the "litmus test" of care coordination rests on the quality of the clinical documentation by all team members. Review one of your patient's clinical records and ask yourself the following: "If I was unable to give a verbal report/update on this child/family's course of care, would a peer be able to pick up and provide the same level of care and know (from the documentation) the current orders, medications, and other details that contribute to effective hospice care?"

This patient population usually has many clinical changes that should be documented. These include weight loss and multiple and changed medication regimens with varying routes. Side effects to the drug regimen should be observed, noted, documented, and reported

Your assessments, observations, and clinical findings are information that assists in painting a picture to support coverage and documentation requirements for hospice care

Document any hospitalizations and changed clinical findings

Document patient changes, symptoms, psychosocial issues impacting the care, and information gathered at the child/family visits and during team meetings

9. **Queries for quality**
   - *Is the child's pain managed adequately?*
   - *Is the child's anxiety managed adequately?*
   - *What are the child's symptoms?*
   - *What support systems are in place for the child/parent(s)/family?*
   - *Have you documented the interdisciplinary POC?*

10. **Resources for hospice care and practice**

    The American Sudden Infant Death Syndrome Institute offers a pamphlet entitled *Coping with Infant Loss Grief and Bereavement* that can be obtained by calling 1-800-232-SIDS or visit online at *www.sias.org*

    The National Easter Seal Society offers brochures about many childhood problems and can be reached at 1-800-221-6827 or visit online at *www.easter-seals.org.*

    The National Information Center for Children and Youth With Disabilities offers information; call 1-800-695-0285.

    The Agency for Health Research and Quality (AHRQ) offers a *Quick Reference Guide for Clinicians: Acute Pain Management in Infants, Children, and Adolescents: Operative and Medical Procedures*, which presents pain assessment tools and pain assessment and management information. This resource can be obtained free by calling 1-800-358-9295 or visit online at *www.ahrq.gov*

    The American Psychiatric Association offers a free 18-page pamphlet entitled *Childhood Disorders*, which addresses information about autism, signs of depression, attention deficit disorder, development disorders, and other conditions. This resource can be obtained by calling 1-800-368-5777 or writing to American Psychiatric Association, Division of Public Affairs, Department SG, 1400 K Street, N.W., Washington, D.C. 20005.

    The Candlelighters Childhood Cancer Foundation offers many services for parents and children, including resources, services, advocacy, and support. Call 1-301-657-8401 or 1-800-366-2223 (CCCF) for information or visit online at *www.candlelighters.org*

5

BOX 5-1

CHILDREN'S HOSPICE INTERNATIONAL
Standards of Hospice Care for Children

Access for Care
Principle
Children with life-threatening, terminal illnesses and their families have special needs. Hospice services for children and their families offer developmentally appropriate palliative and supportive care to any child with a life-threatening condition in any appropriate setting. Children are admitted to hospice services without regard for diagnosis, gender, race, creed, handicap, age, or ability to pay.

Standards
A.C.1. Hospice care services are accessible to children and their families in a setting that is desired and/or appropriate for their needs.

A.C.2. The hospice team is available to provide continuity of care to children and their families in the home and/or in an institutional setting.

A.C.3. The hospice program has eligibility admission criteria for the children and families they serve. Care plans are developed that take into consideration the child's prognosis, and the child and family's needs and desires for hospice services. Admission to the hospice care service does not preclude the child and family from treatment choices or hopeful, supportive therapies.

A.C.4. The hospice program provides information to the community and referral sources about the services that are offered, who qualifies, and how services may be obtained and reimbursed.

Child and Family as a Unit of Care
Principle
Hospice programs provide family-centered care to enhance the quality of life for the child and family as defined by each child-and-family unit. It includes the child and family in the decision making process about services and treatment choices to the fullest degree that is possible and desired.

Standards
C.F.U.1. The unit of care is the child and family. Hospice provides family-centered care. The family is defined as the relatives and/or other significant persons who provide physical, psychological, social, and/or spiritual support for the child.

C.F.U.2. The hospice program recognizes the unique, personal values and beliefs of all children and families. The hospice respects and maintains, as possible, the wishes and dignity of every child and his or her family.

BOX 5-1

CHILDREN'S HOSPICE INTERNATIONAL
Standards of Hospice Care for Children—cont'd

C.F.U.3. The hospice program encourages that children and their families participate in decisions regarding care, including discontinuation of hospice care at any time, and maintains documentation related to consent, advance directives, treatments, and alternative choices of care.

C.F.U.4. The hospice program provides care that considers each child's growth, development, and stage of family life cycle. Children's interests and needs are solicited and considered but are not limited to those related to their illness and disability.

C.F.U.5. The hospice team seeks to assist each child and family to enjoy life as they are able and to continue in their customary lifestyle, functioning, and roles as much as possible, especially helping the child to live as normal a life as is possible.

Policies and Procedures
Principle
The hospice program offers services that are accountable to and appropriate for the children and families it serves.

Standards
P.P.1. The hospice program establishes and maintains accurate and adequate policies and procedures to ensure that the hospice is accountable to children,

their families, and the communities they serve.

P.P.2. The hospice agency is in compliance with all local, state, and federal laws and regulations that govern the appropriate delivery of hospice care services.

P.P.3. The hospice program provides a clear and accessible grievance procedure to families, outlining how to voice complaints or concerns about services and care without jeopardizing services.

Interdisciplinary Team Services
Principle
Seriously ill children with life-threatening conditions and/or facing terminal stages of an illness and their families have a variety of needs that require a collaborative and cooperative effort from practitioners of many disciplines, working together as an interdisciplinary team of qualified professionals and volunteers.

Standards
I.T.1. The hospice program provides care to the child and family by utilizing a core interdisciplinary team, which may include the child, the family and/or significant others, physicians, nurses, social workers, clergy, and volunteers.

5

Continued

BOX 5-1

CHILDREN'S HOSPICE INTERNATIONAL
Standards of Hospice Care for Children—cont'd

I.T.2. Representatives of other appropriate disciplines are involved in the team as needed (i.e., physical therapy, occupational therapy, speech therapy, nutritional consultation, art therapy, music therapy). The team might also include psychologists, child life specialists, teachers, recreation therapists, play therapists, home health aides, nursing assistants, and other specialists or services as needed.

I.T.3. The hospice core team meets on a regular basis, and an integrated plan of care is developed, implemented, and maintained for every child and family.

I.T.4. The hospice staff professionals are qualified in their particular discipline by training, experience, certification, and/or licensure. Complete orientation, training, and continuing education are provided to each hospice staff member.

I.T.5. The hospice have an active volunteer program. All volunteers are carefully and appropriately selected, trained, supervised, and evaluated, at least annually, by hospice professionals.

I.T.6. All hospice personnel receive educational, psychological, and emotional support appropriate to their situational needs and desires.

I.T.7. The hospice core interdisciplinary team meets at least every 2 weeks or sooner if needed to review and update all plans of care.

Continuity of Care
Principle
Hospice is an integrated system of home and inpatient care. Hospice provides a consistent continuum of care in all settings from admission to the final bereavement services.

Standards
CC.1. Hospice services are available to children and their families on a consistent basis: 7 days a week and 24 hours a day in institutions or at home.

C.C.2. Appropriate hospice team members are available to children and their families on an on-call basis when the office is closed.

C.C.3. The hospice program has a communication system that assures confidentiality and privacy and can be used to update team members about each child and family's status so that needs can be addressed as soon as possible.

C.C.4. All children and families receive a timely and comprehensive assessment of their physical, psychosocial, emotional, spiritual, and financial needs.

BOX 5-1

CHILDREN'S HOSPICE INTERNATIONAL
Standards of Hospice Care for Children—cont'd

C.C.5. The hospice team, with the family, develops an integrated, written, interdisciplinary plan of care for each child and family. The plan addresses the unique and individual needs of the child and family, including assessment, identified present and potential problems, interventions, and the type and level of services to be provided.

C.C.6. The hospice team addresses and documents the concerns, needs, and desires of the child and family in developing and implementing the plan of care. This document is updated as indicated by the changing status of the child or family.

C.C.7. The hospice agency maintains appropriate documents and clinical records. The clinical record includes properly executed consents for medical/hospice treatment. Confidentiality of hospice records is maintained.

Pain and Symptom Management
Principle
Children should be as symptom free as possible, and pain and/or other symptoms of their illness should be managed to achieve the greatest possible level of comfort.

Standards
P.S.M.1. The hospice team assists the children in achieving comfort through the most effective treatments available.

P.S.M.2. Palliative therapies are discussed with children and their families and provided to children or ensure the most effective and adequate pain and symptom management.

P.S.M.3. Alternative methods of pain and symptom management are discussed and incorporated into the care of the child as appropriate.

Bereavement Program
Principle
Families of children who die may continue to need appropriate professional and supportive services for a period following the death.

Standards
B.P.1. The hospice program has a structured and active bereavement program. Bereavement services are provided to the surviving family members and/or significant others. Special attention may need to be given to siblings who may not be able to articulate their needs for support.

Continued

BOX 5-1

CHILDREN'S HOSPICE INTERNATIONAL
Standards of Hospice Care for Children—cont'd

B.P.2. The level and type of services provided are determined by the family member(s) and appropriate hospice team members.

B.P.3. Bereavement services are available and provided for at least 13 months following the death of the child, extending throughout the second year if possible.

Utilization Review/Quality Improvement
Principle
The hospice program should monitor and ensure the appropriate allocation and utilization of resources and the effectiveness of services.

Standards
U.R.1. The hospice program has a written continuous quality improvement and utilization review program. The program includes criteria to assess the overall functioning components of the hospice program and the effectiveness of its services.

U.R.2. The continuous quality improvement and utilization review program is an ongoing process and implemented on a regular basis, with results of the evaluation reported to appropriate individuals and/or committees for action.

U.R.3. The hospice program provides a written evaluation tool for all recipients of services to document their satisfaction or dissatisfaction with the services received. A written plan outlining how evaluation information will be used to improve services is available to all consumers.

© 1993 Children's Hospice International, *www.chionline.org/resources/standards*

PART SIX

PAIN
Assessment and Management Resources

6

PAIN ASSESSMENT MONITOR

PAIN ASSESSMENT MONITOR

PAIN ASSESSMENT CODES				
Pain Quality	**Pain Duration**	**Non-Verbal Behaviors**	**Pain Control Therapies/ Treatments (PCT)**	**Side Effects**

A = Ache/dull
N = Nagging
H = Heavy/crushing
S = Sharp/stabbing
Th = Throbbing
R = Radiating
B = Burning
T = Tingling
C = Cramping
O = Other
	C = Continuous
	I = Intermittent
	O = Occasionally
	F = Frequently
		G = Grimacing
		M = Moaning
		R = Restless
		C = Crying
		I = Irritability
		A = Anger
		T = Tense
		V = Change in vital signs
		O = Other
		N = None
			Rx = Medication
			R = Repositioning
			MT = Music therapy
			I = Ice
			H = Heat
			V = Visitors
			D = Diversion/Guided
			      Imagery
			T = Tens unit
			M = Massage
			S = Spiritual (prayer)
			O = Other
				N = Nausea
				V = Vomiting
				S = Sleepy
				CF = Confusion
				C = Constipation
				UR = Urinary retention
				MSD = Motor sensory
				         deficit
				HA = Headache
				J = Itching/rash
				R = Resp. depression
				P = ↑ Pain
				O = Other
				NO = None

PAIN LOCATION	#1 _____	#2 _____	#3 _____	#4 _____
Pain quality				
Pain duration				
What triggers pain?				
Non-verbal behaviors				
Pain intensity before PCT (0-10)				
Pain intensity after PCT (0-10)				
Patient's goal for pain relief (0-10)				
Family's goal for pain relief (0-10)				
Current pain control therapists (PCT)				
Side effects of PCT				

Comments/Plans (e.g. for relief of side effects, improving pain management, pain barriers, family beliefs, concerns)

_____

_____

Wong-Baker FACES Pain Rating Scale

0   1   2   3   4   5   6   7   8   9   10
No Pain   Moderate Pain   Worst Imaginable Pain

Medical Professionals Please Note:
Explain to the person that each face is for a person who feels happy because he has no pain (hurt) or sad because he has some or a lot of pain. **Face 0** is very happy because he doesn't hurt at all. **Face 1** hurts just a little bit. **Face 2** hurts a little more. **Face 3** hurts even more. **Face 4** hurts a whole lot. **Face 5** hurts as much as you can imagine, although you don't have to be crying to feel this bad. Ask the person to choose the face that best describes how he is feeling.

**From Wong D.L., Hockenberry-Eaton M., Wilson D., Winkelstein M.L., Schwartz P.: Wong's Essentials of Pediatric Nursing, ed. 6, St. Louis, 2001, p. 1301. Copyrighted by Mosby, Inc. Reprinted by permission.

Clinician_____   Date_____

Part 1 – Clinical Record	**Part 2 – Care Coordination**

PATIENT NAME–Last, First, Middle Initial	ID#

Form 3459/2P   © BRIGGS, Des Moines, IA 50306 (800) 247-2343 www.BriggsCorp.com
PRINTED IN U.S.A.

PAIN ASSESSMENT MONITOR

(Reprinted with permission of Briggs Health Care Products, Des Moines, Iowa.)

INITIAL PAIN ASSESSMENT TOOL

Initial Pain Assessment Tool

Date _____

Patient's Name _____ Age _____ Room _____

Diagnosis _____ Physician _____

Nurse _____

1. LOCATION: Patient or nurse mark drawing.

2. INTENSITY: Patient rates the pain. Scale used _____

Present: _____
Worst pain gets: _____
Best pain gets: _____
Acceptable level of pain: _____

3. QUALITY: (Use patient's own words, e.g., prick, ache, burn, throb, pull, sharp) _____
_____

4. ONSET, DURATION, VARIATIONS, RHYTHMS: _____

5. MANNER OF EXPRESSING PAIN: _____
_____

6. WHAT RELIEVES THE PAIN? _____
_____

7. WHAT CAUSES OR INCREASES THE PAIN? _____
_____

8. EFFECTS OF PAIN: (Note decreased function, decreased quality of life.)
Accompanying symptoms (e.g., nausea) _____
Sleep _____
Appetite _____
Physical activity _____
Relationship with others (e.g., irritability) _____
Emotions (e.g., anger, suicidal, crying) _____
Concentration _____
Other _____

9. OTHER COMMENTS: _____
_____

10. PLAN: _____
_____

(From McCaffery M, Pasero C: *Pain: Clinical manual,* St. Louis, 1999, Mosby, p. 60. May be duplicated for use in clinical practice.)

6

PAIN INTENSITY SCALES

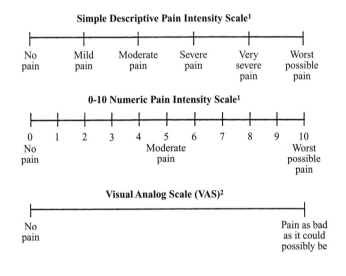

Simple Descriptive Pain Intensity Scale[1]

No pain	Mild pain	Moderate pain	Severe pain	Very severe pain	Worst possible pain

0-10 Numeric Pain Intensity Scale[1]

0   1   2   3   4   5   6   7   8   9   10
No pain   Moderate pain   Worst possible pain

Visual Analog Scale (VAS)[2]

No pain   Pain as bad as it could possibly be

[1]If used as a graphic rating scale, a 10-cm baseline is recommended.
[2]A 10-cm baseline is recommended for VAS scales.

(From Cancer Pain Management Guideline Panel: Management of Cancer pain. Clinical Practice Guideline, AHCPR No. 94-0592, Rockville, MD, 1994, Agency for Health Care Policy and Research, Public Health Services, U.S. Department of Health and Human Services, p. 23.)

Which Face Shows How Much Hurt You Have Now?

0	1	2	3	4	5
No Hurt	Hurts Little Bit	Hurts Little More	Hurts Even More	Hurts Whole Lot	Hurts Worst

FACES PAIN RATING SCALE

Explain to the person that each face is for a person who feels happy because he has no pain (hurt) or sad because he has some or a lot of pain. **Face 0** is very happy because he doesn't hurt at all. **Face 1** hurts just a little bit. **Face 2** hurts a little more. **Face 3** hurts even more. **Face 4** hurts a whole lot. **Face 5** hurts as much as you can imagine, although you don't have to be crying to feel this bad. Ask the person to choose the face that best describes how he is feeling.

This Rating scale is recommended for person's age 3 years and older.
*The brief word instruction under each face can also be used. Point to each face using the words to describe the pain intensity. Ask the child to choose face that best describes own pain and record the appropriate number. NOTE: In a study of 148 children ages 4 to 5 years, there were no differences in pain scores when children used the original or brief word instructions. (From Wong DL, Hockenberry-Eaton M, Wilson D, Winkelstein ML, Schwartz P: *Wong's essentials of Pediatric Nursing*, ed 6, St. Louis, p. 1301. Copyrighted by Mosby Inc. Reprinted by permission.)

6

PAIN CONTROL RECORD

Pain Control Record

This is a record of how your pain medicines are working. Please keep this record until you and your nurse/doctor find the dose and frequency of medicine that provides satisfactory pain relief for you most of the time. After that, you only need to keep this record when you have problems related to your pain medicines.

Name:_____ Date:_____

GOALS Satisfactory pain rating:_____ Activities:_____

My pain rating scale:

```
    |----|----|----|----|----|----|----|----|----|----|
    0    1    2    3    4    5    6    7    8    9    10
    No                      Moderate              Worst
    pain                      pain                possible
                                                   pain
```

Directions: Rate your pain before you take pain medicine and 1 to 2 hours later.

Time:	Pain rating:	Medicine I took:	Side effects (drowsy? upset stomach?)	Other:

If pain is greater than _____ , or if you have other problems with your pain medicine, call:

Nurse: Name/phone _____

Doctor: Name/phone _____

Pain Control Record. (From McCaffery M, Pasero C: *Pain: Clinical manual,* St. Louis, 1999, Mosby, p. 87. May be duplicated for use in clinical practice.)

NURSE'S POWER AND RESPONSIBILITY IN RELATION TO MEDICATION FOR PAIN RELIEF

Nurse Is Expected To:	Comments
1. Determine whether the analgesic is to be given and, if so, when.	1. Many analgesics are on PRN basis (PRN means use clinical judgment). Assess and apply knowledge. Based on this assessment, a PRN analgesic order may be given around the clock (ATC), on a regular basis (e.g., q3h).
2. Choose the appropriate analgesic(s) when more than one is ordered.	2. More than one analgesic is often available. Which one does the nurse give? Two at the same time? Avoid one? This decision is based on pharmacological knowledge along with skills in assessment and evaluation.
3. Be alert to the possibility of certain side effects as a result of the analgesic.	3. Nurse plays key role in identifying life-threatening side effects (e.g., respiratory depression). Identifies constipation, which can seriously influence patient's comfort as much as pain itself.
4. Evaluate effectiveness of analgesic at regular frequent intervals following each administration, but especially the initial dose.	4. This is a vital step in ensuring effective pain control. Assessment and evaluation are continuous processes. A flow sheet is recommended.
5. Report promptly and accurately to the physician when a change is needed.	5. Every new prescription of analgesic for the individual patient is merely a guess that must be evaluated. Too small a dosage should be changed as quickly as too large a dosage.
6. Make suggestions for specific changes (e.g., drug, route, dosage, and interval).	6. The nurse has unique blend of knowledge: pharmacological information and direct observation of patient. The result is that nurse is in ideal position to make an educated guess about what may work better for the individual patient.
7. Advise the patient about the use of analgesics, both prescription and nonprescription.	7. Nurse has a key educational role about dosage, side effects, addressing misconceptions, preventive schedule, and how to talk with physician or nurse about questions or problems with drug.

From McCaffery M, Beebe A: *Pain: Clinical manual for nursing practice*, St Louis, 1989, Mosby, p. 47.

6

BARRIERS TO THE ASSESSMENT
AND TREATMENT OF PAIN

Misconception	Correction
1. The best judge of the existence and severity of a patient's pain is the physician or nurse caring for the patient.	The patient is the authority about his or her pain. The patient's self-report is the most reliable indicator of the existence and intensity of pain.
2. Clinicians should use their personal opinions and beliefs about the truthfulness of the patient to determine the patient's true pain status.	Allowing each clinician to act on personal beliefs presents the potential for different pain assessments by different clinician, leading to different interventions from each clinician. This results in inconsistent and often inadequate pain management. It is essential to establish the patient's self-report of pain as the standard for pain assessment.
3. The clinician must believe what the patient says about pain.	The clinician must accept and respect the patient's report of pain and proceed with appropriate assessment and treatment. The clinician is always entitled to his or her personal opinion, but this cannot be allowed to guide professional practice.
4. Comparable noxious stimuli produce comparable pain in different people. The pain threshold is uniform.	Findings from numerous studies have failed to support the notion of a uniform pain threshold. Comparable stimuli do not result in the same pain in different people. After similar injuries, one person may suffer moderate pain and the other severe pain.
5. Patients with a low pain tolerance should make a greater effort to cope with pain and should not receive as much analgesia as they desire.	A stoic response to pain is valued in this society and many others. Research shows that clinicians often do not like patients with a low pain tolerance. However, imposing these values on the patients and withholding analgesics is inappropriate.

BARRIERS TO THE ASSESSMENT AND TREATMENT OF PAIN—cont'd

Misconception	Correction
6. There is no reason for patients to hurt when no physical cause for pain can be found.	Pain is a new science, and it would be foolish of us to think that we will be able to determine the cause of all the pains that patients report.
7. Patients should not receive analgesics until the cause of pain is diagnosed.	Pain is no longer the clinician's primary diagnostic tool. Symptomatic relief of pain should be provided while the investigation of cause proceeds. Early use of analgesics is now advocated for patients with acute abdominal pain.
8. Visible signs, either physiologic or behavioral, accompany pain and can be used to verify its existence and severity.	Even with severe pain, periods of physiologic and behavioral adaptation occur, leading to periods of minimal or no signs of pain. Lack of pain expression does not necessarily mean lack of pain.
9. Anxiety makes pain worse.	Anxiety is often associated with pain, but the cause-and-effect relationship has not been established. Pain often causes anxiety, but it is not clear that anxiety necessarily makes pain more intense.
10. Patients who are knowledgeable about opioid analgesics and who make regular efforts to obtain them are "drug seeking" (addicted).	Patients with pain should be knowledgeable about their medications, and regular use of opioids for pain relief is not addiction. When a patient is accused of "drug seeking," it may be helpful to ask, "What else could this behavior mean? Might this patient be in pain?"
11. When the patient reports pain relief after a placebo, this means that the patient is a malingerer or that the pain is psychogenic.	About one third of patients who have obvious physical stimuli for pain (e.g., surgery) report pain relief after a placebo injection. Therefore placebos cannot be used to diagnose malingering, psychogenic pain, or any psychologic problem. Sometimes placebos relieve pain, but why this happens remains unknown.

Continued

6

BARRIERS TO THE ASSESSMENT AND TREATMENT OF PAIN—cont'd

Misconception	Correction
12. The pain rating scale preferred for use in daily clinical practice is the VAS.	For patients who are verbal and can count from 0 to 10, the NRS pain rating scale is preferred. It is easy to explain, measure, and record, and it provides numbers for setting pain-management goals.
13. Cognitively impaired elderly patients are unable to use pain rating scales.	When an appropriate pain rating scale (e.g., 0–5) is used and the patient is given sufficient time to process information and respond, many cognitively impaired elderly can use a pain rating scale.

May be duplicated for use in clinical practice. From McCaffery M, Pasero C: *Pain: Clinical manual*, p. 37. Copyright © 1999, Mosby, Inc.

HARMFUL EFFECTS OF UNRELIEVED PAIN

Domains Affected	Specific Response to Pain
Endocrine	↑ Adrenocorticotrophic hormone (ACTH), ↑ cortisol, ↑ antidiuretic hormone (ADH), ↑ epinephrine, ↑ norepinephrine, ↑ growth hormone (GH), ↑ catecholamines, ↑ renin, ↑ angiotensin II, ↑ aldosterone, ↑ glucagon, ↑ interleukin-1; ↓ insulin, ↓ testosterone
Metabolic	Gluconeogenesis, hepatic glycogenolysis, hyperglycemia, glucose intolerance, insulin resistance, muscle protein catabolism, ↑ lipolysis
Cardiovascular	↑ Heart rate, ↑ cardiac output, ↑ peripheral vascular resistance, ↑ systemic vascular resistance, hypertension, ↑ coronary vascular resistance, ↑ myocardial oxygen consumption, hypercoagulation, deep vein thrombosis

Continued

HARMFUL EFFECTS OF UNRELIEVED PAIN—cont'd

6

Domains Affected	Specific Responses to Pain
Respiratory	↓ Flows and volumes, atelectasis, shunting, hypoxemia, ↓ cough, sputum retention, infection
Genitourinary	↓ Urinary output, urinary retention, fluid overload, hypokalemia
Gastrointestinal	↓ Gastric and bowel motility
Musculoskeletal	Muscle spasm, impaired muscle function, fatigue, immobility
Cognitive	Reduction in cognitive function, mental confusion
Immune	Depression of immune response
Developmental	↑ Behavioral and physiologic responses to pain, altered temperaments, higher somatization, infant distress behavior; possible altered development of the pain system, ↑ vulnerability to stress disorders, addictive behavior, and anxiety states
Future pain	Debilitating chronic pain syndromes: postmastectomy pain postthoracotomy pain, phantom pain, posttherapeutic neuralgia
Quality of life	Sleeplessness, anxiety, fear, hopelessness, ↑ thoughts of suicide

Information from Cousins M: Acute postoperative pain. In Wall PD, Melzack R, editors: *Textbook of pain,* ed 3, pp. 357-385, New York, 1994, Churchill Livingstone; Kehlet H: Modification of responses to surgery by neural blockade. In Cousins MJ, Bridenbaugh PO, editors: *Neural blockade*, pp. 129-175, Philadelphia, 1998, Lippincott-Raven; Mcintyre PE, Ready LB: *Acute pain management: A practical guide,* Philadelphia, 1996, WB Saunders.

CLASSIFICATION OF PAIN BY INFERRED PATHOLOGY

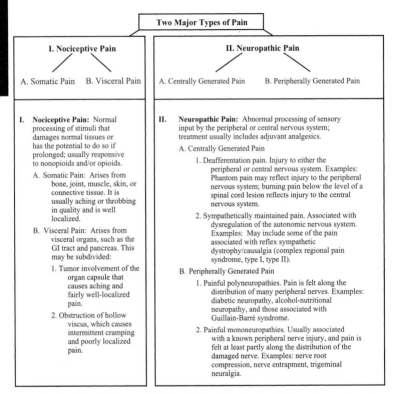

Two Major Types of Pain

I. Nociceptive Pain

A. Somatic Pain   B. Visceral Pain

II. Neuropathic Pain

A. Centrally Generated Pain   B. Peripherally Generated Pain

I. **Nociceptive Pain:** Normal processing of stimuli that damages normal tissues or has the potential to do so if prolonged; usually responsive to nonopioids and/or opioids.

A. Somatic Pain: Arises from bone, joint, muscle, skin, or connective tissue. It is usually aching or throbbing in quality and is well localized.

B. Visceral Pain: Arises from visceral organs, such as the GI tract and pancreas. This may be subdivided:

1. Tumor involvement of the organ capsule that causes aching and fairly well-localized pain.

2. Obstruction of hollow viscus, which causes intermittent cramping and poorly localized pain.

II. **Neuropathic Pain:** Abnormal processing of sensory input by the peripheral or central nervous system; treatment usually includes adjuvant analgesics.

A. Centrally Generated Pain

1. Deafferentation pain. Injury to either the peripheral or central nervous system. Examples: Phantom pain may reflect injury to the peripheral nervous system; burning pain below the level of a spinal cord lesion reflects injury to the central nervous system.

2. Sympathetically maintained pain. Associated with dysregulation of the autonomic nervous system. Examples: May include some of the pain associated with reflex sympathetic dystrophy/causalgia (complex regional pain syndrome, type I, type II).

B. Peripherally Generated Pain

1. Painful polyneuropathies. Pain is felt along the distribution of many peripheral nerves. Examples: diabetic neuropathy, alcohol-nutritional neuropathy, and those associated with Guillain-Barré syndrome.

2. Painful mononeuropathies. Usually associated with a known peripheral nerve injury, and pain is felt at least partly along the distribution of the damaged nerve. Examples: nerve root compression, nerve entrapment, trigeminal neuralgia.

A method of classifying pain is by inferred pathophysiology: 1, nociceptive pain (stimuli from somatic and visceral structure); 2, neuropathic pain (stimuli abnormally processed by the nervous system). ([Information from Max MB, Portenoy RK: Methodological challenges for clinical trials of cancer pain treatments. In Chapman CR, Foley KM, editors: *Current and emerging issues in cancer pain: Research and practice*, pp. 283-299, New York, 1993, Raven Press; Portenoy RK, Neuropathic RK, Kanner RM, editors: *Pain management: Theory and practice,* pp. 83-125, Philadelphia, 1996b, FA Davis.] From McCaffery M, Pasero C: *Pain Clinical manual*, p. 19. Copyright @ 1999, Mosby. May be duplicated for use in clinical practice.)

ROUTES OF OPIOID ADMINISTRATION

6

Route	Comments
Oral	Inexpensive, simple, noninvasive; should be considered before all other routes. Preferred in cancer and chronic nonmalignant pain management. Opioids are subject to extensive hepatic metabolism; slow onset but just as effective as other routes if doses are high enough and given ATC.
Oral transmucosal	Oral transmucosal fentanyl citrate (OTFC) is approved for conscious sedation and use as an anesthetic premedication administered by trained personnel in a monitored setting. A new OTFC has been shown to be effective and convenient in managing breakthrough pain in patients with cancer; awaiting FDA approval. Opioid bypasses significant hepatic metabolism.
Buccal	Supporting data meager; suitable preparations generally unavailable and impractical.
Sublingual	Buprenorphine, fentanyl, and methadone absorbed well; currently only buprenorphine is available in the United States. Morphine is commonly used by the sublingual route, but research is limited.
Rectal	Currently morphine, oxymorphone, and hydromorphone are commercially available in the United States. Alternative for patients unable or unwilling to take analgesics orally. Considerable variation in dose required to produce effect and time to reach effect. Starting dose usually is same dose as oral dose. Any opioid may be compounded by pharmacy for rectal administration or given in an aqueous solution, unmodified tablet, or crushed and placed in gelatin capsule; controlled-release formulations should not be crushed or dissolved.
Vaginal	No commercially available formulations; research lacking, but absorption does occur by this route.
Transdermal	Available in fentanyl citrate drug delivery system incorporated within an adhesive patch. Can provide analgesia for 48-72 h by continuous drug release into the skin. Slow onset, gradual decline after patch is removed. Difficult to titrate; must use IR opioid until analgesia is achieved. Alternative for patients unable or

Continued

ROUTES OF OPIOID ADMINISTRATION—cont'd

6

Route	Comments
	unwilling to take analgesics orally or have failed other opioids and could benefit from a trial. Not suitable for acute pain or severe escalating pain.
Intranasal	Butorphanol is available in the United States but not recommended for cancer or chronic nonmalignant pain. Sufentanil is currently being studied for use as a preanesthetic. Major drawback, especially in children, is burning and stinging on instillation. Bypasses significant hepatic metabolism.
Nebulized	Nebulization is not recommended as a route for analgesia, primarily because current administration techniques result in very small amounts of analgesic being absorbed. However, nebulized morphine is used for management of dyspnea in end-stage terminal illness (e.g., chronic lung disease, heart failure).
Subcutaneous • Single or repetitive bolus • CI with or without PCA	Morphine and hydromorphone most common opioids administered subcutaneously. Alternative when patient is unable to take opioid orally or parenteral route is indicated but venous access is limited. Easy to access, but technique and care require more skill and expertise than oral or rectal administration. Infusion pumps add expense, but are more convenient and allow for CI; newer pumps allow PCA capability.
Intravenous • Single or repetitive bolus • CI with or without PCA	Indicated when rapid titration is required. Provides steady blood levels. Opioids with short half-life recommended. Boluses or PCA commonly used for postoperative pain management. Duration is dose dependent. When steady state is reached by continuous infusion, the various opioids differ little in terms of duration. For long-term CI, permanent venous access is recommended; indicated for cancer and chronic nonmalignant pain when patient has dose-limiting side effects from other systemic routes.
Intraarterial	Direct injection into artery is rarely used; most common use with neonates by indwelling umbilical artery catheter. Requires great care and expertise; first pass is avoided, cleansing effects of lung are not available by this route.

Continued

ROUTES OF OPIOID ADMINISTRATION—cont'd

Route	Comments
Epidural • Single or repetitive bolus • CI with or without PCA • *Chronic*: implanted for CI with side port for bolus injections	Indicated for major abdominal, thoracic, and joint surgeries when severe acute pain is anticipated; rarely indicated for cancer and chronic nonmalignant pain management (e.g., may be alternative for patients with dose-limiting side effects from systemic opioid analgesics). Infusion pumps add expense, but are more convenient and allow for continuous infusion and PCA capability. Duration is dose dependent. When steady state is reached by continuous infusion, the various opioids differ little in terms of duration. May be cost-effective for patients with cancer or chronic nonmalignant pain and long life expectancy; may be administered by external catheter and pump or by implanted infusion pump. Local anesthetics frequently added to opioids by this route.
Intrathecal • *Acute*: single bolus • *Chronic*: implanted for CI with side port for bolus injections	Indicated for some acute pain (single bolus most commonly used because temporary indwelling catheters are difficult to maintain); rarely indicated for cancer and chronic nonmalignant pain management (e.g., may be alternative for patients with dose-limiting side effects from systemic opioid analgesics). May be cost-effective for patients with cancer or chronic nonmalignant pain and long life expectancy; usually administered by implanted infusion pump.

6

ROUTES OF OPIOID ADMINISTRATION—cont'd

ROUTE	COMMENTS
Intraarticular (joint)	Shown to produce adequate analgesia for joint surgeries, but further studies are needed to establish best opioids and local anesthetics to use by this route.
Intracerebroventricular	Rarely indicated. Should be considered investigational.

May be duplicated for use in clinical practice. From McCaffery M, Pasero C: *Pain: Clinical manual*, pp. 195-196. Copyright © 1999, Mosby, Inc.

Opioid analgesics can be administered by a wide variety of routes. Tables 6.6 summarizes the advantages and disadvantages to some of these.

ATC, Around-the-clock; *CI,* continuous infusion; *FDA*, Food and Drug Administration; *IR*, immediate-release; *PCA,* patient-controlled analgesia.

Information from Benet LZ, Kroetz DL, Sheiner LB: Pharmacokinetic. In Hardman JG, Limbird LE, editors: *Goodman and Gilman's the pharmacological basis of therapeutics,* ed 9, pp. 3-27, New York, 1996, McGraw-Hill; Biddle C, Gilliland C: Transdermal and transmucosal administration of pain-relieving and anxiolytic drugs: A primer for the critical care practitioner, *Heart Lung* 12:115-124, 1992; Coyle N, Chemy N, Portenoy RK: Pharmacologic management of cancer pain. In McGuire D, Yarbro CH, Ferrell BR, editors: *Cancer pain management,* ed 2, pp. 89-130, Boston, 1995, Jones and Bartlett; Foley KM, Inturrisi CE: Opioid therapy: General principles, advances, controversies, alternative routes and methods of administration, *Syllabus of the Postgraduate Course,* Memorial Sloan-Kettering Cancer Center, New York, NY, April 2-3, 1992; Joshi GP, McCarroll SM, O'Brien TM et al.: Intraarticular analgesia following knee orthroscopy, *Anesh Analg* 76:333-336, 1993; Kalso E, Tramer MR, Carroll D et al.: Pain relief from intra-articular morphine after knee surgery: A qualitative systemic review, Pain 71:127-134, 1997; Portenoy RK: Opioid analgesics. In Portenoy RK, Kanner RM, editors: *Pain management*: Theory and practice, pp. 249-276, Philadelphia, 1996, FA Davis; Reuben SS, Connelly NR: Postarthroscopic meniscus repair analgesia with intraarticular keloroloc or morphine, *Anesth Analg* 82:1036-1039, 1996; Stanley TH, Ashburn MA: Novel delivery systems: Oral transmucosal and intranasal transmucosal, *J Pain Symptom Manage* 7(3):163-171, 1992; Vranken J, Vissers K, Oosterbosch J et al.: Intra-articular sufentanil analgesia after orthroscopic knee surgery, *Br J Anaesth* 8(1):A400, 1997.

RECTAL ADMINISTRATION OF OPIOID ANALGESICS

1. Position the patient on the left side with the upper leg flexed or in knee-chest position.
2. Lubricate the dosage form with a water-soluble lubricant or a small amount of water. If rectum is dry, instill 5 to 10 ml warm water with a syringe attached to a catheter before inserting tablets or capsules.
3. Do not crush controlled-release preparations.
4. Gently insert the dosage form approximately a finger's length into the rectum at an angle toward the umbilicus so that the medication is placed against the rectal wall. If a suppository is used, the blunted end should be introduced first.
5. Keep liquid volumes of drug preparations at less than 60 ml to prevent spontaneous expulsion. Amounts of 25 ml are usually retained without difficulty. These may be injected into the rectal cavity with a lubricated rubber-tipped syringe or large-bore Foley catheter and balloon. Inflating the balloon may assist in retention.
6. Minimize the number of insertions. When administering multiple tablets for a single dose, enclose them in a single gelatin capsule.
7. Do not split or halve a suppository as this can cause errors in dosing. If it must be halved, cut it lengthwise.
8. After the finger is withdrawn, hold the buttocks together until the urge to expel has ceased.
9. Although rectal irritation is a concern, it need not be a limiting factor when administering commercially prepared suppositories, tablets, or capsules. Irritation may be avoided or treated with lubrication, gentle insertion, and appropriate care topical medications, such as cortisone ointment.
10. Prevent chronic rectal irritation. Avoid repeated rectal instillation of solutions of drugs with alcoholic vehicles or drugs that use glycols as solubilizing agents (parenteral forms of lorazepam, diazepam, chlordiazepoxide, and phenytoin).

May be duplicated for use in clinical practice. From McCaffery M, Pasero C: *Pain: Clinical manual*, p. 205. Copyright © 1999, Mosby, Inc.
cm, centimeter; *F,* French; *ml,* milliliter.

Information from Abd-EI-Maeboud K et al.: Rectal suppository: Common-sense and mode of insertion, *Lancet* 338(8770):798–800, 1991; McCaffery M, Martin L, Ferrell BR: Analgesic administration via rectum or stomo, *J Enterostomal Therapy Nurs* 19(4): 114-121, 1992; Warrent DE: Practical use of rectal medications in palliative care, *J Pain Symptom Manage* 11(6):378-387, 1996; Wong, D: *Wong and Whaley's clinical manual of pediatric nursing*, ed 4, St. Louis, 1996, Mosby.

RECTAL ADMINISTRATION OF OPIOID ANALGESICS—cont'd

6

11. Avoid rectal administration of enteric-coated tablets. The pH of the colon is alkaline and these preparations require an acidic environment to be dissolved and the active drug to be released. The active drug would likely be expelled with the coating intact.

Pediatric Considerations

1. In syringe, combine drug and smallest amount of diluent possible for adequate mixture and for administration using a syringe and catheter.
2. Cut the distal 5 to 10 cm of a 14 F catheter.
3. Attach the syringe of medication solution to the distal end of the catheter.

4. Carefully flush air from catheter without losing medication solution.
5. Lubricate the tip of the catheter.
6. Gently insert catheter tip well into the rectum:
   • Infant: 1 inch (2.5 cm)
   • 2 to 4 years old: 2 inches (5 cm)
   • 4 to 10 years old: 3 inches (7.5 cm)
   • 11 years old: 4 inches (10 cm)
7. Smoothly inject medication solution.
8. Hold buttocks together for 5 to 10 minutes to prevent expulsion.

IMMEDIATE HELP FOR PHARMACOLOGICAL CONTROL OF PAIN

Patient in Home Care Setting Unexpectedly Unable to Take Oral Analgesics

Time involved: Reading time, 4 minutes; implementation time, about 10 minutes.

Situation: Patient of any age being cared for at home with moderate to severe pain controlled with oral analgesics is now unexpectedly unable to swallow or has uncontrolled nausea and vomiting. His next dose of analgesics is due in 1 hour, and he cannot take it orally, even in liquid form. Moderate to severe pain will occur unless analgesics can be administered by another route, but no provision has been made for this (e.g., there are no drugs or equipment for intramuscular, subcutaneous, intravenous, or rectal administration). It would take 2 hours or longer to obtain such drugs or equipment. How can the oral analgesics he has been taking be used to provide pain relief now?

Possible solution: Take all oral forms of analgesics due in the next oral dose, dissolve them in warm water, and administer rectally.

Expected outcome: Pain relief will be satisfactory, but perhaps not ideal. Pain may increase somewhat, but moderate to severe pain will not occur.

HOW TO USE ORAL ANALGESICS RECTALLY IN AN EMERGENCY

- Obtain the physician's approval for changing the route of administration.
- Instruct the patient or family via telephone or do this yourself if you are in the home at the time:
  1. Assemble all the oral analgesics to be given at the next dose, including opioid and nonopioid.
  2. Review the ingredients and formulations.
     Caution: The only known exception to the following instructions concerns sustained-release formulations. Be especially alert to sustained-release morphine (MS Contin, Roxanol SR). If sustained-release morphine is included, administer only a portion of the dose due because dissolving the tablets will convert morphine to immediate-release morphine with a duration of approximately 4 hours. Thus if sustained-release morphine doses are given every 8 hours, each dose would be divided in half and given every 4 hours.
     Although there is no research to support this practice, many home care nurses report that satisfactory analgesia can be obtained

Modified from McCaffery M, Pasero C, *Pain: clinical manual for nursing practice*, St. Louis, 1999, Mosby.

6

from any of the oral analgesics by converting them to the rectal route as explained here. Some medications are more irritating than others, but hopefully this is only a temporary measure. Oral analgesics given rectally with successful pain relief include tablets of oxycodone plus acetaminophen, hydromorphone, liquid or tablets of morphine, methadone, and several of the NSAIDs.

3. Place the tablets in a small but strong container (e.g., cup), and crush them with the bowl of a small spoon.

4. Measure a teaspoon (5 ml), or more if necessary, of very hot tap water. Pour over the crushed tablets. Mix or crush further until fairly well dissolved. Let it sit while you find the equipment needed to insert it into the rectum. It should be about body temperature when it is inserted. Warm again if it gets cold or hardens.

5. Several types of equipment may be improvised for rectal insertion of the liquid. An ideal arrangement is a syringe with a short length of small-lumen rubber catheter attached. If this is not available, any of the following will suffice if the patient is placed in a position where gravity can assist (e.g., bending over or lying on his side):

   • Any equipment used to administer enemas. The main problem is likely to be that the tubing is so long that some of the medication is lost by adhering to the sides of the tubing. Using more water to dissolve the tablets may help.

   • Douche equipment, with some modification of the usual tip for insertion. Again, long tubing may be a problem.

   • Baster (pointed tube with bulb attached, often used for basting turkey) or rubber ear syringe (not used much anymore, but it has a small rubber tip and a bulb). With either of these, immediately before insertion into the rectum, suction up the liquid, point the open end upward, and squeeze out as much air as possible without losing the liquid. Maintain that amount of bulb compression until the tube is inserted in the rectum. Then compress completely and withdraw.

   • Any clean, small-lumen rubber tubing attached to a funnel.

   • If all else fails, a plastic straw may be attached to a funnel shaped of aluminum foil or wax paper.

6. Lubricate the end of the tubing prior to insertion. A water-soluble lubricant (e.g., K-Y Jelly) is best, but if it is not available, use a small amount of any lubricant such as Vaseline, butter, or cooking oil.

7. Slowly insert the tube about $1\frac{1}{2}$ inches into the rectum.

8. After the liquid has been inserted, position the patient on his left side for better absorption.

9. Get a pain rating from the patient at the time the medications is given rectally and then at half-hour intervals. If pain is not relieved or has increased after 1 hour, give another dose rectally. If there is no relief after 1 hour, consider giving 50% to 100% of the previous rectal dose. If there is some relief but not enough, consider giving an additional 25% of the previous dose.

QUICK ALTERNATIVES TO LIQUID FORM OF RECTAL ADMINISTRATION

1. Except for sustained-release tablets, the tablets or capsules themselves may simply be inserted about $1\frac{1}{2}$ inches into the rectum. If lubricant is necessary, moisten with water or use a water-soluble lubricant such as K-Y Jelly. Absorption takes longer, since the tablets must first dissolve, and seems less reliable than the liquid formulation. However, small tablets or those without a coating may work well.
2. If the volume is small, put the crushed tablet in an empty capsule. Simply empty any capsule for use unless the patient is allergic to whatever it contained. Again, absorption may take longer than with the liquid formulation.

IMMEDIATE HELP FOR PHARMACOLOGICAL CONTROL OF PAIN

*Maximal Use of Nonprescription Analgesics When Prescription Analgesics are Unavailable**

Time involved: Reading time, 3 minutes; implementation time, after ingredients are obtained, 5 minutes.

Situation: Unexpected moderate to severe pain of known cause (e.g., dislocated shoulder or broken bone from accidental fall) occurring in a healthy adult patient. A physician is contacted, but it will be 2 hours or longer before the patient can be seen by the physician. Also, due to time, location, and other factors, it is not possible to obtain any prescription analgesic. Using nonprescription analgesics available from a general store, what can be done to obtain maximal analgesia on a one-time-only basis?

Possible solution: Consider a combination of the following, if available, and obtain the physician's consent.

Expected outcome: Significant pain relief, but it may not be sufficient.

Maximal Pain Relief with Nonprescription Drugs

1. Acetaminophen 1000 mg in liquid form, if possible, or tablets (three regular tablets or two "extra strength" tablets)
2. Ibuprofen 800 mg (four tablets of 200 mg each)
3. Antacid (1 teaspoon of a concentrated liqud, if possible)
4. Caffeine 100 to 200 mg (a strong cup of brewed coffee, or one to two "keep awake" nonprescription tablets)
5. Carbonated beverage (e.g., 7-Up) or one with caffeine (e.g., Pepsi)
6. Alcohol (e.g., wine, gin). Many social drinks combine a carbonated beverage with alcohol (e.g., gin and tonic). A social drink may be relaxing or distracting.

Caution: Use of the above should be restricted to emergencies or "one time only." Consult a physician and determine the patient's previous response to each ingredient. Drugs that have produced unwanted side effects should be eliminated.

---

*Or, when the physician won't return your call, when the physician has refused to prescribe anything, when the pharmacy loses the prescription, or in other frustrating situations.

Modified from McCaffery, Beebe A: *Pain: clinical manual for nursing practice*, St. Louis, 1989, Mosby, p. 46.

Rationale: No research supports the safety or effectiveness of the above combination. Separate research studies suggest that these ingredients would be an effective combination and are pharmacologically compatible (i.e., they may be given together). Regarding each item, the rationale is as follows:

1. Acetaminophen relieves pain in a manner different from other nonnarcotics. It is well tolerated (i.e., side effects are unlikely). Combinations of acetaminophen and aspirin have been approved for sale as nonprescription analgesics. Patients on NSAIDs are allowed to take acetaminophen

2. Ibuprofen is an NSAID somewhat similar to aspirin but better tolerated (e.g., fewer GI upsets). The maximal recommended single dose of ibuprogen when it is prescribed by a physician is 800 mg. (The nonprescription recommended dose is limited to 400 mg.) If ibuprofen is unavailable or undesirable for any reason, aspirin can be substituted in a dose of 1000 mg. Aspirin could be given along with ibuprofen and the other ingredients. Omitting it from the above list may be unnecessary, but it could increase the risk of GI upset and decrease the effectiveness of the ibuprofen (probably to a limited extent). There are no data on the combination of ibuprofen and aspirin as a single dose. They are sometimes combined in the treatment of rheumatoid arthritis. The recommendation in this instance to give either aspirin or ibuprofen, but not both, is merely a qualified guess. On a single-dose basis for analgesia only, ibuprofen may do what aspirin does but with fewer side effects. Adding aspirin to the ibuprofen may increase the risks more than the analgesia (possibly is a duplication of effort)

3. Antacids are recommended in combination with NSAIDs to prevent stomach upset. Antacids may also hasten the absorption of NSAIDs

4. Caffeine, in doses of 100 to 200 mg, has been shown to increase the effectiveness of both acetaminophen and aspirin. If patients do not ordinarily consume caffeine beverages, they are probably not tolerant to them, so the dose should be kept to the minimum of 100 mg to prevent side effects such as nervousness. If the patient is a regular user of caffeine (e.g., 4 cups or more of coffee a day), the larger dose of 200 mg may be advisable

5. Carbonation seems to result in a much faster onset of action, probably by helping to dissolve tablets and promoting absorption
6. Alcohol has some analgesic as well as tranquilizing and sedating properties. If the patient drinks alcohol enough to be familiar with his response to it, it can be given in the amount usually tolerated.

However, it does increase the likelihood of GI irritation, especially along with aspirin.

Nausea or anxiety: If the patient has a history of vomiting in response to varied stimuli (a "weak stomach"), give a nonprescription antiemetic or sedative. Most over-the-counter (OTC) antiemetics are sedating. Sedation alone may decrease nausea or anxiety. An OTC product for "motion sickness" or anything for an allergy or cold may help (e.g., one that contains diphenhydramine, or Benadryl). There is some indication that diphenhydramine is analgesic or potentiates analgesia. If needed, give it along with the analgesic combination.

PART SEVEN

HOSPICE DEFINITIONS, ROLES, AND ABBREVIATIONS

KEY HOSPICE DEFINITIONS AND ROLES

Abuse According to Medicare, *abuse* describes practices that, either directly or indirectly, result in unnecessary costs to the Medicare program. An example is providing medically unnecessary services or services that do not meet professionally recognized standards.

Access The availability of health care and the ability of an individual to receive services such as hospice, including all factors related to cost, location, transportation, and ability to receive care.

Accreditation A rigorous process that examines various components of hospice operations and clinical practice. The achievement of accreditation designates that the organization has gone through the accreditation process and meets predetermined standards as measured by on-site survey team "visitors."

A process that an organization or program undertakes to demonstrate it has met established standards or requirements (e.g., the Joint Commission for Accreditation of Healthcare Organizations [JCAHO] and the Community Health Accreditation Program [CHAP]).

Activities of daily living (ADLs) Basic, usually self-care, activities that must be done daily to care for our bodies and overall health. These activities include personal hygiene tasks such as bathing and grooming and obtaining and preparing food. Others include toileting and transferring in and out of bed. These activities are important indicators because they demonstrate the patient's functional status or health care needs.

Advance directives Effective December 1, 1991, participating hospices (and other participating organizations, such as home health agencies and hospitals) must comply with the advance directive provisions of S4206 of the Omnibus Budget Reconciliation Act (OBRA) of 1990. This means the hospice must inform adult patients in writing of state laws regarding advance directives and of their policies regarding the implementation of advance directives. The hospice must document in the individual's clinical record whether the individual has executed an advance directive and cannot impose conditions on the provision of care or otherwise discriminate against an individual based on whether that individual has executed an advance directive (since the law does not require an individual to do so). Moreover, the hospice must educate staff and the community on issues concerning advance directives. Two common forms of advance directives are a living will and a durable power of attorney for health care.

Advocacy A role assumed by a health care professional designed to maximize patient self-determination through education, support and affirmation of patient health care decisions.

Agency for Health Care Policy and Research (AHCPR) An agency of the U.S. Department of Health and Human Services that sponsors research projects and develops clinical practice guidelines related to the delivery of health care services.

Autonomy Respect for patients as individuals who are capable of making their own choices about health care and lifestyle options.

Benchmark A systematic process to measure or quantify; a standard for comparing two similar types of products and services when trying to identify areas for improvement in an organization.

Bereavement Bereavement consists of counseling services provided to the hospice patient's family or survivors after the patient's death. An assessment is usually performed by a bereavement professional or specially trained volunteer to identify families or family members who may be at risk for bereavement problems.

Capitated risk The financial risk involved in not being able to estimate accurately the cost of services and contract appropriately for care or services to a capitated population.

Capitation A set dollar amount established to cover the cost of health care services delivered to an individual. The amount is based on the number of members in the plan, not the amount of services used.

Care plan A plan of action for care that is developed, delivered, and evaluated by a hospice interdisciplinary team. This may also be called the *plan of care*, and the format varies among organizations.

Caregiver Anyone who provides care or services to or for a patient.

Case management A system for overseeing a patient's care across health care settings or systems. Communication among the services and disciplines involved in the care must be documented in the clinical record. In these care conferences, input is given to the case manager to assist the disciplinary team in achieving predetermined or desired patient outcomes. Case management incorporates the principles of managed care. Hospice nurses may also interface with the insurance company nurse who is the care manager.

Case (Care) manager One person who is responsible for the overall care of the patient and use of resources for that care. The case (or care) manager may be a nurse, social worker, or therapist.

The primary person (registered nurse or other health care professional) responsible for developing patient care outcomes for his or her case load. A case manager is accountable for meeting outcomes within an appropriate length of stay, the effective use of resources, and preestablished standards. A case manager collaborates with the health care team and the patient to accomplish those outcomes.

Catheter Any rounded or tubular medical device that is inserted into veins, cavities, or other body passages. The purpose of a catheter is to improve or replace function. Examples include an indwelling urinary catheter in the bladder from which urine drains into a collection bag, suction catheters, and intravenous catheters inserted into the vein that allow for the delivery of fluids.

Centers for Medicare and Medicaid Services (CMS) An agency of the U.S. government under the Department of Health and Human Services (HHS) responsible for the Medicare and Medicaid programs. This direction includes various requirements, policies, payment for services, and many other operational aspects of the programs. CMS sets the coverage policy and payment and other guidelines and directs the activities of government contracts (e.g., carriers and fiscal intermediaries).

Certification Organizations desiring to participate in the Medicare program must meet participation conditions for certification (the Medicare Conditions of Participation). State agencies (such as the Department of Health) certify to the Department of Health and Human Services (DHHS) that the hospice or other types of organizations satisfy, and continue to satisfy, health care quality requirements for participation in the Medicare program.

Chaplaincy services The chaplain serves a population that spans the life continuum, from birth through death. The chaplain, like other hospice team members, interfaces with patients and their families and friends at some of the most difficult times of their lives. Many people who have significant health concerns struggle to come to terms with the meaning of life. The chaplain assists patients and families with this process, regardless of whether they have any formal religious beliefs. The role varies, based on the setting, the patient and family, or other needs. Responsibilities may include patient assessment and support, bereavement counseling, serving on ethics committees, hospice staff support, or performing the sacrament of the sick. The chaplain facilitates the patient's movement toward his or her own resolution of life's questions.

Patients who may benefit from chaplaincy services include those for whom the NANDA International nursing diagnoses *spiritual distress (distress of the human spirit)* and *spiritual well-being (potential for enhanced)* have been identified as appropriate. Other patients may have a need for spiritual care based on their health problems. For example, the elderly patient who is temporarily homebound as a result of a recent fall and fracture and misses going to church services may need a call made to her priest or minister to arrange visits to her home.

Chronic A slow or persistent illness or health problem that must be treated or monitored throughout the patient's life. Examples include diabetes, glaucoma, some cancers, and some chronic lung conditions.

Classification system A system of categorizing elements of similar groups using preestablished criteria.

Client One who receives care. Also called the *patient, customer,* or *consumer* of health care services or products. An individual, customer, consumer, or patient who receives care or services.

Clinical care All the events that encompass the diagnosis and treatment of illness and the attainment of specific patient outcomes; it is the process of the health care team member and the physician working closely with the patient and the patient's family to meet predetermined and patient self-determined clinical outcomes.

Clinical path (CP) A structured plan for care, often categorized by diagnosis or patient problem, that defines specific care interventions, team members, and other information across a time line. Clinical management tools that organize, sequence, and time the major interventions of nursing staff, physicians, rehabilitation therapists, and other health professionals for a particular case type of condition. The pathways describe a standard of practice and are, in essence, a clinical budget.

Coinsurance The amount or percentage of the cost of services that consumers may be required to pay under a cost-sharing agreement with their insurance plan or program. It may also be called a *copayment*.

Collaboration The active process of working together and valuing another's input toward reaching patient goals. The act of working together to achieve a common goal(s). In health care, collaboration is a joint effort by staff from many disciplines planning together to improve the processes, which leads to improved patient care.

Community health nursing A synthesis of nursing practice and public health practice applied to promoting and preserving the health of the population. Health promotion, health maintenance, health education and management, and the coordination and continuity of care contribute to a holistic approach to the management of the health care of individuals, families, and groups within a community.

Continuous quality improvement (CQI) An ongoing process, also called *performance improvement* (PI), that seeks to continuously improve patient care, delivery of services, staff education, and other important parts of operations or other parts of an organization. Accreditation standards demand continuous quality improvement. Home care or hospice team members may be involved in various parts of CQI/PI or be asked to serve on certain committees.

A conceptual framework for evaluating the quality of care that emphasizes an analytical approach to understanding the contributions of all components of the health care system in achieving results and constantly incorporating improvements into the system.

Cost containment Those measures or requirements established by organizations involved in the delivery of health care to control the increases in utilization or expenditures.

Critical path A tool for case management and managed care that is an abbreviated versions of the physician, nursing, rehabilitation therapists, and other service processes that must occur in a timely fashion to achieve an appropriate length of stay. Those key incidents may be categorized according to tests, activities, treatment, medication, diet, discharge planning, teaching and outcomes. This can also be referred to as a *clinical path*. (See *Clinical paths*.)

Data (singular form: *datum*) Products of measurement compiled in such a fashion that discussion can be formulated or inference can be obtained.

Dementia Changes in brain function that cause memory loss, confusion, or the loss of ability to safely function independently.

Diagnoses The identification of problems or diseases. The singular form of the term is *diagnosis*.

Diagnostic-related groups (DRGs) A code of classifying patient illnesses according to principal diagnosis and treatment requirements. Under Medicare, each DRG has its own price (weight) that a hospital is paid regardless of the actual cost of treatment.

Dietitian The role of the registered dietitian (RD) is expanding as more patients are cared for in the community setting. Hospices have professional dietitians available to make home visits and provide consultative services to promote optimal patient nutrition. Another important component of the dietitian's role is as inservice educator for the care team. The RD also explains the nutrition/hydration parts of advanced directives.

Often, after being hospitalized, patients receive instructions on nutrition with regard to their unique needs and medical condition. Some of the common reasons home care patients consult with a dietitian are for enteral/ parenteral nutrition considerations, anorexia, cancer, COPD, pressure ulcers, end-stage renal failure, diabetes, AIDS, and other diseases, as well as assessment and monitoring of nutritional needs. Often, the family or caregiver needs the information from the RD more than the patient does.

More innovative insurers are reimbursing for this care when organizations clearly articulate the patient's need and justify the visits as part of the comprehensive plan.

Documentation The writing of clinical notes that contains information needed for communication and legal and other reasons.

Effective management A health care management style that shares the focus of patient care with administration of the program and effectively seeks improvement through the simplification and review of all systems involved in care or service delivery.

Enteral nutrition Provision of nourishment via a tube inserted into the nose and down to the stomach or through a surgical site through the stomach. A G-tube is one way to administer enteral nutrition.

Enterostomal therapy nurse Some organizations have an enterostomal therapy (ET) nurse, also known as a wound, ostomy, continence nurse (WOCN), available as a consultant and clinical specialist. This role is particularly important in the home care and hospice settings, which have a wound, ostomy continence nurse high volume of patients with ostomy, wound, and skin problems. The clinical specialist role is also important in serving the educational needs of the clinical visiting staff and community.

Equity of care A health care system that differentiates levels of care based on assessed patient needs, not individual or group characteristics (e.g., ability to pay).

Evaluation visit (assessment visit) The first or initial hospice visit to determine whether the patient meets the criteria for admission. It is often the first skilled visit, made when the nurse already has specific physician's orders and is providing a skilled service to the patient.

Extended care services Patient care services provided as an alternative to inpatient hospitalization, in a skilled nursing facility, rehabilitation facility, or subacute facility offered after an acute illness or injury.

Fee for service A health plan in which beneficiaries choose their health care provider and the health plan pays the provider charge for services. This type of plan usually includes some element of utilization review or prior approval by the plan for certain, if not all, services.

Fraud Medicare defines *fraud* as making false statements or representations of material facts in order to obtain some benefit or payment for which no entitlement would otherwise exist. These acts may be committed either for the person's own benefit or for the benefit of some other party. Examples of fraud include billing for services that were not furnished and/or supplies not provided and falsely representing the nature of the services furnished (e.g., describing a noncovered service in a misleading way that makes it appear as if a covered service were actually furnished).

Gatekeeper One who has the overall responsibility for a patient's course of care and reviews, approves, or disapproves all requests for health care services. This rule has traditionally been filled by a physician but may be filled by a managed care provider, a payor, or a subcontracted utilization review group.

Goals The end point of care or the desired results for care. For example, if the goal is to provide safe mobility, everything done should support that goal. The team members work together to achieve the patient goals. The desired result of an action or series of actions an individual or organization might strive for; a goal is different from an objective in that a goal is more broad based, and objectives are more quantifiable and specific and are derived from a goal statement.

G-tube A stomach or gastrostomy tube used to place nutrients into the stomach when the patient cannot safely swallow or eat.

Health maintenance organization (HMO) A health care provider organization that offers a comprehensive health service plan to its beneficiaries through an established network of primary care physicians, specialists, clinics, and hospitals. It provides these services on a prepaid, fixed-cost basis.

Homebound A criterion for meeting Medicare home care requirements. Synonomous with the phrase *confined primarily to the home as a result of medical reasons*, the term connotes that it is a "considerable and taxing effort" for the patient to leave home (applicable only to hospices that are home health agencies).

Home care/Home health A range of health care services and products provided to a patient in his or her place of residence. Medicare home health care currently reimburses skilled nursing, speech-language pathology, physical and occupational therapy, medical social work, and home health aide services.

Home health agency (HHA) An organization that provides care to patients in their homes. The agency may or may not be licensed, depending on state requirements. Medicare-certified agencies must have a survey or a special review to accept Medicare patients.

Home health aide The aide's primary supportive function is to provide personal care and ADL assistance. This role and the associated functions are very important to the patient and family. The aide usually spends more actual time with the patient and family than does any other team member. The aide's contribution is invaluable to both the team process and the achievement of positive patient outcomes.

Home medical equipment (HME) Walkers, wheelchairs, commodes, beds, infusion pumps, TENS units, oxygen, suction machines, and other products related to patient care are HME. Under the Medicare hospice benefit, most medical equipment and supplies are included in the care because the hospice benefit is a managed care payment program. Because Medicare has made many changes to the HME rules, you need to consult your HME representative for specific rules, indications, and coverage requirements. Some equipment requires Certificates of Medical Necessity (CMNs), which are completed by the physician. Most private insurers now provide some coverage for patients needing HME at home. The HME products and supplied needed and used by the hospice patients should be mentioned in the clinical documentation because they may help support the medical necessity and level of needed hospice care.

Hospice care Hospice care is appropriate for patients with a terminal illness. Hospice care focuses on the comfort and quality of life to assist the patient and family in making every remaining day the best that it can be. Hospice is a philosophy, and care can be provided in any setting, such as home, a skilled nursing facility, or an inpatient hospice unit. Palliative care, emotional support, and control of pain and other symptoms are some of the areas of expertise addressed by the hospice team. Through team meeting and individual visits, the physician, the spiritual counselor, the primary nurse, the hospice volunteers, the social worker, the hospice clinical specialist, and others assist the patient and family in meeting their unique needs.

After death, bereavement support services are provided to the family as a key component of continued hospice care.

Hospice nursing Hospice nursing uses knowledge gained as a professional nurse to execute skills, render judgments, and evaluate process and outcome while supporting and caring for a diverse group of patients and families. Teaching, assessment, pain management, support, presence, active listening, and evaluation skills are some of the many areas of expertise that are hallmarks of hospice nursing practice. For Medicare, nursing care is provided by or under the supervision of a registered nurse.

ICD-9 code A coding method developed to identify specific clinical diagnoses for the purpose of data collection and payment. DRGs are assigned an ICD-9 code.

Instrumental care (IADLS) The provision of assistance with instrumental activities of daily living, such as shopping, cooking, transportation, financial management, homemaking, and home maintenance.

Integrated delivery network A provider of health care services that offers a wide continuum of services to its customer population. It usually comprises one or more acute care hospitals, skilled and intermediate nursing facilities, outpatient and ambulatory surgery centers, home health care agencies, hospices, and physicians who either are employees of the group or are tightly controlled by utilization management techniques.

Intermediary (also called the *Regional Home Health Intermediary [RHHI]*—The Medicare Part A RHHI is an organization that has entered into an agreement with the Centers for Medicare and Medicaid Services (CMS) to process Medicare claims and make payment determinations or adjudications for home care and hospice organizations. Hospices are generally assigned to the RHHI based on their geographic location.

Length of stay/service (LOS) The number of hospice days for each patient. Each patient's care is subject to review to determine the appropriateness of the length of stay (ALOS, average length of stay).

Managed care Care that is organized to achieve specific patient outcomes within fiscally responsible time frames (length of stay) using resources that are appropriate in amount and sequenced to the specific case type and population of the individual patient. Care is structured by case management care plans and clinical paths that are based on knowledge by case type regarding usual length of stay, critical events and their timing, anticipated outcomes, and resource utilization.

Managed care plan or organization (MCP or MCO) Any organization providing a network of patient care services, including physician and clinic or hospital care, for a set, agreed-upon payment. These plans employ a variety of cost-containment measures, discounts, and utilization review services in an effort to control or manage the risk of providing health care.

Medicaid A health program that is administered at the state level for patients who qualify. The basis for qualification is financial. Medicaid coverage varies by state. Sometimes even the name is different; for example, in California it is called *MediCal*.

Medical Social Services (MSS) Social services in hospice provide support to the patient and family and are related to the patient's medical condition. When social concerns impede the effective implementation of the POC, a social worker is appropriate. These concerns may include family, finances, grief work, housing, and caregiver issues. The social worker has an important role in assisting hospice patients and families through their unique situation and journey.

Medicare A federal program for people who are over age 65 or disabled or who have end-stage renal disease (ESRD). Medicare is complex but has two main parts, Part A and Part B, that cover different services, such as inpatient hospitalization (after the Medicare beneficiary pays a deductible), home care, and hospice. Medicare is a medical insurance program, and like all insurance programs, it has exclusions, eligibility, and coverage rules.

Medicare health maintenance organization (HMO) An alternative insurance product for Medicare beneficiaries that allows commercial insurers to contract with the CMS to provide similar Medicare covered services. Providers must have a contract with such insurers to provide beneficiary care. The advantages of such a program are that beneficiaries do not have to submit paperwork for payment, do not have to pay a copayment or deductible, and may appear to have a richer benefit package. However, beneficiaries are limited in the number of providers to whom they may go for services and the number or types of services allowed.

Medicare hospice The Medicare definition of hospice is that a hospice is a public agency or private organization that is primarily engaged in providing care to terminally ill individuals, meets the conditions of participation for hospices, and has a valid provider agreement. An individual may elect to receive Medicare coverage of election periods for hospice care. For patients to be eligible for Medicare hospice care, they must be entitled to Medicare Part A and be certified as being terminally ill. An individual is considered to be terminally ill if the individual has a medical prognosis that his or her life expectancy is 6 months or less if the terminal illness runs its normal course. The patient "elects" the benefit and is the one who can "revoke" or decide to discontinue the Medicare benefit, thus reverting to traditional Medicare benefits. There are four levels of care and reimbursement through the Medicare hospice benefit: (1) routine home care, (2) continuous home care, (3) impatient respite care, and (4) general impatient care.

Occupational therapy (OT) OT services are usually based on the loss of function and not the specific diagnosis. Occupational therapy services may include but are not limited to patients who have a decreased ability to perform ADLs, have impaired cognition, required joint protection techniques and energy conservation techniques, and who regime care-giver support and instruction.

Occupational Safety and Health Administration (OSHA) All clinicians have heard much in recent years about the need for practice of universal or standard precautions. Clinicians are well aware of the dangers of hepatitis B and HIV. Employees must create infection-control policies that support the use of these precautions. In addition, nurses, home health aides, and other team members must be educated about the policy. In practice, this means that hepatitis B immunizations are available when the job requires exposure to blood or other potentially infectious body fluids. The hospice must also provide protective equipment and supplies, including gloves, face masks or other protective shields, fluidproof aprons, gowns, and other needed protection. These should be provided by the organization free of charge to the hospice nurses and staff. OSHA also issues guidelines on blood or other body fluid transport, blood spill clean up, and the safe disposal of infectious waste.

Outcomes Outcomes are quantifiable or measurable goals of care to be achieved in a specific time frame (e.g., the patient, by a certain date, can name all medications and the times to take them).

Outcome, clinical The results or effects of clinical processes on patients. The results may be described by outcome criteria.

Outcomes criteria The ends to be achieved. From a knowledge of the usual course of events and the factors relevant to the patient group involved, that clinician should be able to determine the desired results for a given patient at the end of a program or service of care. Services should have been carried out in a fashion adequate to achieve the purpose of the outcome criteria.

Payor The payor or insurance company financially responsible for the services or care provided to patients. Examples include Medicare or other insurance companies.

The organization responsible for paying a health care provider for the health care products and/or services provided to a patient or beneficiary.

Performance Improvement See Continuous quality improvement (CQI).

Performance measure A quantifiable standard or measurement to determine how successful a health care provider has been in meeting established outcomes or goals of care.

Personal emergency response systems (PERSs) PERSs are a unique technology that links the frail or elderly with community resources, neighbors, or a friend at the push of a button or through voice-activated mechanisms. Although different types exist, all are telephone service dependent. PERSs may be appropriate for single patients returning home after surgery, patients who live alone or spend many hours at home alone, or patients at risk from falls. PERSs allow subscribers to signal for help at the push of a button. For the system to be effective, the emergency device must be worn at all times. Hospice nurses are in a unique position to identify this safety need in the community setting so that a referral can be initiated.

Pharmacist The role of the clinical pharmacist in hospice and home care is growing as the emphasis on quality and addressing patient needs from an interdisciplinary model continues. In practice, nurses are acutely aware of many patients who are inappropriately mediated or overmedicated.

Traditionally, the pharmacist has been considered the provider of a product—drugs. While this is certainly true, the pharmacist can offer many other services to the home care team.

Many patients are elderly and have multiple risk factors for therapeutic misadventures secondary to drug therapy. These patients may have multiple pathological conditions and different prescribers. They may exhibit polypharmacy (both prescription and nonprescription medications) and are at a greater risk for adverse effects from medications because of altered physiology secondary to aging and disabilities (e.g., poor eyesight, impaired hearing, arthritic fingers). Don't forget that a pharmacist can offer more than the provision of drugs; the pharmacist is the drug expert. This discipline is an excellent position to review medication regimens and screen for drug interactions (i.e., drug-drug, drug-disease, drug-food), adverse drug reactions, and incorrect doses or dosage forms and make recommendations. The pharmacist can suggest simplifying the patient's medication regimen by altering drug delivery systems or medication administration scheduling or by suggesting ways to monitor and assess the therapeutic or toxic effect of drugs. Hospice providers can always turn to a pharmacist for drug information, the provision of inservice education, or participation in case conferences and home care/hospice rounds.

Physical therapy (PT) PT services are usually based on the loss of function and not the specific diagnosis. Physical therapy services may include but are not limited to patients who are at risk for falling, have decreased bed mobility, decreased gait ability, functional loss of ROM or extremity strength as well as caregiver support and instruction.

Physician certification The physician is an important member of the hospice care team. Medicare requires that the physician certify that the patient is terminally ill. The timeline for signature varies, depending on state licensure, but must be obtained before billing (Balanced Budget Act of 1997).

In subsequent hospice periods the organization must obtain written certification no later than 2 calendar days after the first day of each period. The certification includes: (1) the statement that the individual's medical prognosis includes a life expectancy of 6 months or less, (2) the signatures of the physicians.

Preferred provider organization (PPO) A health services program that provides its members with services from contracted providers of care. Beneficiaries receive better cost coverage by using a contracted provider; they can use a noncontracted provider but will be responsible for a copayment or additional fee for service.

Pressure sore An area of redness or skin breakdown, possibly affecting surrounding tissues, usually over a bony prominence and related to immobility.

Process A series of activities or events that are related and sequenced in such a fashion as to effect a prescribed or established patient outcome.

Quality A degree of excellence. The achievement of individualized outcomes. *Quality* is defined by the organization and also by the patient/family.

Quality assessment The measurement or assessment of care provided to an individual or a group.

Quality assurance The systematic review of all activities included in the provision of services or the production of a product that meets preestablished criteria, which provides a sense of confidence that a certain level of quality has been achieved.

Quality improvement The achievement of a level of performance or quality status that has not been met before in this process.

Respiratory therapy Respiratory therapy services usually involve patients who need oxygen or have other respiratory problems or illnesses.

Sentinel event A significant or serious patient event or outcome that needs to be evaluated immediately. Sentinel events are commonly risk management issues.

Speech-language pathology (S-LP) S-LP services are usually based on the loss of function and not the specific diagnosis. Speech-language pathology services may include but are not limited to patients with decreased communication abilities, impaired cognition, dysphagia, and apraxia, as well as caregiver support and instruction.

Standard A level of performance or set of conditions considered acceptable by some authority or by the individual or individuals engaged in performing or maintaining the set of conditions in question.

Structure The framework of an organization that supports and defines how the components of a process are bound together to meet or achieve a given outcome (e.g., in hospice organizations the policies, procedures, and clinical competency checklists and standards define in part how patient care will be delivered).

Time line Identifies when an event or a series of event should occur, following a preestablished and agreed-upon framework for those events to happen or specific outcomes to be achieved.

Total quality management A system of continuous quality improvement that empowers employees to review and concentrate on the system or processes affecting group achievements and that is directed from senior management.

Variance The difference between what is expected and what actually happens. Variances are differential by system (internal or external), practitioner, and patient.

Volunteers Volunteers are the backbone of hospice services and provide respite and advocacy services. Some programs are solely volunteer driven, although this model is changing as reimbursement and costs make significant changes in health care generally. Volunteers are specially trained and selected for multifaceted skills that include well-honed listening skills and the ability to demonstrate empathy and provide support. Activities or duties in which volunteers may participate are as varied as hospice but may include bereavement, direct care, and transportation assistance.

7

KEY HOSPICE ABBREVIATIONS

The following abbreviations are those most commonly used in the practice of hospice and home care. Please refer to your hospice's own designated list of approved abbreviations for daily use in documentation.

ADLs	Activities of daily living
ADR	Adverse drug reaction; additional development request
ALS	Amyotrophic lateral sclerosis (Lou Gehrig's disease)
APHA	American Public Health Association
ASCVD	Arteriosclerotic cardiovascular disease
ASD	Atrial septal defect
ASHD	Arteriosclerotic heart disease
BP	Blood pressure
BPH	Benign prostatic hypertrophy
BRP	Bathroom privileges
BS	Blood sugar
CA	Cancer
CABG	Coronary artery bypass graft
CBC	Complete blood count
CDC	Centers for Disease Control and Prevention
CHAP	Community Health Accreditation Program
CHF	Congestive heart failure
CHPN	Certified Hospice and Palliative Nurse
CHPNA	Certified Hospice and Palliative nursing Assistant
CLIA	Clinical Laboratory Improvement Act
CMS	Centers for Medicare and Medicaid Services
CNA	Certified nursing assistant
CNS	Clinical nurse specialist; Central nervous system
COPD	Chronic obstructive pulmonary disease
COPs	(Medicare) Conditions of Participation
CPM	Continuous passive motion
CPR	Cardiopulmonary resuscitation
CVA	Cerebral vascular accident
CXR	Chest x-ray (film)
DJD	Degenerative joint disease
DM	Diabetes mellitus
DME	Durable medical equipment
DNI	Do not intubate
DNR	Do not resuscitate
DOE	Dyspnea on exertion
DRG	Diagnosis-related group
DX	Diagnosis
ET	Enterostomal therapist
FBS	Fasting blood sugar
FMR	Focused medical review
FX	Fracture
HHA	Home health agency or home health aide

HHC	Home health care
HHS	Health and Human Services
HME	Home medical equipment
IDDM	Insulin-dependent diabetes mellitus
IDG	Interdisciplinary group
IDT	Interdisciplinary team
IG	Inspector General
IM	Intramuscular
IV	Intravenous
JCAHO	Joint Commission on Accreditation of Healthcare Organizations
LLE	Left lower extremity
LLL	Left lower lung
LUE	Left upper extremity
MI	Myocardial infarction
MOW	Meals on Wheels
MSS	Medical social services
NHP	Nursing home placement
NIDDM	Non-insulin–dependent diabetes mellitus
NIH	National Institutes of Health
OIG	Office of Inspector General
OSHA	Occupational Safety and Health Administration
OT	Occupational therapy
PC	Pastoral care
PCA	Patient-controlled analgesia
PERLA	Pupils equal, react to light and accommodation
PICC (line)	Peripherally inserted central catheter
PO	By mouth (orally)
POC	Plan of care
PRE	Progressive resistive exercises
PRN	As needed
PT	Physical therapy
PVD	Peripheral vascular disease
RHHI	Regional home health intermediary
RLE	Right lower extremity
RLL	Right lower lung
ROM	Range of motion
RUE	Right upper extremity
SKN or SN	Skilled nursing
S-LP	Speech-language pathology
SNF	Skilled nursing facility
SNV	Skilled nursing visit
SOB	Shortness of breath
S/P	Status post
SQ	Subcutaneous
SX	Symptoms
TC	Telephone call
TENS	Transcutaneous electrical nerve stimulation

7

TF	Tube feeding
TIA	Transient ischemic attack
Title XVIII	The Medicare section of the Social Security Act
Title XIX	The Medicaid section of the Social Security Act
Title XX	The Social Services section of the Social Security Act
TO	Telephone order
TPN	Total parenteral nutrition
TPR	Temperature, pulse, and respiration
TURP	Transurethral resection of prostate
TX	Treatment
UA/C&S	Urinalysis/culture and sensitivity
UE	Upper extremity
URI	Upper respiratory infection
UTI	Urinary tract infection
VO	Verbal order
WNL	Within normal limits

7

PART EIGHT

DIRECTORY OF RESOURCES

RESOURCES

1.	Administration
2.	Advance Directives
3.	Aides
4.	AIDS/HIV
5.	Book Resources
6.	Clinical Resources
7.	End-of-Life Issues
8.	Ethics
9.	Fraud and Abuse
10.	Government
11.	Hospice Nursing Certification
12.	Internet Sites
13.	Journals
14.	Medicare
15.	National Organizations
16.	Nutrition Resources
17.	Orientation
18.	Other Resources
19.	Pain
20.	Patient Resources
21.	Pediatric
22.	Spiritual
23.	Volunteers

8

ADMINISTRATION

Kilburn L: *Hospice operations manual: hospice for the next century*. To order, call 800-646-6460, or write to the following address for further information: NHPCO Marketplace, Dept. 929, Alexandria, VA 22334-0929 or visit online at *www.nhpco.org*

Marrelli T: The *nurse manager's survival guide: practical answers to every-day problems*, ed 2, St. Louis 2004, Mosby. Call 800-993-6397 or 941-697-2900 for more information.

Medical guidelines for determining prognosis in selected non-cancer diseases, ed 2, Arlington, Va, 1996, National Hospice & Palliative Care Organization (NHPCO). This book can be obtained by writing to NHPCO Marketplace, Dept. 929, Alexandria, VA 22334-0929 or visit online at *www.nhpco.org*

National Hospice & Palliative Care Organization (NHPCO). This book can be obtained by writing to NHPCO Marketplace, Dept. 929, Alexandria, VA 22334-0929 or visit online at *www.nhpco.org*

ADVANCE DIRECTIVES (SEE ALSO "END-OF-LIFE ISSUES")

The American Bar Association
Commission on Legal
Problems of the Elderly
1800 M Street, NW
Washington, DC 20036

American Health Decisions
319 E. 46th Street #9V
New York, NY 10017
212-268-8900

Hastings Center
Institute of Society, Ethics,
and the Life Sciences
255 Elm Road
Briarcliff Manor, NY 10510
914-478-0500

Pacific Center for Health Policy
and Ethics
444 Law Center
University of Southern California
Los Angeles, CA 90089
213-740-2541

U.S. Department of Health
and Human Services
Office of Public Affairs
Centers for Medicare & Medicaid
Services (CMS)
6325 Security Boulevard
Baltimore, MD 21207
202-245-6977

AIDES (HOSPICE AIDE, HOME HEALTH AIDE, CERTIFIED NURSING ASSISTANT [CNA])

Home Health Aide Digest. For subscriptions, write to 404 Parkwood Ave, Kalamazoo, MI 49001 (800-340-3356; fax 616-344-8274).

Home Health Aide Video Series, Marrelli and associates, Inc, call 800-993-6397 or 941-697-2900

Marrelli T, Whittier S: *Home health aide: guidelines for care*, Englewood, Fla, 1996, Marrelli and Associates. For more information, call 800-993-6397 or 941-697-2900.

Marrelli T, Friend L: *Home health aide: guidelines for care instructor manual*, Englewood, Fla, 1997, Marrelli and Associates. For more information, call 800-993-6397 or 941-697-2900.

AIDS/HIV

A Clinical Guide to Supportive and Palliative Care for HIV/AIDS, Health and Human Services, available online at *http://hab.hrsd.gov* or order from HRSA Information Center at 888-275-4772.

Carr D, editor: *Pain in HIV/AIDS*, Washington, DC, 1994, France-USA Pain Society. Available from Roxane Pain Institute, Cail 800-335-9100.

Flaskerud JH, Ungvarski PJ: *HIV/AIDS: a guide to nursing care*, ed 3, Philadelphia, 1997, WB Saunders.

Ross Labs offers a free videotape entitled *Taking charge: managing the symptoms of HIV*. This videotape addresses interventions for pain and fatigue in patients with AIDS. Ask your local Ross representative for the tape, or call 800-227-5767 if you do not know who the representative in your area is. Ask for Tape #H358V.

Visit online at *www.AIDS.org,* for information about HIV infection and prevention.

Visit online at *www.AIDSaction.org*, works in HIV/AIDS policy arena.

BOOK RESOURCES

Aspen Reference Group: *Palliative care patient and family counseling manual*, Gaithersburg, MD., 1996, Aspen.

Berger AM, Portenoy RK and Weissman DE (eds) (2002). *Principles and practice of palliative care and supportive oncology*. Hagerstown, MD: Lippincott, Williams & Wilkins.

Byock I: *Dying well: the prospect for growth at the end of life*, New York, 1997, Riverhead Books.

Callahan M, Kelley P: *Final gifts*, New York, 1993, Bantam.

Doyle D, Hanks GWC, McDonald N, (eds): *The Oxford textbook of palliative medicine*, New York, 2003, Oxford University Press.

Ferrell BR and Coyle N (eds) (2001). *The textbook of Palliative Nursing*. New York: Oxford University Press.

Finkelman AW: *Psychiatric home care*, 1997, 3rd ed. Jones and Bartlett.

Forman WB, Sheehan DC, et al (eds) (2003): *Hospice and palliative care: concepts and practice*, Sudbury, MA: Jones and Bartlett.

Irish DP, Lundquist KF, Nelson VJ: *Ethnic variations in dying, death, and grief*, 1993, Taylor and Franas.

Kübler-Ross E: *Death: the final stage of growth*, Englewood Cliffs, NJ, 1975, Prentice-Hall

Larson DG: *The helper's journey: working with people facing grief, loss, and life-threatening illness*. Champaign, III, 1993, Research Press.

Lipman AG, Jackson KC, Tyler LS (eds): *Evidence based symptom control in palliative care: Systemic reviews and validated clinical practice guidelines for 15 common problems in patients with life limiting disease*, Binghamton, NY, 2000, The Haworth Press.

Marrelli T: *Handbook of home health standards and documentation guidelines for reimbursement*, ed 4, St. Louis, 2001, Mosby. For more information, call 800-993-6397 or 941-697-2900.

Marrelli T, Friend L: *Home health aide: guidelines for care instructor, 2000, manual*, Englewood, Calif, 1997, Marrelli and Associates. For more information, call 800-993-6397 or 941-697-2900.

Marrelli T, Whittier S: *Home health aide: guidelines for care*, Englewood, Calif, 1996, Marrelli and Associates. For more information, call 800-993-6397 or 941-697-2900.

Matzo ML and Sherman DW: *Palliative care nursing: quality care to the end of life*. New York, 2001, Springer Publishing Company.

Medical guidelines for determining prognosis in selected non-cancer diseases, ed 2, Arlington, VA, 1996, National Hospice Organization (NHO). For information, write NHPCO at 1700 Diagonal Rd, Suite 625, Alexandria, VA 22314, or call 703-837-1500 or visit online at *www.nhpco.org*.

Robert D: *Profits of death: an insider exposes the death care industries*, Chandler, AZ, 1997, Five Star Publications.

Storey P: *Primer of palliative care*, ed 2, Glenview, IL, 1996, American Academy of Hospice and Palliative Medicine. For more information, write the American Academy of Hospice and Palliative Medicine at 4700 W. Lake Avenue, Glenview, IL 60025, 847-375-4712, *www.aahpm.org*.

Yarbro CH, Frogge MH, Goodman M, Groenwald SL (eds): *Cancer Nursing: Principles and Practice*. Sudbury, MA, 2000, Jones and Bartlett Publishers.

CLINICAL RESOURCES

After Diagnosis
Communicating with Friends and Relatives About You
A Message of Hope: Coping with Cancer in Everyday Life
Sexuality and Cacner

The American Cancer Society provides several cancer information pamphlets and booklets free of charge to people with cancer and their families and friends. They can be obtained by calling the American Cancer Society (ACS) at 800-227-2345 or visit online at *www.cancer.org*.

The Cancer Survivor's Toolbox, a set of six audiotapes is available free of charge by calling 877-866-5748 or visit online at *www.cansearch.org/programs/toolbox.htm*.

Home Care of the Hospice Patient is an informational/instructional booklet for caregivers in the home. For more information, write Purdue Frederick Company, 100 Connecticut Avenue, Norwalk, CT 06850-3590 or call 1800-733-1333.

How to Find Resources in Your Own Community if You Have Cancer
Taking Time
Facing Forward

The National Cancer Institute (NCI) provides information on coping with cancer. This information can be obtained free of charge by calling 1800-4CANCER or visit online at *www.cancer.gov.*

National Hospice and Palliative Care Organization (NHPCO): *NHPCO medical guidelines for determining prognoses in selected non-cancer diseases.* These guidelines may be obtained by calling the NHPCO or by writing the NHPCO Store, 1700 Diagonal Rd, Suite 625, Alexandria, VA, 223141 or call 1703-837-1500 or online at *www.nhpco.org.*

Pressure ulcer treatment: Clinical practice guideline, No. 15, Rockville, Md, 1994, U.S. Department of Health and Human Services, Public Health Service, Agency for Health Care Policy and Research. AHCPR Pub. No. 95-0653.

END-OF-LIFE ISSUES

8

The Center to Improve Care of the Dying (CICD), *http://gwu.edu/~cicd.* Research, advocacy, and educational activities to improve the care of the dying.

Commission on Aging with Dignity offers the "Five Wishes" living will free of charge. It can be obtained by writing to P.O Box 11180, Tallahassee, FL 32302-3180 or by calling toll-free 1888-5-WISHES.

Webb M: *The good death: the new American search to reshape the end of life*, New York, 1997, Bantam.

ETHICS

National Hospice and Palliative Care Organization (2002). *Vital Bonds: Ethical Principles and Guidelines for Organizational Conduct.* Alexandria, VA: Author, To order, contact NHPCO at 1800-646-6460, visit online at *www.nhpco.org,* or Department 929, Alexandria, VA 22334-0929.

Hastings Center report. Call 1-845-424-4040 or visit online at *www.Thehastingcenter.org*

The Institute of Ethics Journal. Call 1-800-548-1784 or visit online at *www.press.jhu.edu*

FRAUD AND ABUSE

The Department of Health and Human Services has a toll-free hotline to report fraud and abuse by providers in the Medicare and Medicaid programs: 800-447-8477. Their mailing address is Office of Inspector

General, Department of Health and Human Services, HHS-TIPS Hot Line, P.O. Box 23489, Washington, DC 20026.

GOVERNMENT

Centers for Medicare and Medicaid Services (CMS) (800-638-6833) or visit online at *cms.gov*
  Medicare Hospice Benefits (free flyer)
  Medicare Handbook (free, includes detailed information about Medicare programs, including hospice)
Centers for Medicare and Medicaid Services (CMS) manuals are available through the following subscription services:
  Government Printing Office
  Superintendent of Documents (Sup Docs)
  Washington, DC 20402
  202-512-1800
  web site: www.gpoaccess.gov

  National Technical Information Services (NTIS)
  Department of Commerce
  5285 Port Royal Road
  Springfield, VA 22161
  1-888-584-8332
  web site: www.ntis.gov

Medicare Hospice Benefits is a free brochure (Publication No. HCFA 02154). For more information, call the Centers for Medicare and Medicaid Services (CMS) at 800-638-6833.
Medicare Hospice Manual (CMS Pub. 21) is available by calling the U.S. Department of Commerce's National Technical Information Service (NTIS) at 888-584-8332. Medicare-certified hospices will receive the manual from their designated regional home health intermediary (RHHI). (The RHHIs process and adjudicate the hospice and home care claims.)

HOSPICE NURSING CERTIFICATION

The National Board for Certification of Hospice and Palliative Nurses (NBCHPN®) promotes a certification process that advances quality in the provision of end of life care. Current certifications include those for RNs (CHPN) and nursing assistants (CHPNA). A certification for LPNs/LVNs will be implemented September 2004. For more information, contact NBCHPN® at Penn Center West One, Suite 229, Pittsburgh, PA 15276; email online at *nbchpn@hpna.org;* or phone 412-787-1057.

INTERNET RESOURCE SITES

AHRQ (Agency for Healthcare Research and Quality)
web site: *http://www.ahcpr.gov*

Alzheimer's Disease Education and Research
web site: *http://www.alzheimers. org/adear*

American Academy of Hospice and Palliative Medicine
web site: *http://www.aahpm.org*

American Cancer Society
web site: *http://www.cancer.org*

American Pain Society
web site: *http://ampainsoc.org*

American Society for Pain Management Nurses
web site: *http://www.aspmn.org*

Last Acts
web site: *http://www.lastacts.org*

Food and Drug Administration
web site: *http://www.fda.gov*

Health and Human Services, Department of (DHHS)
web site: *http://www.dhhs.gov*

Hospice and Palliative Nurses Association
web site: *http://www.hpna.org*

House of Representatives
web site: *http://www.house.gov*

Innovations in End-of-Life Care
web site: *http://www.edc.org/ lastacts*

Institute for Safe Medication Practices, Nurse Advise-ERR
web site: *http://www.ismp.org*

Library of Congress
web site: *http://www.loc.gov*

Marrelli and Associates, Inc.
web site: *http://www.marrelli.com*

National Committee for Quality Assurance (HMOs)
web site: *http://www.ncqa.org*

National Hospice and Palliative Care Organization (NHPCO)
web site: *http://nhpco.org*

National Institute of Health (NIH)
web site: *http://www.nih.gov*

Occupational Safety and Health Administration
web site: *http://www.osha.gov*

Social Security Administration
web site: *http://www.ssa.gov*

U.S. Senate
web site: http://www.senate.gov

White House
web site: *http://www.whitehouse.gov*

JOURNALS

AJN publishes bimonthly articles on hospice and palliative care. Visit online at *www.nursingcenter.com*

American Journal of Hospice and Palliative Care is a multiprofessional journal published bimonthly by Prime National Publishing Corporation,

470 Boston Post Road, Weston, MA 02493. Call 781-899-2702 to order, or get more information online at *www.pnpco.com.*

Clinical Journal of Oncology Nursing, official journal of the Oncology Nursing Society, *www.ons.org.*

Healing Ministry is a peer-reviewed quarterly publication available from Prime National Publishing Corporation, 470 Boston Post Road, Weston, MA 02493. Call 781-899-2702 to order, or get more information online at *www.pnpco.com.*

Home Healthcare Nurse, The Journal for the Home Care and Hospice Professional, is published monthly by Lippincott, Williams & Wilkins, 16522 Hunters Green Parkway, Hagerstown, MD 21740. Call 301-223-2300 or get information online at *www.lww.com.*

Journal of Health Care Chaplaincy is a biannual publication available from The Haworth Press, Inc., 10 Alice Street, Binghamton, NY 13904-1580. Call 800-3-HAWORTH (342-9678) or fax 1-607-722-6362 for more information.

Journal of Hospice and Palliative Nursing, the official journal of the Hospice and Palliative Nursing Association, is a quarterly publication available from Lippincott, Williams & Wilkins, 16522 Hunters Green Parkway, Hagerstown, MD 21740. Call 301-223-2300 or get information online at *www.lww.com.*

Journal of Pain and Palliative Care Pharmacotherapy is a quarterly publication available from The Haworth Press, 10 Alice Street, Binghamton, NY 13904-1350. Call 1-800-429-6784 or order online at *www.haworth-press.com.*

Journal of Pain and Symptom Management (Including Supportive and Palliative Care) is a monthly publication available from Elsevier. Visit online at *www.elsevier.com* for more information.

Journal of Palliative Medicine, the official journal of the American Academy of Hospice and Palliative Medicine, is a bimonthly interdisciplinary journal published by Mary Ann Liebert, Inc. Publishers, 2 Madison Ave., Larchmont, NY 10538-1962. Call 914-834-3100 or get information online at *www.liebertpub.com.*

MEDICARE

Centers for Medicare and Medicaid Services (CMS) (1-800-638-6833)
   Medicare Hospice Benefits (free flyer)
   Medicare Handbook (free; includes detailed information about Medicare programs, including hospice)

Centers for Medicare and Medicaid Services (CMS) manuals are available through the following subscription services:
   CMS Open Door Forum e-newsletter, *http://www.cms.hhs.gov/opendoor/*

Government Printing Office
Superintendent of Documents (Sup Docs)
Washington, DC 20402
202-512-1800
web site: *http://www.fedbbs.access.gpo.gov*

National Technical Information Services (NTIS)
Department of Commerce
5285 Port Royal Road
Springfield, VA 22161
800-553-NTIS (6847)
web site: *www..fedworld.gov/NTIShome.html*

Dear Marci is a free, weekly newsletter about health care benefits, rights and options for older and disabled Americans. It is a service of the Medicare Rights Center (MRC) at *www.medicarerights.org.*

Medicare Hospice Benefits is a free brochure (Publication No. CMS 02154). Call 800-638-6833.

Medicare Hospice Manual (HCFA Pub. 21) can be ordered by calling the U.S. Department of Commerce's National Technical Information Service (NTIS) at 703-487-4630. Medicare-certified hospices will receive the Manual from their designated regional home health intermediary (RHHI). (The RHHIs process and adjudicate the hospice and home care claims.)

NATIONAL ORGANIZATIONS

American Academy of Hospice and Palliative Medicine (AAHPM)
  4700 W. Lake Avenue
  Glenview, IL 60025
  847-375-4712
  website: *www.aahpm.org*
Hospice Association of America
  228 Seventh St., SE
  Washington, DC 20003
  202-547-7424
  web site: *http:www.nahc.org/haa*
Hospice Foundation of America
  2001 S St., NW, #300
  Washington, DC 20009
  800-854-3402
  web site: *www.hospicefoundation.org*
Hospice and Palliative Nurses Association
  Penn Center West One, Suite 229
  211 North Whitfield St.
  Pittsburgh, PA 15276
  412-787-9301
  web site: *www.hpna.org*

National Association for Home Care and Hospice (NAHC)
   228 Seventh St., SE
   Washington, DC 20003
   202-547-7424
   web site: *http://www.nahc.org*
National Family Caregivers Association (NCFA)
   10400 Connecticut Ave, #500
   Kensington, MD 20895-3944
   800-896-3650
   web site: *http://www.nfcacares.org*
National Funeral Directors Association
   13625 Bishop's Drive
   Brookfield, WI 53005-6607
   800-228-6332 or 414-541-2500
National Prison Hospice Association (NPHA)
   P.O. Box 3769
   Boulder, CO 80307-3769
   303-447-8051
   web site: *http://npha.org*
National Hospice and Palliative Care Organization (NHPCO)
   1700 Diagonal Road #300
   Alexandria, VA 22314
   703-837-1500
   website: *www.nhpco.org*
Oncology Nursing Society (ONS)
   125 Enterprise Drive
   Pittsburgh, PA 15275-1214
   866-257-4ONS
   web site: *www.ons.org*

8

NUTRITION RESOURCES

Gallagher-Allred CR: *Nutritional care of the terminally ill.* Sudbury, MA: 1989, Jones and Bartlet Publishers.

Gallagher-Allred C, Amenta MO, editors: *Nutrition and hydration in hospice care: needs, strategies, ethics.* New York, 1993, The Haworth Press.

ORIENTATION

Marrelli T: *Handbook of home health orientation.* St Louis, 1998, Mosby. Call 800-993-6397 or 941-697-2900 for more information.

Marrelli T, Hilliard L: *Manual of home health practice: guidance for effective clinical operations.* St. Louis, 1998, Mosby. Call 800-993-6397 or 941-697-2900 for more information.

OTHER RESOURCES

Access to Hospice Care: Expanding Boundaries, Overcoming Barriers, a special supplement to the Hastings Center Report, The Hastings Center, 21 Malcolm Gordon Road, Garrison, NY 10524-5555 (845-424-4040), or visit online at *www.thehastingscenter.org*

Center to Advance Palliative Care (CAPC), 125 Fifth Avenue, Suite C-2, New York, NY 10029 (212-201-2670) or visit online at *www.capc.org.*

Hospice Helpline (800-658-8898), provided by the National Hospice and Palliative Care Organization (NHPCO), offers information about hospice care in general and hospices in the caller's community.

Hospice Link (800-331-1620) is a nationwide toll-free service provided by the Hospice Education Institution to the general public and to health care professionals seeking referrals to local hospices and palliative care services or bereavement groups.

National Hospice and Palliative Care Organization (2001). *Hospice Service Guidelines.* Alexandria, VA: Author. To order, contact NHPCO at 800-646-6460, or visit online at *www.nhpco.org,* or Department 929, Alexandria, VA 22334-0929.

National Hospice and Palliative Care Organization (2001). *Competency-Based Education for Social Workers.* Alexandria, VA: Author. To order, contact NHPCO at 800-646-6460, or visit online at *www.nhpco.org,* or Department 929, Alexandria, VA 22334-0929.

National Hospice and Palliative Care Organization (2001). *Total Sedation: A Hospice and Palliative Care Resource Guide.* Alexandria, VA: Author. To order, contact NHPCO at 800-646-6460, or visit online at *www.nhpco.org,* or Department 929, Alexandria, VA 22334-0929.

National Hospice and Palliative Care Organization (2002). *Guidelines for Bereavement Care in Hospice.* Alexandria, VA: Author. To order, contact NHPCO at 800-646-6460, or visit online at *www.nhpco.org,* or Department 929, Alexandria, VA 22334-0929.

National Hospice and Palliative Care Organization (2000). *standards of Practice for Hospice Programs.* Alexandria, VA: Author. To order, contact NHPCO at 800-646-6460, or visit online at *www.nhpco.org*, or Department 929, Alexandria, VA 22334-0929.

National Hospice and Palliative Care Organization (2000). *Guidelines for Nursing in Hospice Care.* Alexandria, VA: Author. To order, contact NHPCO at 800-646-6460, or visit online at *www.nhpco.org,* or Department 929, Alexandria, VA 22334-0929.

National Hospice and Palliative Care Organization (NHPCO) store offers a catalog of consumer education brochures, books, technical materials, videos, posters, and promotional items. For more information, write to NHPCO store at 200 State Road, South Deerfield, MA 01373-0200 (800-646-6460; Fax 800-499-6464).

NHPCO Standards and Accreditation Committee, Medical Guidelines Task Force: *Medical guidelines for determining prognosis in selected non-cancer diseases*, Arlington, VA, 1996, National Hospice Organization.

Wrede-Seaman, L. (1999). *Symptom Management Algorithms: A Handbook for Palliative Care.* Yakima, WA: Intellicard. To order, contact Intellicard, P.O. Box 8255, Yakima, WA 98908 or visit online at *http://intellicard.com.*

PAIN

Agency for Healthcare Policy and Research (AHCPR) (800-358-9295 or 301-495-3453) or visit online at *www.ahrq.gov*
   Clinical Practice Guideline Number 9: *Management of Cancer Pain; Quick Reference Guide for Clinicians; Management of Cancer Pain: Adults; Patient Guide Managing Cancer Pain.*

Cancer Information Service of National Cancer Institute (800-4-CANCER [422-6237]):
   Get Relief from Cancer Pain (free pamphlet)
   Questions and Answers about Pain Control (free 76-page booklet)
   AHCPR Cancer Pain Guidelines (free)

Competency Guidelines for Cancer Pain Management in Nursing Education and Practice Developed by the Wisconsin Center Cancer Pain Initiative (WCPI). Single laser-printed copy available free of charge by writing the WCPI at 1300 University Avenue, Room 4720, Madison WI 53706 or calling 608-262-0978.

DuPen, Inc., online at *www.painconsult.com,* for a decision tree/algorithm for managing cancer pain.

Ferrell BR: *Suffering,* Boston, 1996, Jones and Bartlett.

International Association for the Study of Pain (IASP), 909 NE 43rd St, Suite 306, Seattle, WA 98150-6020 (206) 547-6409, or visit online at *www.iasp-pain.org* and *www.painbooks.org* newsletter: PAIN Clinical Updates.

Kaye P: *Notes on symptom control in hospice & palliative care*, Essex, Conn. 1990, Hospice Education Institute.

Management of cancer pain. Clinical practice guideline No. 9, Rockville, MD. 1994, Agency for Health Care Policy Research, Public Health Service, U.S. Department of Health and Human Services. AHCPR Publication No. 94-0592.

McCaffery, M, Pasero, C: *Pain: Clinical Manual,* ed. 2, St. Louis, 1999, Mosby.

Principles of analgesic use in the treatment of acute pain and cancer pain, ed. 3, Skokie, III, 1992, American Pain Society. For more information, write to the American Pain Society at 5700 Old Orchard Road, First Floor, Skokie, IL 60077-1057 (708-966-5595)

For the "Patient Comfort Assessment," write to The Purdue Frederick Company, 100 Connecticut Avenue, Norwalk, CT 06850-3590. Ask for a listing of free resources related to pain and its management available to home care and hospice nurses.

The Roxane Pain Institute for Cancer and AIDS has a 24-hour toll-free number for services to both professional and patients. For information and reference materials, such as AHCPR materials, call 800-335-9100.

8

PATIENT RESOURCES

American Brain Tumor Association, 2720 River Road, Des Plaines, IL 60018 (847-827-9910 or 800-886-2282 [patient line]; fax 847-827-9918) or visit online at *www.abta.org*. Patient education booklets, listings of support groups, referrals to support organizations, and information about treatment facilities.

Chemotherapy and You: A Guide to Self-Help During Treatment (NIH Publication No. 96-1136; free booklet). Published by the National Cancer Institute of the National Institutes of Health (800-4-CANCER) or online at *www.cancer.gov*.

Eating Hints for Cancer Patients (NIH Publication No. 95-2079; free booklet). Published by the National Cancer Institute of the National Institutes of Health (800-4-CANCER) or online at *www.cancer.gov*.

Caregiving at Life's End is a program that teaches a framework for caregiving training provided by The Hospice Institute of the Florida Suncoast. Call 727-586-4432 or get information online at *www. thehospice.org*.

Gone from My Sight: The Dying Experience. This pamphlet may be obtained by writing to Barbara Karnes, RN, P.O. Box 189, Depoe Bay, OR 97341.

Heads Up, The Newsletter of The Braintumor Society, 124 Watertown Street, Suite 3H, Watertown, MA 02472-2500, or visit online at *www.tbts.org*.

Hungry for Air: Sharing the Grief about COPD is a free informational card about Chronic Obstructive Pulmonary Disease available from The American Lung Association®, 61 Broadway, 6th Floor, NY, NY 10006, 212-315-8700, or visit online at *www.lungusa.org*.

The Leukemia and Lymphoma Society, 1311 Mamaroneck Ave., White Plains, NY 10605, 914-949-5213, or visit online at *www.leukemia.org*.

My Friend, I Care: The Grief Experience. This pamphlet may be obtained by writing to Barbara Karnes, RN, P.O. Box 189, Depoe Bay, OR 97341.

News from SPOHNC, a publication of Support for People with Head and Neck Cancer, or visit online at *http://www.spohnc.org*.

Radiation Therapy and You: A Guide to Self-Help During Treatment (NIH Publication No. 95-2227; free booklet). Published by the National Cancer Institute of the National Institutes of Health (800-4-CANCER) or visit online at *www.cancer.gov*.

A Time to Live: Living with a Life-Threatening Illness. This pamphlet may be obtained by writing to Barbara Karnes, RN, P.O. Box 189, Depoe Bay, OR 97341.

"tlc" Catalog of hats, scarves, hairpieces, and mastectomy bras and clothing from the American Cancer Society. To request a catalog, call (800-850-9445), or visit online at *www.tlccatalog.org*

Traveling with Oxygen (air, land, sea, international travel) are informational items available from the American Lung Association website, *http://www.lungusa.org/support/traveloxygen.html*.

PEDIATRIC

Acute Pain Management in Infants, Children, and Adolescents: Operative and Medical Procedures (AHCPR 92-0020). U. S. Department of Health and Human Services, Agency for Health Care Policy and Research (800-358-9295 or 301-495-3453).

Alex's Journey: *The Story of a Child with a Brain Tumor* is a video from the American Brain Tumor Association, 2720 River Road, Des Plaines, IL 60018 (847-827-9910 or 800-886-2282).

Armstrong-Daily A, Zarbock S, editors: *Hospice care for children*, New York, 1993, Oxford University Press. Available from Children's Hospice Inter-national: 800-2-4-CHILD or 703-684-0330.

Children's Hospice International (902 North Pitt Street, Suite 230, Alexandria, VA 22314, 800-2-4-CHILD or 703-684-0330) offers information, a referral network, and numerous resources and publications. For more information, call or visit online at *www.chionline.org*.

CHIPACC (*CHI Program for All-Inclusive Care for Children and their families®*) is a federally funded program created by Children's Hospice International with technical assistance from CMS, or visit online at *www.chionline.org*.

ELNEC – Pediatric Palliative Care Training Program (ELNEC-PPC) is a national educational curriculum to prepare nurses in end-of-life, or visit online at *www.aach.nche.edu/elnec/ELNECPediatric.htm*.

Funletter is a national activities letter for kids and families living with cancer published by Friends Network, P.O. Box 4545, Santa Barbara, CA 93140. For more information, call 805-565-7031; or visit online at *www.kidscancernetwork.org*

Harriet Lane Handbook: A Manual for Pediatric House Officers (2002), edited by The Johns Hopkins Hospital, Christian Nechyba, MD, and Veronica L. Gunn, MD, is published by Mosby.

Home Care For Seriously Ill Children: A Manual For Parents, by I.M. Martinson and D.G. Moldow, is available from Children's Hospice International (800-2-4-CHILD or 703-684-0330).

Implementation Manual: Establishing Hospice Programs to Serve Children and their Families, by Paul Brenner and Sarah Zarbock, is a manual that focuses on application of hospice and palliative care philosophy, planning and model of care for children. Available from Children's Hospice International, 901 North Pitt Street, Suite 230, Alexandria, VA 22314, 800-2-4-CHILD, 703-684-0330.

Interdisciplinary Clinical Manual for Pediatric Hospice and Palliative Care, Edited by Susan M. Huff, RN, MSN, and Stacy Orloff, LCSW, EdD, Focuses on the role of the clinicians in the provision of care to children with life-threatening conditions and their families. Available from Children's Hospice International, 800-2-4-CHILD or or visit online at *www.chioniline.org*.

8

SPIRITUAL

Carson VB, editor: *Spiritual dimensions of nursing practice*, Philadelphia, 1989, WB Saunders.

Fitchett G: *Assessing spiritual needs: a guide for caregivers*, (2002) Academic Renewal Press.

Johnson C, McGee M: How different religions view death and afterlife, Philadelphia, 1998, The Charles Press.

Journal of Health Care Chaplaincy is a biannual publication available from The Haworth Press, Inc., 10 Alice Street, Binghamton, NY 13904-1580 (800-3-HAWORTH [342-9678]; fax 607-722-6362).

Kalina K: *Midwife for souls: spiritual care for the dying*, Boston, 1994, Pauline Books and Media. A guide for hospice care workers and all who live with the terminally ill. For more information, write the publisher at 50 St. Paul's Avenue, Boston, MA 02130.

National Hospice and Palliative Care Organization (2001). *Guidelines for Spiritual Care in Hospice*, Alexandria, VA: Author. To order, contact NHPCO at 800-646-6460, or visit online at *www.nhpco.org,* or Department 929, Alexandria, VA 22334-0929.

Reanney D: *After death, a new future for human consciousness*, New York, 1996, Avon.

Spiritual Assessment in Pastoral Care: A Guide to Selected Resources by G. Fitchett, is published by The Journal of Pastoral Care Publications (404-320-0195).

VOLUNTEERS

National Hospice and Palliative Care Organization (2001). *Hospice Volunteer Program Resource Manual.* Alexandria, VA: Author. To order, contact NHPCO at 800-646-6460, or visit online at *www.nhpco.org,* or Department 929, Alexandria, VA 22334-0929.

APPENDIX

NANDA INTERNATIONAL–APPROVED NURSING DIAGNOSES

Activity intolerance
Activity intolerance, risk for
Adjustment, impaired
Airway clearance, ineffective
Allergy response, latex
Allergy response, latex, risk for
Anxiety
Anxiety, death
Aspiration, risk for
Attachment, impaired parent/infant/child, risk for
Autonomic dysreflexia
Autonomic dysreflexia, risk for
Body image, disturbed
Body temperature, imbalanced, risk for
Bowel incontinence
Breastfeeding, effective
Breastfeeding, ineffective
Breastfeeding, interrupted
Breathing pattern, ineffective
Cardiac output, decreased
Caregiver role strain
Caregiver role strain, risk for
Comfort, impaired
Communication, verbal, impaired
Communication, readiness for enhanced
Conflict, decisional (specify)
Conflict, parental role
Confusion, acute
Confusion, chronic
Constipation
Constipation, perceived
Constipation, risk for
Coping, ineffective
Coping, readiness for enhanced
Coping, community, ineffective
Coping, community, readiness for enhanced
Coping, defensive
Coping, family, compromised
Coping, family, disabled
Coping, family, readiness for enhanced
Death syndrome, sudden infant, risk for
Denial, ineffective
Dentition, impaired
Development, delayed, risk for

From North American Nursing Diagnoses Association International: *Nursing diagnoses: definitions and classification, 2003-2004*, Philadelphia, 2003, the Association.

Diarrhea
Disuse syndrome, risk for
Diversional activity, deficient
Energy field, disturbed
Environmental interpretation syndrome, impaired
Failure to thrive, adult
Falls, risk for
Family processes: alcoholism, dysfunctional
Family processes, interrupted
Family processes, readiness for enhanced
Fatigue
Fear
Feeding pattern, infant, ineffective
Fluid balance, readiness for enhanced
Fluid volume, deficient
Fluid volume, excess
Fluid volume, deficient, risk for
Fluid volume, imbalanced, risk for
Gas exchange, impaired
Grieving
Grieving, anticipatory
Grieving, dysfunctional
Growth and development, delayed
Growth disproportionate, risk for
Health maintenance, ineffective
Health-seeking behaviors
Home maintenance, impaired
Hopelessness
Hyperthermia
Hypothermia
Identity, personal, disturbed
Incontinence, urinary, functional
Incontinence, urinary, reflex
Incontinence, urinary, stress
Incontinence, urinary, total
Incontinence, urinary, urge
Incontinence, urinary, urge, risk for
Infant behavior, disorganized
Infant behavior, disorganized, risk for
Infant behavior, organized, readiness for enhanced
Infection, risk for
Injury, risk for
Injury, perioperative positioning, risk for
Intracranial adaptive capacity, decreased
Knowledge, deficient
Knowledge of (Specify), readiness for enhanced
Loneliness, risk for
Memory, impaired

A

Mobility, bed, impaired
Mobility, physical, impaired
Mobility, wheelchair, impaired
Nausea
Neglect, unilateral
Noncompliance
Nutrition, readiness for enhanced
Nutrition: less than body requirements, imbalanced
Nutrition: more than body requirements, imbalanced
Nutrition: more than body requirements, risk for imbalanced
Oral mucous membrane, impaired
Pain, acute
Pain, chronic
Parenting, readiness for enhanced
Parenting, impaired
Parenting, impaired, risk for
Peripheral neurovascular dysfunction, risk for
Poisoning, risk for
Post-trauma syndrome
Post-trauma syndrome, risk for
Powerlessness
Powerlessness, risk for
Protection, ineffective
Rape-trauma syndrome
Rape-trauma syndrome: compound reaction
Rape-trauma syndrome: silent reaction
Relocation stress syndrome
Relocation stress syndrome, risk for
Role performance, ineffective
Self-care deficit, bathing/hygiene
Self-care deficit, dressing/grooming
Self-care deficit, feeding
Self-care deficit, toileting
Self-concept, readiness for enhanced
Self-esteem, chronic low
Self-esteem, situational low
Self-esteem, situational low, risk for
Self-mutilation
Self-mutilation, risk for
Sensory perception, disturbed
Sexual dysfunction
Sexuality patterns, ineffective
Skin integrity, impaired
Skin integrity, impaired, risk for
Sleep deprivation
Sleep patterns, disturbed
Sleep, readiness for enhanced
Social interaction, impaired

A

Social isolation
Sorrow, chronic
Spiritual distress
Spiritual distress, risk for
Spiritual well-being, readiness for enhanced
Suffocation, risk for
Suicide, risk for
Surgical recovery, delayed
Swallowing, impaired
Therapeutic regimen management, effective
Therapeutic regimen management, ineffective
Therapeutic regimen management, readiness for enhanced
Therapeutic regimen management, community, ineffective
Therapeutic regimen management, family, ineffective
Thermoregulation, ineffective
Thought processes, disturbed
Tissue integrity, impaired
Tissue perfusion ineffective
Transfer ability, impaired
Trauma, risk for
Urinary elimination, readiness for enhanced
Urinary elimination, impaired
Urinary retention
Ventilation, spontaneous, impaired
Ventilatory weaning response, dysfunctional
Violence, other-directed, risk for
Violence, self-directed, risk for
Walking, impaired
Wandering

A

INDEX

A

AAHPM (American Academy of Hospice and Palliative Medicine), 492

Abbreviations, 480-482
dangerous, 66b, 67t-70t

Abuse
defined, 468
resources on, 488

Access to care
by children, 438b
defined, 468

Access to Hospice Care, 493

Accreditation, 35, 57, 468

Acetaminophen, 464, 465

Acquired immunodeficiency syndrome (AIDS), 89-104
bereavement counselor for, 96-97, 100
children with, 402-413
bereavement counselor for, 407, 410
comfort and symptom control for, 403-404
diagnoses and codes for, 402-403
educational needs of, 410-411
elimination in, 405
emotional/spiritual considerations for, 405, 406, 409
equipment and supply needs for, 402
general considerations for, 402
home health aide or certified nursing assistant for, 405, 409
Hospice nursing for, 403-405, 407-409
hydration/nutrition in, 405, 406, 409
music, massage, art, or other therapies or services for, 407, 410
occupational therapist for, 406, 409-410

Acquired immunodeficiency syndrome (AIDS) *(Continued)*
other considerations for, 405
outcomes for care of, 407-410
pharmacist for, 407, 410
physical therapist for, 407, 410
resources for, 413
safety considerations for, 402, 404
skills and services for, 403-407
skin care for, 405
social worker for, 406, 409
speech-language pathologist for, 407, 410
therapeutic/medication regimens for, 405
tips for quality and reimbursement for, 411-413
volunteers for, 406, 409
comfort and symptom control for, 91-92
diagnoses and codes for, 89-91
educational needs with, 101
elimination with, 93
emotional/spiritual considerations with, 92, 95-96, 99
epidemiology of, 89
equipment and supply needs for, 89
focus of care for, 89
home health aide or certified nursing assistant for, 95, 99
Hospice nursing for, 91-95, 97-99
hydration/nutrition with, 93-94, 96, 100
mobility considerations with, 92
music, massage, art, or other therapies or services for, 97, 101
occupational therapist for, 96, 100
other considerations with, 94-95
outcomes for care with, 97-101
pharmacist for, 97, 101
physical therapist for, 96, 100
resources for, 104, 486
safety considerations with, 89, 92

*Page numbers followed by f indicate figures; those followed by t indicate tables; those followed by b indicate boxed material.

505

Acquired immunodeficiency syndrome
        (AIDS) *(Continued)*
    skills and services for, 91-97
    skin care with, 92-93
    social worker for, 95, 99
    specific tips for quality and
            reimbursement for, 102-104
    speech-language pathologist for, 96,
            100
    therapeutic/medication regimens for,
            94
    volunteers for, 95, 99
Activities of daily living (ADLs), 468
    instrumental, 474
Administration, resources on, 485
Administrative staff, 7
Advance directives, 48, 468, 485
Advocacy, 468
Agency for Health Care Policy and
        Research (AHCPR), 468
Aides
    resources on, 485-486
    services provided by, 20-21
AIDS. *See* Acquired immunodeficiency
        syndrome (AIDS).
Alcohol, for pain, 464, 466
ALOS (average length of stay), 475
ALS. *See* Amyotrophic lateral sclerosis
        (ALS).
Alzheimer's disease, 105-116
    bereavement counselor for, 110, 113
    comfort and symptom control for,
            106-107
    diagnoses and codes for, 105-106
    educational needs with, 113-114
    elimination with, 108
    emotional/spiritual considerations
            with, 107, 109-110, 112-113
    equipment and supply needs for, 105
    general considerations with, 105
    home health aide or certified nursing
            assistant for, 109, 112
    Hospice nursing for, 106-109,
            110-112
    hydration/nutrition with, 108, 110,
            113
    mobility considerations with, 107
    music, massage, art, or other
            therapies or services for, 110,
            113

Alzheimer's disease *(Continued)*
    occupational therapist for, 110, 113
    other considerations with, 109
    outcomes for care with, 110-113
    physical therapist for, 110, 113
    resources for, 115-116
    safety considerations with, 105, 107
    skills and services for, 106-110
    skin care with, 107-108
    social worker for, 109, 112
    therapeutic/medication regimens for,
            108-109
    tips for quality and reimbursement
            for, 114-115
    volunteers for, 109, 112
American Academy of Hospice and
        Palliative Medicine (AAHPM),
        492
Amyotrophic lateral sclerosis (ALS),
        117-128
    bereavement counselor for, 122, 124
    comfort and symptom control for,
            117-118
    diagnoses and codes for, 117
    educational needs with, 125-126
    elimination with, 119
    emotional/spiritual considerations
            with, 118-119, 121, 123
    equipment and supply needs for, 117
    general considerations with, 117
    home health aide or certified nursing
            assistant for, 120, 123
    Hospice nursing for, 117-120,
            122-123
    hydration/nutrition with, 119-120,
            121, 123
    mobility considerations with, 118
    music, massage, art, or other therapies
            or services for, 122, 124
    occupational therapist for, 121, 124
    other considerations with, 120
    outcomes for care with, 122-125
    physical therapist for, 122, 124
    resources for, 128
    safety considerations with, 117, 118
    skills and services for, 117-122
    skin care with, 119
    social worker for, 120-121, 123
    speech-language pathologist for, 122,
            124

Amyotrophic lateral sclerosis (ALS)
  (Continued)
    therapeutic/medication regimens for, 120
    tips for quality and reimbursement for, 126-128
    volunteers for, 121, 123
Analgesics
  nonprescription, 464-466
  nurse's power and responsibility in relation to, 449*t*
  opioid, 455*t*-460*t*
  rectal administration of oral, 461-463
Antacids, with NSAIDs, 464, 465
Anxiety, and pain, 451*t*
Apothecary symbols, 67*t*
ARAdgA, 67*t*
Around the clock (ATC) medications, 449*t*
Aseptic technique, 50*b*
Assessment visit, 472
Associations, national, 492-493
AU, 67*t*
Automation, 75
Autonomy, 36, 469
Average length of stay (ALOS), 475
AZT, 67*t*

B
Bedbound patient, 129-143
  bereavement counselor for, 137, 140
  comfort and symptom control for, 132-133
  diagnoses and codes for, 130-132
  educational needs with, 140-141
  elimination by, 134
  emotional/spiritual considerations with, 133, 136, 139
  equipment and supply needs for, 129
  general considerations with, 129
  home health aide or certified nursing assistant for, 135-136, 139
  Hospice nursing for, 132-135, 138-139
  hydration/nutrition of, 135, 136-137, 140
  mobility considerations with, 133
  music, massage, art, or other therapies or services for, 137, 140

Bedbound patient *(Continued)*
  occupational therapist for, 137, 140
  other considerations with, 135
  outcomes for care with, 138-140
  physical therapist for, 137, 140
  resources for, 143
  safety considerations with, 129-130, 133
  skills and services for, 132-137
  skin care for, 133-134
  social worker for, 136, 139
  speech-language pathologist for, 137, 140
  therapeutic/medication regimens for, 135
  tips for quality and reimbursement for, 141-143
  volunteers for, 136, 139
Bedsores. *See* Pressure ulcers.
Benchmark, 469
Bereavement, 469
Bereavement assessment tool, 12, 13*f*-14*f*
Bereavement counselors, services provided by, 12, 13*f*-15*f*
Bereavement follow-up tool, 12, 15*f*
Bereavement program, for children, 441*b*-442*b*
Bisacodyl (Dulcolax), for constipation, 216*t*
Bolus administration, of opioids, 456*t*, 457*t*
Book resources, 486-487
Brain tumor, 144-156. *See also* Head and neck cancer.
  bereavement counselor for, 150, 153
  comfort and symptom control for, 145-146
  diagnoses and codes for, 145
  educational needs with, 154
  elimination with, 147
  emotional/spiritual considerations with, 146, 149, 152
  equipment and supply needs for, 144
  general considerations with, 144
  home health aide or certified nursing assistant for, 148, 152
  Hospice nursing for, 145-148, 150-152

Brain tumor *(Continued)*
 hydration/nutrition with, 147, 149,
  152-153
 mobility considerations with, 146
 music, massage, art, or other
  therapies or services for, 150,
  153-154
 occupational therapist for, 149, 153
 other considerations with, 148
 outcomes for care with, 150-154
 pharmacist for, 150, 153
 physical therapist for, 150, 153
 resources for, 155-156
 safety considerations with, 144, 146
 skills and services for, 145-150
 skin care with, 147
 social worker for, 148-149, 152
 speech-language pathologist for, 150,
  153
 therapeutic/medication regimens for,
  147-148
 tips for quality and reimbursement
  for, 154-155
 volunteers for, 149, 152
Breast cancer, 157-169
 bereavement counselor for, 163, 166
 comfort and symptom control for,
  158-159
 diagnoses and codes for, 157-158
 educational needs with, 167
 elimination with, 160
 emotional/spiritual considerations
  with, 159, 162, 165
 equipment and supply needs for, 157
 general considerations with, 157
 home health aide or certified nursing
  assistant for, 161, 165
 Hospice nursing for, 158-161, 163-
  165
 hydration/nutrition with, 160, 162,
  166
 mobility considerations with, 159
 music, massage, art, or other
  therapies or services for, 163,
  166
 occupational therapist for, 162-163,
  166
 other considerations with, 161
 outcomes for care with,
  163-166
 physical therapist for, 163, 166
 resources for, 169
 safety considerations with, 157, 159
 skills and services for, 158-163
 skin care with, 159-160
 social worker for, 161-162, 165
 therapeutic/medication regimens for,
  160-161
 tips for quality and reimbursement
  for, 167-169
 volunteers for, 162, 165
Breathing, during dying, 29*b*
"Bridge" program, 30
BT, 69*t*
Buccal administration, of opioids, 455*t*
Buprenorphine, sublingual
  administration of, 455*t*
Butorphanol, intranasal administration
  of, 456*t*

C
Caffeine, with nonprescription pain
  medications, 464, 465
Cancer, 170-184
 bereavement counselor for, 177, 181
 brain. *See* Brain tumor.
 breast. *See* Breast cancer.
 children with, 414-425
  bereavement counselor for, 418,
   422
  comfort and symptom control for,
   415
  diagnoses and codes for, 414-415
  educational needs of, 422-423
  elimination in, 416
  emotional/spiritual considerations
   for, 416, 417-418, 421
  equipment and supply needs for,
   414
  general considerations for, 414
  home health aide or certified
   nursing assistant for, 417,
   420
  Hospice nursing for, 415-417,
   419-420
  hydration/nutrition in, 416, 418,
   421
  music, massage, art, or other
   therapies or services for,
   419, 422

Cancer *(Continued)*
    occupational therapist for, 418, 421
    other considerations for, 417
    outcomes for care in, 419-422
    pharmacist for, 418-419, 422
    physical therapist for, 418, 421
    resources for, 424-425
    safety considerations for, 414, 416
    skills and services for, 415-419
    skin care for, 416
    social worker for, 417, 420
    speech-language pathologist for, 418, 421
    therapeutic/medication regimens for, 416-417
    tips for quality and reimbursement for, 423-424
    volunteers for, 417, 420-421
  comfort and symptom control for, 172-173
  diagnoses and codes for, 170-172
  educational needs with, 181
  elimination with, 174
  emotional/spiritual considerations with, 173, 176, 180
  equipment and supply needs for, 170
  general considerations with, 170
  of head and neck. *See* Head and neck cancer.
  home health aide or certified nursing assistant for, 175, 179
  Hospice nursing for, 172-175, 178
  hydration/nutrition with, 174, 176, 180
  mobility considerations with, 173
  music, massage, art, or other therapies or services for, 177-178, 181
  occupational therapist for, 177, 180
  other considerations with, 175
  outcomes for care with, 178-181
  pain management for, 178, 179*b*
  pharmacist for, 177, 181
  physical therapist for, 177, 180
  prostate. *See* Prostate cancer.
  resources for, 184
  safety considerations with, 170, 173
  skills and services for, 172-178
  skin care with, 174

Cancer *(Continued)*
  social worker for, 175-176, 179
  speech-language pathologist for, 177, 180-181
  therapeutic/medication regimens for, 174-175
  tips for quality and reimbursement for, 181-183
  volunteers for, 176, 180
CAPC (Center to Advance Palliative Care), 493
Capitated risk, 469
Capitation, 469
Car, 36, 52*b*-53*b*
Carbonated beverage, with nonprescription pain medications, 464, 466
Cardiac disease, 185-199
  bereavement counselor for, 192, 196
  comfort and symptom control for, 187-188
  diagnoses and codes for, 185-187
  educational needs with, 196
  elimination with, 189
  emotional/spiritual considerations with, 188, 191, 195
  equipment and supply needs for, 185
  general considerations with, 185
  home health aide or certified nursing assistant for, 190, 194
  Hospice nursing for, 187-190, 192-194
  hydration/nutrition with, 189-190, 191, 195
  mobility considerations with, 188
  music, massage, art, or other therapies or services for, 192, 196
  occupational therapist for, 192, 195
  other considerations with, 190
  outcomes for care with, 192-196
  pharmacist for, 192, 196
  physical therapist for, 192, 195-196
  resources for, 199
  safety considerations with, 185, 188
  skills and services for, 187-192
  skin care with, 189
  social worker for, 190-191, 194-195
  therapeutic/medication regimens for, 190

Cardiac disease *(Continued)*
    tips for quality and reimbursement
      for, 197-199
    volunteers for, 191, 195
Cardiovascular effects, of pain, 452t
Care guidelines, outline for, 88
Care manager, 469
Care plan, 8, 10, 65, 469
Care standards, 2-3, 35, 62-64
Caregiver, 469
Cascara, for constipation, 217t
Case management, 469
Case manager, 469
Catheter, 352-381
    bereavement counselor for, 368, 375
    comfort and symptom control for,
      354-356
    defined, 469
    diagnoses and codes for, 353
    educational needs with, 376-377
    elimination with, 357
    emotional/spiritual considerations
      with, 356, 367, 375
    equipment and supply needs for, 352
    general considerations with, 352
    home health aide or certified nursing
      assistant for, 366, 374
    Hospice nursing for, 354-358,
      369-370
    hydration/nutrition with, 357,
      367-368, 375
    music, massage, art, or other
      therapies or services for, 368,
      376
    occupational therapist for, 368, 375
    other considerations with, 358
    outcomes for care with, 369-370,
      374-376
    pharmacist for, 368, 375-376
    physical therapist for, 368, 375
    resources for, 381
    safety considerations with, 352, 356
    skills and services for, 354-358,
      360-368
    skin care with, 356
    social worker for, 366-367, 374
    speech-language pathologist for, 368,
      375
    therapeutic/medication regimens for,
      357-358

Catheter *(Continued)*
    tips for quality and reimbursement
      for, 377-378, 380-381
    volunteers for, 367, 374
cc, 69t
Center to Advance Palliative Care
    (CAPC), 493
Centers for Medicare and Medicaid
    Services (CMS), 10, 64, 469-470,
    475
Centrally generated pain, 454f
Cerebral vascular accident (CVA),
    200-214
    bereavement counselor for, 207, 210
    comfort and symptom control for,
      201-202
    diagnoses and codes for, 200-201
    educational needs with, 211
    elimination with, 203-204
    emotional/spiritual considerations
      with, 203, 206, 210
    equipment and supply needs for, 200
    general considerations with, 200
    home health aide or certified nursing
      assistant for, 205, 209
    Hospice nursing for, 201-205,
      207-209
    hydration/nutrition with, 204, 206,
      210
    mobility considerations with, 202
    music, massage, art, or other
      therapies or services for, 207,
      211
    occupational therapist for, 206, 210
    other considerations with, 205
    outcomes for care with, 207-211
    pharmacist for, 207
    physical therapist for, 206, 210
    resources for, 214
    safety considerations with, 200, 202
    skills and services for, 201-207
    skin care with, 203
    social worker for, 205, 209
    speech-language pathologist for, 206,
      210
    therapeutic/medication regimens for,
      204-205
    tips for quality and reimbursement
      for, 211-214
    volunteers for, 205, 209

Certificates of Medical Necessity
(CMNs), 474
Certification
defined, 470
hospice nursing, 9, 489
physician, 478
Certified nursing assistants (CNAs),
services provided by, 20-21
CHAP (Community Health
Accreditation Program), 35, 57,
468
Chaplains, services provided by, 13-16,
16*f*, 470
Cheyne-Stokes breathing, 29*b*
Children
access to care by, 438*b*
with AIDS, 402-413
bereavement counselor for, 407,
410
comfort and symptom control for,
403-404
diagnoses and codes for, 402-403
educational needs of, 410-411
elimination in, 405
emotional/spiritual considerations
for, 405, 406, 409
equipment and supply needs for,
402
general considerations for,
402
home health aide or certified
nursing assistant for, 405,
409
Hospice nursing for, 403-405,
407-409
hydration/nutrition in, 405, 406,
409
music, massage, art, or other
therapies or services for,
407, 410
occupational therapist for, 406,
409-410
other considerations for, 405
outcomes for care in, 407-410
pharmacist for, 407, 410
physical therapist for, 407, 410
resources for, 413
safety considerations for, 402, 404
skills and services for, 403-407
skin care for, 405

Children *(Continued)*
social worker for, 406, 409
speech-language pathologist for,
407, 410
therapeutic/medication regimens
for, 405
tips for quality and reimbursement
for, 411-413
volunteers for, 406, 409
bereavement program for, 441*b*-442*b*
with cancer, 414-425
bereavement counselor for, 418,
422
comfort and symptom control for,
415
diagnoses and codes for, 414-415
educational needs of, 422-423
elimination in, 416
emotional/spiritual considerations
for, 416, 417-418, 421
equipment and supply needs for,
414
general considerations for, 414
home health aide or certified
nursing assistant for, 417,
420
Hospice nursing for, 415-417,
419-420
hydration/nutrition in, 416, 418,
421
music, massage, art, or other
therapies or services for,
419, 422
occupational therapist for, 418,
421
other considerations for, 417
outcomes for care in, 419-422
pharmacist for, 418-419, 422
physical therapist for, 418, 421
resources for, 424-425
safety considerations for, 414, 416
skills and services for, 415-419
skin care for, 416
social worker for, 417, 420
speech-language pathologist for,
418, 421
therapeutic/medication regimens
for, 416-417
tips for quality and reimbursement
for, 423-424

Children *(Continued)*
  volunteers for, 417, 420-421
  continuity of care for, 440b-441b
  family-centered care for, 438b-439b
  hospice policies and procedures for, 439b
  interdisciplinary team services for, 439b-440b
  medically fragile, 426-437
    bereavement counselor for, 431, 435
    comfort and symptom control for, 427-428
    diagnoses and codes for, 426-427
    educational needs of, 435
    elimination in, 429
    emotional/spiritual considerations for, 429, 430-431, 434
    equipment and supply needs for, 426
    general considerations for, 426
    home health aide or certified nursing assistant for, 430, 433
    Hospice nursing for, 427-430, 432-433
    hydration/nutrition in, 429, 431, 434
    music, massage, art, or other therapies or services for, 432, 435
    occupational therapist for, 431, 434
    other considerations for, 430
    outcomes for care in, 432-435
    pharmacist for, 431-432, 435
    physical therapist for, 431, 434
    resources for, 437
    safety considerations for, 426, 428-429
    skills and services for, 427-432
    skin care for, 429
    social worker for, 430, 433
    speech-language pathologist for, 431, 434
    therapeutic/medication regimens for, 429-430
    tips for quality and reimbursement for, 436-437
    volunteers for, 430, 433

Children *(Continued)*
  outline for care guidelines for, 401
  pain and symptom management in, 441b
  rectal administration of opioids in, 460
  resources on, 496-497
  standards of hospice care for, 438b-442b
  utilization review/quality improvement for, 442b
Children's Hospice International, standards of hospice care for children by, 438b-442b
Chronic, defined, 470
Chronic obstructive pulmonary disease (COPD), 291-306
  bereavement counselor for, 297, 300-301
  comfort and symptom control for, 292-294
  diagnoses and codes for, 291-292
  educational needs with, 301-302
  elimination with, 295
  emotional/spiritual considerations with, 294, 296, 300
  equipment and supply needs for, 291
  general considerations with, 291
  home health aide or certified nursing assistant for, 296, 299
  Hospice nursing for, 292-295, 298-299
  hydration/nutrition with, 295, 296-297, 300
  mobility considerations with, 294
  music, massage, art, or other therapies or services for, 297-298, 301
  occupational therapist for, 297, 300
  other considerations with, 295
  outcomes for care with, 298-301
  pharmacist for, 297, 301
  physical therapist for, 297, 300
  resources for, 305-306
  safety considerations with, 291, 294
  skills and services for, 292-298
  skin care with, 294-295
  social worker for, 296, 299
  therapeutic/medication regimens for, 295

Chronic obstructive pulmonary disease
  (COPD) *(Continued)*
  tips for quality and reimbursement
    for, 302-305
  volunteers for, 296, 299-300
Chronulac (lactulose), for constipation,
  216*t*
CI (continuous infusion), of opioids,
  456*t*, 457*t*
Classification system, 470
Client, 470
Clinical care, 470
Clinical outcomes, 476
Clinical path (CP), 74-75, 470-471
Clinical record, importance of, 57-59
Clinical resources, 487-488
Clinicians, role of, 9, 22
Clinician's bag, 49*b*-50*b*
CMNs (Certificates of Medical
  Necessity), 474
CMS (Centers for Medicare and
  Medicaid Services), 10, 64, 469-
  470, 475
CNAs (certified nursing assistants),
  services provided by, 20-21
Cognitive effects, of pain, 453*t*
Coinsurance, 471
Collaboration, 471
Communication skills, 23-28, 36
Community Health Accreditation
  Program (CHAP), 35, 57, 468
Community health care, 471
Community resources, 48-51
Competency assessment and validation,
  40-41
Computerization, 75
Conditions of Participation (COPs), 10,
  38, 65
Confusion, during dying, 29*b*
Consent form, 44-45, 47*f*
Constipation, 215-226
  bereavement counselor for, 221, 223
  bowel regimen to prevent narcotic-
    induced, 215, 216*t*-217*t*
  comfort and symptom control for,
    217-218
  diagnoses and codes for, 215-217
  educational needs with, 223-224
  elimination with, 219
  equipment and supply needs for, 215

Constipation *(Continued)*
  general considerations with, 215
  home health aide or certified nursing
    assistant for, 219, 222
  Hospice nursing for, 217-219,
    221-222
  hydration/nutrition with, 219,
    220-221, 223
  mobility considerations with, 218
  music, massage, art, or other
    therapies or services for, 221,
    223
  other considerations with, 219
  outcomes for care with, 221-223
  pharmacist for, 221, 223
  resources for, 226
  safety considerations with, 215, 218
  skills and services for, 217-221
  skin care with, 218-219
  social worker for, 220, 222
  spiritual counseling for, 220, 222
  tips for quality and reimbursement
    for, 224-226
  volunteers for, 220, 222
Consumer, 470
Contamination, 50*b*
Continuity of care, for children,
  440*b*-441*b*
Continuous infusion (CI), of opioids,
  456*t*, 457*t*
Continuous quality improvement (CQI),
  471
Copayment, 471
COPD. *See* Chronic obstructive
  pulmonary disease (COPD).
COPs (Conditions of Participation), 10,
  38, 65
Cost containment, 471
Cost issues, 82
Counseling, 11
  bereavement, 12, 13*f*-15*f*
  dietary, 11-12
  spiritual, 13-16, 16*f*
CP (clinical path), 74-75, 470-471
CPZ, 67*t*
CQI (continuous quality improvement),
  471
Critical path, 471
Cross-contamination, 50*b*
Cross-infection, 50*b*

Customer, 470
CVA. *See* Cerebral vascular accident
  (CVA).

D
Data, 471
D/C, 67*t*
Deafferentation pain, 454*f*
Death and dying
  knowledge of concepts related to, 23
  signs of approaching, 28, 29*b*
Decubitus ulcers. *See* Pressure ulcers.
Definitions, 468-479
Dementia, 105-116
  bereavement counselor for, 110, 113
  comfort and symptom control for,
    106-107
  defined, 471
  diagnoses and codes for, 105-106
  educational needs with, 113-114
  elimination with, 108
  emotional/spiritual considerations
    with, 107, 109-110, 112-113
  equipment and supply needs for, 105
  general considerations with, 105
  home health aide or certified nursing
    assistant for, 109, 112
  Hospice nursing for, 106-109,
    110-112
  hydration/nutrition with, 108, 110,
    113
  mobility considerations with, 107
  music, massage, art, or other
    therapies or services for, 110,
    113
  occupational therapist for, 110, 113
  other considerations with, 109
  outcomes for care with, 110-113
  physical therapist for, 110, 113
  resources for, 115-116
  safety considerations with, 105,
    107
  skills and services for, 106-110
  skin care with, 107-108
  social worker for, 109, 112
  therapeutic/medication regimens for,
    108-109
  tips for quality and reimbursement
    for, 114-115
  volunteers for, 109, 112

Depression, 227-240
  bereavement counselor for, 233-234,
    237
  comfort and symptom control for,
    228-229
  diagnoses and codes for, 227-228
  educational needs with, 237-238
  elimination with, 230-231
  emotional/spiritual considerations
    with, 229-230, 233, 236-237
  equipment and supply needs for, 227
  general considerations with, 227
  home health aide or certified nursing
    assistant for, 232, 236
  Hospice nursing for, 228-232,
    234-236
  hydration/nutrition with, 231, 233,
    237
  music, massage, art, or other therapies
    or services for, 234, 237
  occupational therapist for, 233, 237
  other considerations with, 232
  outcomes for care with, 234-237
  pharmacist for, 234, 237
  resources for, 240
  safety considerations with, 227, 229
  skills and services for, 228-234
  skin care with, 230
  social worker for, 232-233, 236
  therapeutic/medication regimens for,
    231-232
  tips for quality and reimbursement
    for, 238-240
  volunteers for, 233, 236
Developmental effects, of pain, 453*t*
Diabetes mellitus, 241-257
  bereavement counselor for, 249, 253
  comfort and symptom control for,
    243-244
  diagnoses and codes for, 242-243
  educational needs with, 254
  elimination with, 246
  equipment and supply needs for, 241
  general considerations with, 241
  home health aide or certified nursing
    assistant for, 247, 252
  Hospice nursing for, 243-247,
    249-252
  hydration/nutrition with, 246, 248,
    252

Diabetes mellitus *(Continued)*
music, massage, art, or other
therapies or services for, 249,
253-254
occupational therapist for, 248-249,
253
other considerations with, 247
outcomes for care with, 249-254
pharmacist for, 249, 253
physical therapist for, 249, 253
resources for, 257
safety considerations with, 241,
244-245
skills and services for, 243-249
skin care with, 245-246
social worker for, 247-248, 252
speech-language pathologist for,
249, 253
spiritual counseling for, 248, 252
therapeutic/medication regimens for,
246-247
tips for quality and reimbursement
for, 254-256
volunteers for, 248, 252
Diagnosis(es), 471
nursing, 499-503
Diagnosis-related groups (DRGs), 79,
471
Dialysis. *See* Renal disease.
Dietitians/dietary counselors, services
provided by, 11-12, 472
Dioctyl sodium sulfosuccinate plus
casanthranol (Peri-Colace), for
constipation, 216*t*
Directions, 52*b*, 53-54
Documentation, 57-76
abbreviations not to use in, 66*b*,
67*t*-70*t*
automation in, 75
basics of, 65-72
checklist approach to, 72-74
clinical path considerations in, 74-75
defined, 472
factors contributing to more
emphasis on, 60-64
hospice chart audit tool in, 57,
58*f*-61*f*
importance of clinical record in, 57-59
importance of hospice record in,
64-65

Documentation *(Continued)*
as key to coverage, compliance, and
quality, 65
for Medicare, 72
tips for, 65, 66*b*
Docusate calcium plus danthron
(Doxidan), for constipation, 216*t*
Docusate sodium plus senna (Senokot-S),
for constipation, 216*t*
Dose designations, dangerous
abbreviations or symbols in,
68*t*-70*t*
DPT, 67*t*
DRGs (diagnosis-related groups), 79,
471
"Drug seeking" behavior, 451*t*
Dulcolax (bisacodyl), for constipation,
216*t*

E
Effective management, 472
Effectiveness, 64
Efficiency, 64
Election of Medicare hospice benefit
form, 31, 32*f*
Emergency preparedness, 51, 53*b*
Endocrine effects, of pain, 452*t*
End-of-life issues, resources on, 488
Enteral nutrition. *See also* Feeding tube.
defined, 472
Enterostomal therapy (ET) nurse, 472
Epidural administration, of opioids,
457*t*
Equipment, infection control for, 49*b*
Equity of care, 472
Ethics, resources on, 488
Evaluation visit, 472
Exercise program, 17
Extended care services, 472
Extremities, cooling of, 29*b*

F
Faces Pain Rating Scale, 444*f*, 446,
447*f*
Family-centered care, for children,
438*b*-439*b*
Fecal impaction. *See* Constipation.
Federal Patient Self-Determination Act,
48
Fee for service, 472-473

Feeding tube, 352-381
  bereavement counselor for, 368, 375
  comfort and symptom control for,
     358-360
  diagnoses and codes for, 353
  educational needs with, 376, 377
  elimination with, 361
Feeding tube *(Continued)*
  emotional/spiritual considerations
     with, 360, 367, 375
  equipment and supply needs for, 352
  general considerations with, 352
  home health aide or certified nursing
     assistant for, 366, 374
  Hospice nursing for, 358-362,
     370-372
  hydration/nutrition with, 361,
     367-368, 375
  music, massage, art, or other
     therapies or services for, 368,
     376
  occupational therapist for, 368, 375
  other considerations with, 362
  outcomes for care with, 370-372,
     374-376
  pharmacist for, 368, 375-376
  physical therapist for, 368, 375
  resources for, 381
  safety considerations with, 352, 360
  skills and services for, 358-362,
     366-368
  skin care with, 360-361
  social worker for, 366-367, 374
  speech-language pathologist for, 368,
     375
  therapeutic/medication regimens for,
     361-362
  tips for quality and reimbursement
     for, 377-379, 380-381
  volunteers for, 367, 374
Fentanyl, sublingual administration of,
    455*t*
Fentanyl citrate
  oral mucosal, 455*t*
  transdermal, 455*t*-456*t*
Fleet enema, for constipation, 217*t*
Flexibility, in care and care planning,
    28, 36
Fluid build-up, during dying, 29*b*
Form 485, 10

Fraud
  defined, 473
  resources on, 488

G

Gastrointestinal effects, of pain, 453*t*
Gatekeeper, 473
Genitourinary effects, of pain, 453*t*
Glycerin suppository, for fecal
    impaction, 217*t*
Goals, 473
Government services, resources on, 489
G-tube, 473. *See also* Feeding tube.

H

Handwashing, 48, 49*b*
Hazardous waste management, 49*b*
HCl, 68*t*
HCT, 68*t*
HCTZ, 68*t*
Head and neck cancer, 258-272. *See
    also* Brain tumor.
  bereavement counselor for, 265, 268
  comfort and symptom control for,
     259-261
  diagnoses and codes for, 258-259
  educational needs with, 269
  elimination with, 262
  emotional/spiritual considerations
     with, 261, 264, 267
  equipment and supply needs for, 258
  general considerations with, 258
  home health aide or certified nursing
     assistant for, 263, 267
  Hospice nursing for, 259-263,
     265-268
  hydration/nutrition with, 262, 264,
     267
  music, massage, art, or other
     therapies or services for, 265,
     268-269
  occupational therapist for, 264,
     267-268
  other considerations with, 263
  outcomes for care with, 265-269
  pharmacist for, 265, 268
  physical therapist for, 264, 268
  resources for, 272
  safety considerations with, 258, 261
  skills and services for, 259-265

Head and neck cancer *(Continued)*
  skin care with, 261-262
  social worker for, 263, 267
  speech-language pathologist for, 264, 268
  therapeutic/medication regimens for, 262-263
  tips for quality and reimbursement for, 269-271
  volunteers for, 263, 267
Health Care Financing Administration, 10, 64
Health care reform, 82
Health Insurance Portability and Accountability Act (HIPAA), 39, 44
Health maintenance organization (HMO), 473
  Medicare, 475
Hearing, during dying, 29b
Heart disease. *See* Cardiac disease.
HIV (human immunodeficiency virus). *See* Acquired immunodeficiency syndrome (AIDS).
HME (home medical equipment), 474
Home care, 473
  vs. hospice nursing, 28-31
Home exercise program (HEP), 17
Home health, 473
Home health agencies (HHAs), 35, 473
Home health aides (HHAs), services provided by, 20-21, 473-474
Home Health Certification and Plan of Care, 10
Home medical equipment (HME), 474
Homebound, 473
Homemakers, services provided by, 21
Hospice
  defined, 2-3
  eligibility for, 65-72
  growth of, 3-6, 4f-5f
  Medicare, 476
  NHPCO standards for, 2-3, 35
  patients seen in, 6
  safety in, 51, 52b-53b
Hospice aides, services provided by, 20-21
Hospice and Palliative Nurses Association (HPNA), 9, 492

Hospice Association of America, 492
Hospice benefit certification form, 33, 33f
Hospice brochure, 42-43
Hospice care
  defined, 3, 474
  hallmarks of effective, 22-28, 24f-27f
  interdisciplinary team for. *See* Interdisciplinary team (IDT).
  planning and managing, 79-85, 80b-81b
    examples of, 83-85
  skills and knowledge needed in, 35-38
  standardization of, 2-3, 35, 62-64, 82
Hospice chart audit tool, 57, 58f-61f
Hospice documentation, 57-76
  abbreviations not to use in, 66b, 67t-70t
  automation in, 75
  basics of, 65-72
  checklist approach to, 72-74
  clinical path considerations in, 74-75
  factors contributing to more emphasis on, 60-64
  hospice chart audit tool in, 57, 58f-61f
  importance of clinical record in, 57-59
  importance of hospice record in, 64-65
  as key to coverage, compliance, and quality, 65
  for Medicare, 72
  tips for, 65, 66b
Hospice Foundation of America, 492
Hospice Helpline, 494
Hospice Link, 494
Hospice medical director, responsibilities of, 10-11
Hospice Medicare benefit revocation form, 33-34, 34f
Hospice nursing
  defined, 22, 474
  vs. home care, 28-31
Hospice nursing certification, 489
Hospice organizations, types of, 6-7

Hospice orientation, 38-51
 community resources in, 48-51
 competency assessment and
   validation in, 40-41
 considerations for, 39-40
 emergency preparedness in, 51
 HIPAA and notice of privacy
   practice in, 39, 44
 hospice brochure in, 42-43
 infection control in, 46-48, 49b-50b
 information included in, 38-39
 mission, vision, values, and
   philosophy in, 42
 office information in, 43
 organizational chart in, 43
 outcomes or goals of, 40
 patient consent for hospice care in,
   44-45, 47f
 patient rights and responsibilities in,
   44, 45f-46f
 personnel or human resource
   information in, 43
 policies and procedures in, 44-51
 position description in, 43-44
 self-determination/advance directives
   in, 48
 staff involved in, 42
 tips for going through, 41, 41b
 topics covered in, 41-51
Hospice record, importance of, 64-65
Hospice satisfaction survey, 62, 63f
Hospice settings, 6
Hospice visits, appropriate frequency
   and length of, 79-85, 80b-81b
HPNA (Hospice and Palliative Nurses
   Association), 9, 492
h.s., 69t
Human immunodeficiency virus (HIV).
   See Acquired immunodeficiency
   syndrome (AIDS).
Human resources (HR) information, 43
Humor, sense of, 28, 37
Hydromorphone
 rectal administration of, 455t
 subcutaneous administration of, 456t

I
IADLs (instrumental activities of daily
   living), 474
Ibuprofen, 464, 465

ICD-9 code, 474
IDG (interdisciplinary group) meetings,
   7-8, 8f
IDT. See Interdisciplinary team (IDT).
Immobility. See Bedbound patient.
Immune effects, of pain, 453t
Immunosuppressed patients, infection
   control in, 50b
Infection control, 46-48, 49b-50b
Infusion(s), 273-290
 bereavement counselor for, 281, 285
 comfort and symptom control for,
   275-276
 diagnoses and codes for,
   274-275
 educational needs with, 286
 elimination with, 277-278
 emotional/spiritual considerations
   with, 277, 280, 284
 equipment and supply needs for, 273
 general considerations with, 273
 home health aide or certified nursing
   assistant for, 279, 284
 Hospice nursing for, 275-279,
   281-284
 hydration/nutrition with, 278, 280,
   284-285
 mobility considerations with, 277
 music, massage, art, or other
   therapies or services for, 281,
   286
 occupational therapist for, 280, 285
 other considerations with, 279
 outcomes for care with, 281-286
 pharmacist for, 281, 285
 physical therapist for, 280-281, 285
 resources for, 289-290
 safety considerations with, 273-274,
   277
 skills and services for, 275-281
 skin care with, 277
 social worker for, 279, 284
 speech-language pathologist for, 281,
   285
 therapeutic/medication regimens for,
   278-279
 tips for quality and reimbursement
   for, 287-289
 volunteers for, 280, 284
Infusion pumps, for opioids, 456t, 457t

Initial Pain Assessment Tool, 445*f*
Instrumental activities of daily living (IADLs), 474
Instrumental care, 474
Integrated delivery network, 474
Interdisciplinary group (IDG) meetings, 7-8, 8*f*
Interdisciplinary team (IDT), 7-22
   administrative staff on, 7
   bereavement counselors on, 12, 13*f*-15*f*
   for children, 439*b*-440*b*
   clinicians on, 9
   dietitians/dietary counselors on, 11-12
   home health or hospice aides on, 20-21
   homemakers on, 21
   medical social workers on, 9
   meetings of, 7-8, 8*f*
   occupational therapists on, 18-19
   other services provided by, 22
   overview of, 7-9
   pharmacists on, 21-22
   physical therapists on, 17
   physicians on, 9-11
   speech-language pathologists on, 20
   spiritual counselors/chaplains on, 13-16, 16*f*
   volunteers on, 17, 18*f*, 19*f*
Intermediary, 475
Internet sites, 489-490
Intraarterial administration, of opioids, 456*t*
Intraarticular administration, of opioids, 458*t*
Intracerebroventricular administration, of opioids, 458*t*
Intranasal administration, of opioids, 456*t*
Intrathecal administration, of opioids, 457*t*
Intravenous (IV) administration, of opioids, 456*t*
Intravenous (IV) care. *See* Infusions.
IU, 69*t*

J
Job description, 43-44
Joint Commission on Accreditation of Healthcare Organizations (JCAHO), 35, 57, 468
Journals, 490-491

K
Kidney disease. *See* Renal disease.

L
Lactulose (Chronulac), for constipation, 216*t*
Laryngectomy care, 271
Length of stay/service (LOS), 475
Licensed physical therapists (LPTs), services provided by, 17
Lou Gehrig's disease. *See* Amyotrophic lateral sclerosis (ALS).
Lung disease, 291-306
   bereavement counselor for, 297, 300-301
   comfort and symptom control for, 292-294
   diagnoses and codes for, 291-292
   educational needs with, 301-302
   elimination with, 295
   emotional/spiritual considerations with, 294, 296, 300
   equipment and supply needs for, 291
   general considerations with, 291
   home health aide or certified nursing assistant for, 296, 299
   Hospice nursing for, 292-295, 298-299
   hydration/nutrition with, 295, 296-297, 300
   mobility considerations with, 294
   music, massage, art, or other therapies or services for, 297-298, 301
   occupational therapist for, 297, 300
   other considerations with, 295
   outcomes for care with, 298-301
   pharmacist for, 297, 301
   physical therapist for, 297, 300
   resources for, 305-306
   safety considerations with, 291, 294
   skills and services for, 292-298
   skin care with, 294-295
   social worker for, 296, 299
   therapeutic/medication regimens for, 295
   tips for quality and reimbursement for, 302-305
   volunteers for, 296, 299-300

M

Magnesium citrate, for constipation, 216*t*
Managed care, 475
Managed care organization (MCO), 475
Managed care plan (MCP), 475
Map reading, 53-54
Mastectomy care. *See* Breast cancer.
Medicaid, 30, 31, 475
Medical advisor, responsibilities of, 10
Medical director, responsibilities of, 10-11
Medical Social Services (MSS), 475
Medical social workers, services provided by, 9
Medically fragile children, 426-437
  bereavement counselor for, 431, 435
  comfort and symptom control for, 427-428
  diagnoses and codes for, 426-427
  educational needs of, 435
  elimination in, 429
  emotional/spiritual considerations for, 429, 430-431, 434
  equipment and supply needs for, 426
  general considerations for, 426
  home health aide or certified nursing assistant for, 430, 433
  Hospice nursing for, 427-430, 432-433
  hydration/nutrition in, 429, 431, 434
  music, massage, art, or other therapies or services for, 432, 435
  occupational therapist for, 431, 434
  other considerations for, 430
  outcomes for care in, 432-435
  pharmacist for, 431-432, 435
  physical therapist for, 431, 434
  resources for, 437
  safety considerations for, 426, 428-429
  skills and services for, 427-432
  skin care for, 429
  social worker for, 430, 433
  speech-language pathologist for, 431, 434
  therapeutic/medication regimens for, 429-430
  tips for quality and reimbursement for, 436-437
  volunteers for, 430, 433

Medicare
  defined, 475
  documentation for, 65-72
  eligibility for, 31
  forms for, 32*f*-34*f*, 33-34
  home care covered by, 30
  hospice care covered by, 30, 31-35, 32*f*-34*f*, 476
  information on, 491-492
  physician services covered by, 10
Medicare Conditions of Participation, 35
Medicare health maintenance organization, 475
Medicare hospice, 30, 31-35, 32*f*-34*f*, 476
Medicare hospice benefit (MHB), 31-35, 32*f*-34*f*
  qualification for, 65-72
Medicare Hospice Manual, 35
Metabolic effects, of pain, 452*t*
Methadone, sublingual administration of, 455*t*
mg, 68*t*
MgSO₄, 68*t*
MHB (Medicare hospice benefit), 31-35, 32*f*-34*f*
  qualification for, 65-72
Milk of magnesia, for constipation, 216*t*, 217*t*
Mineral oil, for constipation, 217*t*
Mission statement, 42
Mononeuropathies, painful, 454*f*
Morphine
  nebulized, 456*t*
  rectal administration of, 455*t*
  rectal administration of oral, 461
  subcutaneous administration of, 456*t*
  sublingual administration of, 455*t*
MSO₄, 68*t*
MSS (Medical Social Services), 475
MTX, 68*t*
Musculoskeletal effects, of pain, 453*t*

N

NANDA (North American Nursing Diagnosis Association), 82, 499-503
National Association for Home Care (NAHC), 492

National Board for Certification of Hospice and Palliative Nurses, 9

National Family Caregivers Association (NFCA), 492-493

National Funeral Directors Association, 493

National Hospice and Palliative Care Organization (NHPCO), 2-3, 35, 71, 493, 494

National organizations, 492-493

National Prison Hospice Association (NPHA), 493

Nebulization, of opioids, 456*t*

Neck cancer. *See* Head and neck cancer.

Needles, precautions with, 49*b*

Neuromuscular disorders, 117-128

  bereavement counselor for, 122, 124

  comfort and symptom control for, 117-118

  diagnoses and codes for, 117

  educational needs with, 125-126

  elimination with, 119

  emotional/spiritual considerations with, 118-119, 121, 123

  equipment and supply needs for, 117

  general considerations with, 117

  home health aide or certified nursing assistant for, 120, 123

  Hospice nursing for, 117-120, 122-123

  hydration/nutrition with, 119-120, 121, 123

  mobility considerations with, 118

  music, massage, art, or other therapies or services for, 122, 124

  occupational therapist for, 121, 124

  other considerations with, 120

  outcomes for care with, 122-125

  physical therapist for, 122, 124

  resources for, 128

  safety considerations with, 117, 118

  skills and services for, 117-122

  skin care with, 119

  social worker for, 120-121, 123

  speech-language pathologist for, 122, 124

  therapeutic/medication regimens for, 120

  tips for quality and reimbursement for, 126-128

  volunteers for, 121, 123

Neuropathic pain, 454*f*

Neuropathies, 454*f*

NFCA (National Family Caregivers Association), 492-493

NHPCO (National Hospice and Palliative Care Organization), 2-3, 35, 71, 493, 494

"Nitro" drip, 68*t*

Noah's Ark approach, 38

Nociceptive pain, 454*f*

Nonsteroidal anti-inflammatory drugs (NSAIDs), 465

"Norflox," 68*t*

North American Nursing Diagnosis Association (NANDA), 82, 499-503

Notice of Privacy Practice (NPP), 39, 44

NPHA (National Prison Hospice Association), 493

NRS pain rating scale, 452*t*

Nurses, role of, 9, 22

Nurse's notes, 62

Nursing diagnoses, 499-503

Nutrition

  enteral, 472. *See also* Feeding tube.

  parenteral. *See* Infusions.

  resources on, 493

Nutritional services, 11-12

O

OBRA (Omnibus Budget Reconciliation Act), 48, 468

Occupational Safety and Health Administration (OSHA), 39, 46, 476

Occupational therapy (OT), 18-19, 476

OD, 68*t*

o.d., 68*t*

Office information, 43

Oil retention enema, for fecal impaction, 217*t*

Omnibus Budget Reconciliation Act (OBRA), 48, 468

Oncology Nursing Society (ONS), 493

Opioid administration, routes of, 455*t*-460*t*

Oral administration, of opioids, 455*t*

Oral analgesics, rectal administration of, 461-463

Oral transmucosal administration, of
opioids, 455*t*
Oral transmucosal fentanyl citrate
(OTFC), 455*t*
Organic brain syndrome. *See* Dementia.
Organization(s), national, 492-493
Organizational chart, 43
Orientation, 38-51
community resources in, 48-51
competency assessment and
validation in, 40-41
considerations for, 39-40
emergency preparedness in, 51
HIPAA and notice of privacy
practice in, 39, 44
hospice brochure in, 42-43
infection control in, 46-48, 49*b*-50*b*
information included in, 38-39
mission, vision, values, and
philosophy in, 42
office information in, 43
organizational chart in, 43
outcomes or goals of, 40
patient consent for hospice care in,
44-45, 47*f*
patient rights and responsibilities in,
44, 45*f*-46*f*
personnel or human resource
information in, 43
policies and procedures in, 44-51
position description in, 43-44
resources on, 493
self-determination/advance directives
in, 48
staff involved in, 42
tips for going through, 41, 41*b*
topics covered in, 41-51
OSHA (Occupational Safety and Health
Administration), 39, 46, 476
Ostomy, 352-381
bereavement counselor for, 368, 375
comfort and symptom control for,
362-363
diagnoses and codes for, 353-354
educational needs with, 376, 377
elimination with, 364-365
emotional/spiritual considerations
with, 364, 367, 375
equipment and supply needs for, 352
general considerations with, 352

Ostomy *(Continued)*
home health aide or certified nursing
assistant for, 366, 374
Hospice nursing for, 362-365,
372-374
hydration/nutrition with, 365,
367-368, 375
music, massage, art, or other
therapies or services for, 368,
376
occupational therapist for, 368, 375
other considerations with, 366
outcomes for care with, 372-376
pharmacist for, 368, 375-376
physical therapist for, 368, 375
resources for, 381
safety considerations with, 352, 363
skills and services for, 362-368
skin care with, 364
social worker for, 366-367, 374
speech-language pathologist for, 368,
375
therapeutic/medication regimens for,
365-366
tips for quality and reimbursement
for, 377-378, 379-381
volunteers for, 367, 374
OT (occupational therapy), 18-19, 476
OTFC (oral transmucosal fentanyl
citrate), 455*t*
Outcomes, 476
clinical, 476
Outcomes criteria, 476
Oxymorphone, rectal administration of,
455*t*

P
Pain, 307-320, 443-466
analgesics for
nonprescription, 463-464
nurse's power and responsibility
in relation to, 449*t*
opioid, 455*t*-460*t*
rectal administration of oral,
461-463
anxiety and, 451*t*
assessment of, 444*f*-447*f*, 446
barriers to, 450*t*-452*t*
barriers to management of, 450*t*-452*t*
bereavement counselor for, 313, 317

Pain *(Continued)*
  centrally generated, 454*f*
  in children, 441*b*
  classification of, 454*f*
  comfort and symptom control for,
    308-309
  deafferentation, 454*f*
  diagnoses and codes for, 307
  educational needs with, 317
  elimination with, 310
  emotional/spiritual considerations
    with, 309, 312, 316
  equipment and supply needs for, 307
  future, 453*t*
  general considerations with, 307
  harmful effects of unrelieved,
    452*t*-453*t*
  home health aide or certified nursing
    assistant for, 311, 315
  Hospice nursing for, 308-311, 314-315
  hydration/nutrition with, 310,
    312-313, 316
  low tolerance for, 450*t*
  mobility considerations with, 309
  music, massage, art, or other
    therapies or services for, 313
  neuropathic, 454*f*
  nociceptive, 454*f*
  occupational therapist for, 313, 316
  other considerations with, 311
  outcomes for care with, 314-317
  pathophysiology of, 454*f*
  peripherally generated, 454*f*
  pharmacist for, 313, 317
  physical therapist for, 313, 317
  resources for, 320, 494-495
  safety considerations with, 307, 309
  skills and services for, 308-313
  skin care with, 309-310
  social worker for, 311-312, 316
  somatic, 454*f*
  speech-language pathologist for, 313,
    317
  sympathetically maintained, 454*f*
  therapeutic/medication regimens for,
    310-311
  tips for quality and reimbursement
    for, 317-320
  visceral, 454*f*
  volunteers for, 312, 316

Pain Assessment Monitor, 444*f*
Pain Control Record, 448*f*
Pain intensity scales, 446*f*
Pain management skills, 22-23
Pain rating scales, 444*f*, 446, 447*f*, 452*t*
Pain threshold, 450*t*
Palliative care, hallmarks of effective,
  22-28, 24*f*-27*f*
Parenteral therapy. *See* Infusions.
Pathogens, 50*b*
Patient, 470
Patient consent form, 44-45, 47*f*
Patient resources, 495-496
Patient Rights and Responsibilities
  policy, 44, 45*f*-46*f*
Patient Self-Determination Act, 48
Patient-controlled analgesia (PCA),
  456*t*, 457*t*
Payor, 476-477
Pediatric patients. *See* Children.
per os, 68*t*
Perdiem (psyllium and senna), for
  constipation, 216t
Perdiem rate, 30
Performance improvement (PI), 39,
  61-62, 471
Performance measure, 477
Peri-Colace (dioctyl sodium
  sulfosuccinate plus casanthranol),
  for constipation, 216*t*
Peripheral vascular disease, 241-257
  bereavement counselor for, 249, 253
  comfort and symptom control for,
    243-244
  diagnoses and codes for, 242-243
  educational needs with, 254
  elimination with, 246
  equipment and supply needs for, 241
  general considerations with, 241
  home health aide or certified nursing
    assistant for, 247, 252
  Hospice nursing for, 243-247,
    249-252
  hydration/nutrition with, 246, 248,
    252
  music, massage, art, or other
    therapies or services for, 249,
    253-254
  occupational therapist for, 248-249,
    253

Peripheral vascular disease *(Continued)*
    other considerations with, 247
    outcomes for care with, 249-254
    pharmacist for, 249, 253
    physical therapist for, 249, 253
    resources for, 257
    safety considerations with, 241,
        244-245
    skills and services for, 243-249
    skin care with, 245-246
    social worker for, 247-248, 252
    speech-language pathologist for, 249,
        253
    spiritual counseling for, 248, 252
    therapeutic/medication regimens for,
        246-247
    tips for quality and reimbursement
        for, 254-256
    volunteers for, 248, 252
Peripherally generated pain, 454f
Personal emergency response systems
    (PERSs), 477
Personnel information, 43
Pharmacists, 21-22, 477
Physical therapy (PT), 17, 477
Physician(s)
    certification of, 478
    services provided by, 9-11
PI (performance improvement), 39,
    61-62, 471
Placebo, pain relief after, 451t
Plan of care (POC), 8, 10, 65, 469
Pneumocystis carinii/pneumonia, in
    AIDS, 89
Policies and procedures, 44-51
    for children, 439b
    standardization of, 62
Polyneuropathies, painful, 454f
Position description, 43-44
PPSs (prospective payment systems), 79
Preceptor, 40-41
Preferred provider organization (PPO),
    478
"Pre-hospice" program, 30
Pressure ulcers, 382-399
    bereavement counselor for, 390, 394
    comfort and symptom control for,
        384-386
    defined, 478
    diagnoses and codes for, 382-384

Pressure ulcers *(Continued)*
    educational needs with, 395
    elimination with, 387
    emotional/spiritual considerations
        with, 386, 389, 393
    equipment and supply needs for, 382
    general considerations with, 382
    home health aide or certified nursing
        assistant for, 388, 393
    Hospice nursing for, 384-388,
        390-393
    hydration/nutrition with, 387, 389,
        393-394
    music, massage, art, or other
        therapies or services for, 390,
        394-395
    occupational therapist for, 389, 394
    other considerations with, 388
    outcomes for care with, 390-395
    pharmacist for, 390, 394
    physical therapist for, 390, 394
    resources for, 399
    safety considerations with, 382, 386
    skills and services for, 384-390
    skin care with, 386
    social worker for, 388-389, 393
    speech-language pathologist for, 390,
        394
    therapeutic/medication regimens for,
        387-388
    tips for quality and reimbursement
        for, 395-399
    volunteers for, 389, 393
Privacy practice, 39, 44
PRN basis, 449t
Procedures, 44-51
    for children, 439b
    standardization of, 62
Process, 478
Prospective payment systems (PPSs),
    79
Prostate cancer, 321-335
    bereavement counselor for, 327, 331
    comfort and symptom control for,
        322-323
    diagnoses and codes for, 321-322
    educational needs with, 331-332
    elimination with, 324
    emotional/spiritual considerations
        with, 323, 326, 330

Prostate cancer *(Continued)*
  equipment and supply needs for, 321
  general considerations with, 321
  home health aide or certified nursing
      assistant for, 325, 329
  Hospice nursing for, 322-325,
      327-329
  hydration/nutrition with, 324, 326,
      330
  mobility considerations with, 323
  music, massage, art, or other
      therapies or services for, 327,
      331
  occupational therapist for, 326, 330
  other considerations with, 325
  outcomes for care with, 327-331
  pharmacist for, 327, 331
  physical therapist for, 327, 331
  resources for, 334-335
  safety considerations with, 321, 323
  skills and services for, 322-327
  skin care with, 323-324
  social worker for, 325-326, 330
  speech-language pathologist for, 327,
      331
  therapeutic/medication regimens for,
      324-325
  tips for quality and reimbursement
      for, 332-334
  volunteers for, 326, 330
Psychiatric disorders, 227-240
  bereavement counselor for, 233-234,
      237
  comfort and symptom control for,
      228-229
  diagnoses and codes for, 227-228
  educational needs with, 237-238
  elimination with, 230-231
  emotional/spiritual considerations
      with, 229-230, 233, 236-237
  equipment and supply needs for, 227
  general considerations with, 227
  home health aide or certified nursing
      assistant for, 232, 236
  Hospice nursing for, 228-232, 234-236
  hydration/nutrition with, 231, 233,
      237
  music, massage, art, or other
      therapies or services for, 234,
      237

Psychiatric disorders *(Continued)*
  occupational therapist for, 233, 237
  other considerations with, 232
  outcomes for care with, 234-237
  pharmacist for, 234, 237
  resources for, 240
  safety considerations with, 227, 229
  skills and services for, 228-234
  skin care with, 230
  social worker for, 232-233, 236
  therapeutic/medication regimens for,
      231-232
  tips for quality and reimbursement
      for, 238-240
  volunteers for, 233, 236
Psychosocial assessment tool, 23,
      24f-27f
Psyllium and senna (Perdiem), for
      constipation, 216t
PT (physical therapy), 17, 477
Pulmonary disease. *See* Lung disease.

Q
QD, 69t
q.d., 69t
qhs, 69t
qn, 69t
QOD, 69t
q.o.d., 69t
Quality, 478
Quality assessment, 478
Quality improvement, 478
  for children, 442b
  continuous, 471
Quality initiatives, 61-62
Quality management, total, 479
Quality of life, effect of unrelieved pain
      on, 453t

R
Rectal administration
  of opioids, 455t, 459-460
  of oral analgesics, 461-463
Regional Home Health Intermediaries
      (RHHIs), 64-65, 71, 475
Registered dietitian (RD), 472
Renal disease, 336-351
  bereavement counselor for, 343, 347
  comfort and symptom control for,
      338-339

Renal disease *(Continued)*
  diagnoses and codes for, 336-338
  educational needs with, 348
  elimination with, 340-341
  emotional/spiritual considerations
      with, 339-340, 342, 346
  equipment and supply needs for, 336
  general considerations with, 336
  home health aide or certified nursing
      assistant for, 342, 346
  Hospice nursing for, 338-341, 344-346
  hydration/nutrition with, 341,
      342-343, 346
  music, massage, art, or other
      therapies or services for, 344,
      347
  occupational therapist for, 343,
      346-347
  other considerations with, 341
  outcomes for care with, 344-347
  pharmacist for, 343, 347
  physical therapist for, 343, 347
  resources for, 350-351
  safety considerations with, 336, 339
  skills and services for, 338-344
  skin care with, 340
  social worker for, 342, 346
  speech-language pathologist for, 343,
      347
  therapeutic/medication regimens for,
      341
  tips for quality and reimbursement
      for, 348-350
  volunteers for, 342, 346
Resources, 483-498
  on administration, 485
  on advance directives, 485
  on aides, 485-486
  on AIDS/HIV, 486
  books, 486-487
  clinical, 487-488
  on end-of-life issues, 488
  on ethics, 488
  on fraud and abuse, 488
  on government services, 489
  on hospice nursing certification, 489
  on Internet sites, 489-490
  journals, 490-491
  on Medicare, 491-492

Resources *(Continued)*
  national organizations, 492-493
  on nutrition, 493
  on orientation, 493
  other, 493-494
  on pain, 494-495
  patient, 495-496
  on pediatric care, 496-497
  on spiritual care, 497-498
  on volunteers, 498
Respiratory disease. *See* Lung disease.
Respiratory effects, of pain, 453*t*
Respiratory therapy, 478
Restlessness, during dying, 29*b*
RHHIs (Regional Home Health
    Intermediaries), 64-65, 71, 475
Routes of administration
    emergency change in, 461-463
    for opioids, 455*t*-460*t*

S
Safety, in hospice, 51, 52*b*-53*b*
SC, 69*t*
Self-determination, 48
Self-direction, 36
Senna (Senokot), for constipation,
    216*t*, 217*t*
Senokot-S (docusate sodium plus
    senna), for constipation, 216*t*
Sentinel event, 478
Sleeping, during dying, 29b
Social workers, services provided by, 9
Somatic pain, 454*f*
Speech-language pathologists
    (S-LPs), 20, 478
Spiritual assessment tool, 16, 16*f*
Spiritual care, resources on, 497-498
Spiritual counselors, services provided
    by, 13-16, 16*f*
Spiritual distress, 470
Spiritual well-being, potential for
    enhanced, 470
ss, 69*t*
Standard, 478
Standard Precautions, 46, 49*b*
Standardization, of care, policies and
    procedures, and processes,
    62, 82
Standardized care plans, 82

iStandards of a Hospice Program of Care/i, 2-3, 35
Standards of care, 2-3, 35, 62-64
Sterile technique, 50*b*
Stress management skills, 23
Stroke. *See* Cerebral vascular accident (CVA).
Structure, 478
sub q, 69*t*
Subcutaneous administration, of opioids, 456*t*
Sublingual administration, of opioids, 455*t*
Sufentanil, intranasal administration of, 456*t*
Supportive care. *See* Catheter, Feeding tube, Ostomy.
Suppository, opioid administration via, 459
Sympathetically maintained pain, 454*f*
Symptom management, in children, 441*b*
Symptom management skills, 22-23

T
TAC, 68*t*
Time line, 479
Time-management skills, 38
TIW, 68*t*
tiw, 68*t*
Total quality management, 479
Tracheostomy care, 271
Transdermal administration, of opioids, 455*t*-456*t*
Transmucosal administration, of opioids, 455*t*
Transportation, 36
Tube feeding. *See* Feeding tube.

U
U, 69*t*
u, 69*t*
Ulcers, pressure. *See* Pressure ulcers.
Utilization management, 61
Utilization review, 61
for children, 442*b*

V
Vaginal administration, of opioids, 455*t*

Variance, 479
Vascular access devices. *See* Infusions.
Visceral pain, 454*f*
Visual analog scale (VAS), for pain, 446*f*, 452*t*
Volunteer(s)
resources on, 498
services provided by, 17, 18*f*, 19*f*, 479
Volunteer activity record, 19*f*
Volunteer assessment care plan, 18*f*

W
"Waterless wash," 48
Web pages, 489-490
Wong-Baker Faces Pain Rating Scale, 444*f*, 446, 447*f*
Wound(s), 382-399
bereavement counselor for, 390, 394
comfort and symptom control for, 384-386
diagnoses and codes for, 382-384
educational needs with, 395
elimination with, 387
emotional/spiritual considerations with, 386, 389, 393
equipment and supply needs for, 382
general considerations with, 382
home health aide or certified nursing assistant for, 388, 393
Hospice nursing for, 384-388, 390-393
hydration/nutrition with, 387, 389, 393-394
music, massage, art, or other therapies or services for, 390, 394-395
occupational therapist for, 389, 394
other considerations with, 388
outcomes for care with, 390-395
pharmacist for, 390, 394
physical therapist for, 390, 394
resources for, 399
safety considerations with, 382, 386
skills and services for, 384-390
skin care with, 386
social worker for, 388-389, 393
speech-language pathologist for, 390, 394

therapeutic/medication regimens
    387-388
tips for quality and reimbursement
    for, 395-399
Wound(s) *(Continued)*
    volunteers for, 389, 393
Wound, ostomy, continence nurse
    (WOCN), 472

x3d, 69t

Z
ZnSO$_4$, 68t

AAP-1279